Medical Laboratory Management and Supervision 2nd Edition

Lionel A. Varnadoe, Jr., M.B.A., Ph.D.
MT(ASCP)H, HT(ASCP)

PriorityEd (*PriorityEd.com*)
Lionel A. Varnadoe, Jr.

PriorityEd (PriorityEd.com)
Lionel A. Varnadoe, Jr.
Fort Pierce, Florida
Lvarnadoe@aol.com

ISBN – (13#) 9781605855479
(10#) 1605855472

Last digit indicate print Number: 10 9 8 7 6 5 3 2

This book is presented as a 2nd edition, revision, update, additional text content, and sequential of: Varnadoe, Lionel A; Medical Laboratory Management and Supervision: *Operations, Review, and Study Guide*; F. A. Davis Company, Philadelphia; 1996.

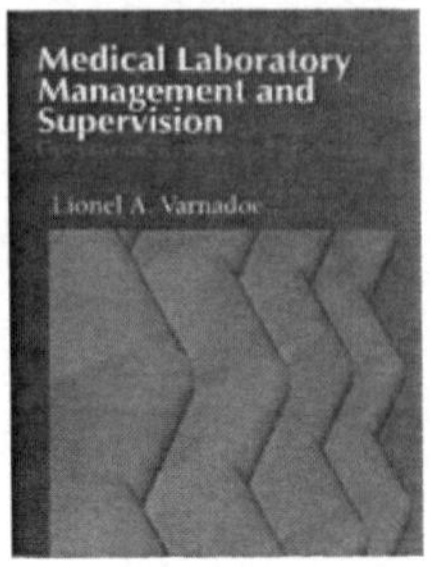

To my wife, Veselka

The joy and spirit of my life

Preface

Preface to original (1st) edition of Medical Laboratory Management and Supervision: *Operations, Review and Study Guide (1996)*

Medical laboratory practitioners are finding themselves under increasing pressure from many sources in the competitive battle that is today's marketplace for all health care services. These include not only the familiar and welcome advances in technology, which is the life blood of our profession, but also assaults that challenge the very survival of the traditional laboratory as a viable financial and health care delivery entity. This book is designed to help laboratorians acquire the management tools with which to deal with these forces and prepare for the challenges of tomorrow.

Laboratory Management Supervision is directed toward the laboratorian who may be an expert in the technical and professional operations of the laboratory but who has no previous knowledge of the administrative and management aspects of running a laboratory. The book is intended to be used as:

- A textbook for college-level courses preparing students to take leadership positions in the medical laboratory
- A study guide for those preparing to take professional examinations for certification as laboratory supervisors and directors
- A self-contained study course for those in need of training in management skills to deal with the increasing pressures of the business of laboratory medicine
- A resource for those who may need a ready desk reference or review of management topics

To meet these objectives the book is organized into four sections, each covering a specific part of laboratory management. The text covers the basic theory of each area with emphasis on the application of the principles presented.

1. *Management of Organizations.* This section covers the theory and application of general management concepts to the laboratory as a business organization. Bureaucratic, scientific, and systems approaches to management are introduced, along with management by objectives and operational research. Leadership of groups and organizations is also discussed.
2. *Management of Human Resources.* Theories of human and work motivation are reviewed in this section, again with heavy emphasis on application to the medical technologist and the laboratory environment. Job design, job descriptions, job performance, appraisal, and the personnel process make up the chapters in this section.
3. *Management of Financial Resources.* The basic accounting model, operations budget, capital budgeting, and productivity measurement are in-

cluded in this section. Examples of the application of these topics to the medical laboratory are presented.

4. *Management of Laboratory Operations.* Specific issues unique to the medical laboratory are reviewed in this section. Safety concerns, regulatory and professional requirements, quality management, work flow and laboratory design, and staff scheduling are examples of the chapters found in this section.

2008

The objectives and ambitions of this edition of the book have not changed. There are, however, several revisions. Most notable, is that there are no questions and answer key for each part. This is replaced by a case study for each chapter, which is designed to reinforce the reader's learning experience.

Given the new world of publishing, especially Print-on-Demand programs readily available through the internet; the book can continually be updated with each printing. While normal corrections (misspelled words, grammatical errors, etc.) will not be noted; new updates and additions may be edited which no not change the 2nd edition content, and will be reflected in the print number listed on the copyright page.

Medical Laboratory Management and Supervision

Contents

Part I: Management of Organizations

Part 3: Management of Financial Resources

Chapter 13: Revenue and Cost Accounting for Medical Laboratories

Part 4: Management of Operations

Chapter 21: Quality Assessment and Performance Improvement

Medical Laboratory Management and Supervision

Part 1: Management of Organizations

[1]

Management

— Chapter One —

What is management? Who qualifies as a manager? Is management different than supervision or administration? Are managers "born," or can these skills be acquired? These are some of the questions this chapter addresses. For this purpose, management is examined from the following four perspectives.

1. A definition of management.
2. Managers, their roles and skills.
3. Historical and current management philosophies.
4. The functions and processes of management

OBJECTIVES

After completion of this chapter, the reader will be able to demonstrate accomplishment of the following objectives.

1. Define "management" and the conditions necessary for its success.
2. Identify the roles and skills associated with being a manager.
3. Compare and contrast the four major schools of management philosophies within the context of their historical development and contribution to current knowledge.
4. Describe the management process and the functions of management.
5. Apply management principles to the medical laboratory through the introduction of a MBO program.

Chapter Highlights and Glossary of Key Terms

I. DEFINING MANAGEMENT (ADMINISTRATION)

***Management**: The implementation of the four conditions that must be present for management to succeed: mission; authority; resources; and, accountability.*

***Mission**: The purpose or reason for the existence of an organization.*

II. MANAGERS

A. Roles of a Manager

***Professional Manager**: A person employed to manage someone else's business.*

1. The manager as a person: Talents and knowledge

   ***Chief Executive Officer (CEO):** The top administrator or manager of an organization, usually reports directly to the board of directors.*

2. The manager as a servant
3. The Manager as a representative

B. Skills of a Manager

III. MAJOR MANAGEMENT THEORIES

A. Scientific Management

Scientific Management: *The application of a systematic or scientific approach to the study of organizations.*

B. Bureaucracy The Study of Organizational Structure

Bureaucracy: *The process of examining the organizational aspects of companies and their work flow to explain how institutions function and how to improve their performance.*

C. Organizational Behavior Management

Organizational Behavior Management: *A management approach that looks at the performance and interaction of people within the organization.*

D. Systems Analysis Management

Systems Analysis Management: *The analytical view of an organization as a complete, self-contained unit that interacts within itself and with it environment in a continuous process of interchange and renewal.*

IV. THE MANAGEMENT PROCESS

Planning: *The thought and analysis process that result in a formal strategy for realizing the goals of the organization*

Organizing: *The process of assembling the necessary resources and people for implementing a plan of action.*

Directing: *Leading in achieving the day-to-day tasks necessary to implement the management plan and ensure a smooth running facility.*

Controlling: *The process of monitoring the standards, measurement, and feedback mechanism that were set in place to ensure implementation of the management plan.*

A. Planning
1. Identify goals

   Goals: *A broad, long-term ambition of the organization.*
2. Evaluating the current situation
3. Establishing a time frame
4. Setting objectives

   Objective: *A measurable standard or task sent in a designated time frame.*
5. Forecasting resources needs
6. Implementing the plan
7. Creating feedback mechanisms

B. Organizing

C. Directing

D. Controlling

V. MANAGEMENT BY OBJECTIVES (MBO)

Management by Objectives (MBO): *A program for managing an organization by setting and monitoring performance objectives.*

A. Setting Objectives

B. Implementing a MBO program

Defining Management (Administration)

Throughout the history of the study of organizations and their operation and functions, there have been many attempts to codify **management** into a single sentence or phrase. Although these efforts have provided significant insight into the process, they have failed to clearly define just what is included in the term "management." "*Working with and through people to accomplish a common mission*" is usually the core of the short descriptions that have been proposed. However, placing the focus primarily on *people* and their role in the organization, discounts the other resources and skills managers must balance in their job.

Generally, the following conditions must be present for management to succeed. As you will notice, these terms are closely interwoven and often overlapping with blurred boundaries as to where one condition may end and the other begins. This demonstrates the complete process which is "management."

1. A *mission*, or goal, that the organization or sub-unit expects to accomplish.
2. Leaders with the *authority* to direct the team toward the goal.
3. Necessary *resources* (people, equipment, supplies, and money).
4. *Responsibility* for achieving the goals assigned.
5. *Accountability* for using the resources established.

With these ingredients present, management can be defined **as the process of coordinating and implementing these five functions**.

Managers

Since human beings first began to join together into groups, there have been leaders. Chiefs, kings, cardinals, military captains, business owners, coaches, and presidents have all overseen various groups and organizations. The arrival of professional managers employed to "manage" someone else's business, however, is largely a phenomenon of the last century.

Management's ascendancy as a profession has paralleled the Industrial Revolution, when specific knowledge in operating an enterprise became increasingly crucial to the success of a business endeavor. Organizing the work flow, requisitioning supplies, accounting for the financial resources, selling products, and assuring delivery to the customer all required increasing specialization and commitment as the economy and means of production increased in sophistication.

As stewards of the assets entrusted to them, managers must recognize the many roles they are asked to play and obtain the expertise and skills necessary to accomplish the mission for which they are held accountable.

Roles of a Manager

Professional managers are called on the wear many hats in performing their duties. Managers must preside over events that have a direct impact on the well-being of the organization and its individual members. As leaders of organizations, managers are required to play three basic roles: people (or person), servants, and representatives. This emphasis on human factors forms the core for all management theories.

The Manager as a Person: Talent and Knowledge

The manager is first and foremost a person—responsible for, and to, other people with similar fears, dreams, hopes, life problems, aspirations, potential, and expectations. Like the people they supervise, managers bring with them their own individual talents, training, and weaknesses.

Some people may appear to be "natural leaders" with inborn people skills. However, without an understanding of the management process, they soon fail when placed in situations demanding extensive planning or technical knowledge. There may also be "born organizers" who thrive in situations that require exacting attention to detail. They too may quickly run into trouble when required to interact with, or direct a group of people. The ability to deal with both people and things is essential to management. This ability can be developed only through proper training programs. *In other words ...* ***managers are made, not born!***

In management the emphasis is on the development of the person. This is crucial at all levels of the organization, from the entry-level worker to the **chief executive officer (CEO)**, because the organization is people, and every link in the chain must be strong. If the people fail, so does the company. As we explore the workings and goal of an organization and its objectives, the people theme will be repeatedly highlighted. All authors build their definition of management around this foundation. This concept is even more pronounced in health care, were the direct, hands-on recipients of our efforts are also people ... our patients.

The Manager as a Servant

The second role of a manager is that of servant. This part of the definition may contradict common notions about managers, but the primary role of the manager is one of instrumentality: *seeing that the person who actually performs the tasks and work of the institution has the resources necessary to effectively and efficiently accomplish his or her duties.* This is the responsibility of every manager, from the CEO to the immediate supervisor. The product must be manufactured, sold, and delivered. The patient's needs, diagnosis and treatment must be attended to promptly. The manager is responsible for making certain that the person performing these tasks has the training and resources necessary to accomplish these duties. To illustrate this point, use Figure 1 – 1 to complete the following exercise.

TRADITIONAL	PATIENT—FOCUSED
↓	→ ↑
Board of Directors	(Patient/Customer)
↓	↑
Chief Executive Officer/Administrator	Line Worker
↓	↑
Vice President/Assistant Administrator	Section Supervisor
↓	↑
Department Manager	Department Manager
↓	↑
Section Supervisor	Vice President/Assistant Administrator
↓	↑
Line Worker	Chief Executive Officer/Administrator
→ ↓	↑
(Patient/Customer)	Board of Directors

→ place where the patient interacts with the institution

FIGURE 1—1. Organizational Chart

- Locate the place on the traditional organizational chart where the patient or customer comes into contact with the business.
- Note that the patient or client interfaces with, and receives services from the person at the bottom the traditional chart.
- Because patients and clients are the reason for the organization's existence, should they not be the top priority of any enterprise?
- Now place "*patient*" at the point of contact with a person in the laboratory, and then flip the organizational chart upside down. This creates a patient–focused organizational

chart. This concept is so important that some companies have published this *bottom up* approach as their organizational chart, in an effort to emphasize how crucial to their success is this contact person's interface with their customer.

Managers must become supporters of their staff if their organization is to prosper. This exercise illustrates how manager act as servants as they provide the means for the employees to meet the needs of their patients and customers.

The Manager as a Representative

The manager is a paid representative of the owners (private or board-of-directors) in both for-profit and not-for-profit organizations. Managers also represent those they supervise, as they are responsible for supplying their needs and presenting their concerns to the owners. This crucial coordination and communication link is magnified at each level of the business as information flows back and forth between management and staff. Some experts have argued that this representation function is the most important role of a manager in the successful operation of any business.

Skillsof a Manager

For manager to succeed in their roles, they need specific skills in each area. Like management roles, the competencies needed center around people, things, and their coordination. The mission of an organization is to produce either material goods (e.g., cars, chemicals, televisions, pencils) or services (e.g., health care, insurance, loans, police protections, laboratory tests). Managers must have a basic understanding of the organization's product and be proficient in organizing the physical and human resources of the corporation to deliver a high-quality product. *....this job requires management skills.*

The closer to the production process the manager, the greater the dependency on technical competence, as compared with the ability to work with people. As managers advance up the hierarchy, they become more dependent on people skills and detailed knowledge of every aspect of the technical process becomes less important. Each level of supervision, however, requires some degree of competence and skill in every area of management.

Management skills can be divided into four groups, each of which is the focus of a section of this book.

also the course, *Transition to Management*; a management and supervision competency certification and credentialing program for medical laboratory professionals: *PriorityEd.com*.

Organizational skills include the ability to conceptualize and apply the management process, systematize work flow, make decisions, and communicate with coworkers. These are covered in **Part 1: Management of Organizations**.

People skills are the topic of **Part 2: Management of Human Resources**. An understanding of the basic theories of human needs and work motivation is essential to accomplishing the goals of the individual and the organization.

Financial management skills are discussed in **Part 3: Management of Financial Resources**. These skills involve the effective use of, and accounting for the monetary assets of the laboratory.

Technical skills involve the synthesis of the first three skills and the management of physical resources (supplies, equipment, and facilities) into the operational parameters (products/services) unique to each origination. These skills are covered in **Part 4: Management of Laboratory Operations**.

Major Management Theories

With the advent of railroads, banks, and other modern large-scale institutions in the 19th century, there has been an interest in the operation and administration of these organizations. Of the schools of management and management theories that developed, four theories have achieved particular prominence among management experts. Each school claims important basic concepts specific to its discipline, and each one should be examined for its contribution to the overall understanding of the dimensions of management.

Here is a list of the four major groups of management thought.

1. *Scientific Management*, which attempts to apply a systematic or scientific approach to the study of organizations.
2. *Bureaucracy Management*, which examines the organizational aspects of the company and its work flow to explain how institutions function and how to improve their structural process.
3. *Behavioral Science (Organizational Behavior)*, which focuses on the performance and interaction of people within the organization.
4. *Systems Analysis*, an outgrowth of management science, which views the organization as a continuous process interacting within itself and with its environment.

A brief overview of the historical development of and major contribution to these four management perspectives follows. This review will lay the groundwork for an understanding of current management theories.

Scientific Management

Scientific management represents the first orderly effort to examine the functioning of complex organizations. The idea was to apply the scientific method of cause-and-effect analysis, used in the study of natural phenomena, to the examination of business enterprises.

Henri Fayol (1941-1925) first introduced the concept that management should be an orderly process of tasks and duties, of which planning was the most important. Fayol's thesis provides the base for the theory call the *functions of management*, or *management process*, presented later in this chapter.

Frederick Taylor (1856-1945), often called the father of scientific management, broke down each task into segments that could be analyzed for ways to improve efficiency. Many of the principles and concepts proposed by modern theorist can be traced to Taylor.

Frank Gilbreth (1856-1924) and Lillian Gilbreth (1878-1972) perfected Taylor's motion study method and developed methods analysis. Performance standards, such as those that were used by the College of American Pathologist (CAP) during the time when it sponsored a work-load units (WLU) program, are dependent on the procedures developed by the Gilbreths.

Other important scientific management innovators include Mary Parker Follett (1868-1933) who pointed out that management is essentially *coordination*, and Lyndall Urwick (1891-1983), who introduced the role of the management consultant and attempted to classify and codify the work done on management theories. Scientific management has since spawned many sub disciplines and has now been absorbed and succeed by the systems theory.

Bureaucracy: The Study of Organizational Structure

Many students of management have used the hierarchical chain of command to examine the working of organizations. This field of investigation is referred to as **bureaucracy management**: it exams the organizational aspects and work flow of companies to explain how institutions function and how to improve the process. Particular attention is given to the bureaucratic characteristics of organizations as they relate to rules, regulations, impersonality, and the division of labor.

Bureaucracy is often spoken of negatively, for example, "bureaucrat" or "red tape." In spite of this view, however, most academic and business consultant's recommendations focus on the structure of the institution and propose that implementing modifications in this area will improve management performance. For example, too many management layers may hinder communication and cause huge amounts of red tape, but too few layers may result in loss of control, thereby hindering management effectiveness.

The majority of management principles, despite claims to the contrary, are developed around a specific bureaucratic model. For example, the scalar (as in "*ladder*" or "*steps*") principle (*see Part 2, chapter 7*), which deals with the chain of command in an organization, states that each person should have only one boss.

The search for the perfect organizational structure is an ongoing process, and much discussion has been generated in the literature. From Adam Smith (1723-1790) and Tom Peters (b. 1942), an understanding has developed of how companies should be organized to more effectively pursue their operational goals. Even commentators who claim allegiance to other management disciples, such as Chester I. Barnard (1886-1961), James D. Mooney (18884-1957), and Alan C. Riley (1896-1947), made major contributions to the bureaucratic management of organizations.

Organizational Behavior Management

Looking at people and how they function in groups is another approach to examining how organizations perform. This approach uses concepts from psychology and sociology as well as management theories. The origins of these efforts lie in the studies conducted by Elton Mayo (1880-1949) between 1924 and 1932 at the Hawthorne Western Electric plant in Chicago. Mayo's lead was followed by Douglas McGregor (1906-1964), who developed assumptions about the basic nature of man; Rensis Likert (1903-1981), whose writings encouraged managers to be supportive in their relationships; and Barnard, who recommended that executives encourage a climate of cooperation. Part 2 of this book, *Management of Human Resources*, presents the theories that have developed from the ideas of these early researchers.

Systems Analysis Management

"Systems" is a term that permeates our language. We speak about school systems, banking systems, government systems, ecological systems, the circulatory system, computer systems, and blood bank systems. Given its universality, is not surprising that nearly all management theories include the concept in some form. Analyzing businesses as a system was a natural evolution of scientific management. The systems approach has been claimed by researchers who rely heavily on mathematical models, scientific methodology, and computer simulations to investigate management problems and recommend solutions. These specialties include operations research, management science, and systems (computer) analysis. Systems theory as applied to organizations is reviewed in chapter 2.

The Management Process

Management pioneer Henri Fayol first proposed that the management process was a continuum of functions that the manager must perform to ensure the smooth operations of an organization.

Fayol's initial analysis has been elaborated upon by many authors, including Peter Drucker, a recognized modern authority on management who stated: "There are five basic operations in the work of the manager. Together they result in the integration of resources into a viable growing organization (Drucker: *Management: Tasks, Responsibilities, Practices*, p. 400). Drucker's five basic management operations are: setting objectives; organizing; motivating and communicating; establishing standards or measurement of performance; and, developing people, including the managers themselves.

The actual number of management functions cited by different theorists varies from four to six, depending on how the operations are grouped. For example, because of their importance to the success of the enterprise, staffing and decision making are often listed as separate functions. In these cases staffing is set apart for the organizing function, and decision making is separated from controlling. Most management texts, however, distill the management process into four main functions: **planning**, **organizing**, **directing**, and **controlling**.

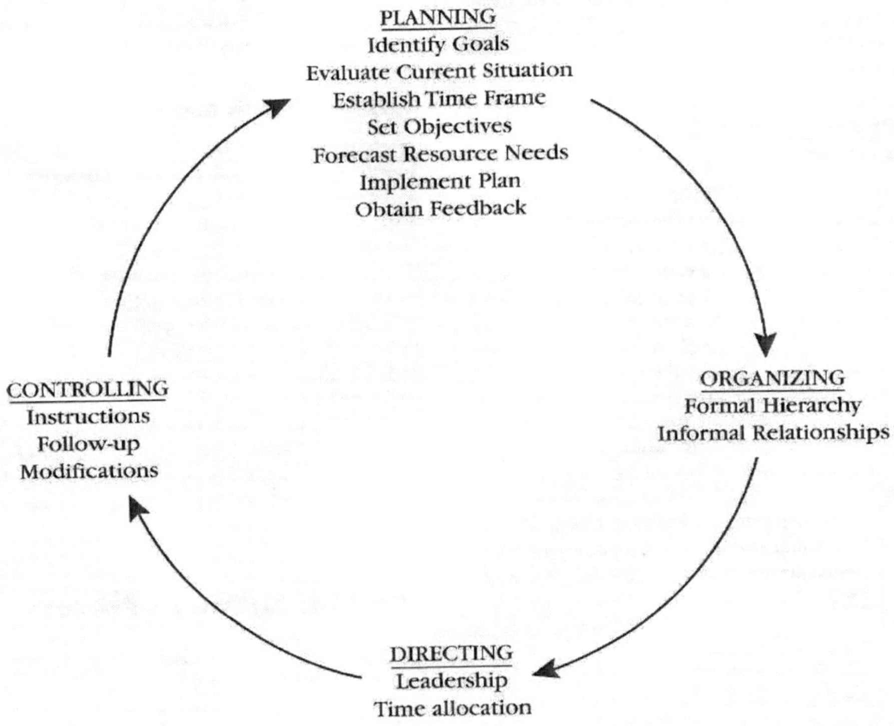

FIGURE 1–2. The management process cycle.

The concept of management as a continuous process of interacting functions, each dependent on the success of the other, is an additional example of the theory of organizations as systems, or "viable growing organisms." The management process and functions are illustrated in Figure 1 – 2 and reviewed in the following sections.

Planning

"*Before you can begin a journey, you must know where you are going.*" This axiom applies to running a business as well as to going on a vacation. During the planning phase, managers attempt to anticipate the future and shape it to their own ends or prepare for the coming changes. Planning is the thinking and analyzing portion of the management process; the other three phases (organizing, directing, and controlling) focus on implementation of the plan developed in this initial stage. Another saying illustrate the importance of planning: "*The manager must plan to succeed or plan on failing.*"

The management planning process can be divided into seven steps.

1. Determine the goals the organization wishes to accomplish.
2. Collect information and evaluate the current situation.
3. Compared with where the enterprise wishes to be.
4. Establish a time frame or period in which to achieve the goals.
5. Set objectives that will move the company toward the desired future.
6. Forecast needs and the use of resources, and determine the steps necessary to implement the plan.
7. Provide for a feedback mechanism to continually review the success of the plan and to implement necessary revisions.

Identify Goals

Where, or what, does the institution wish to be? It cannot be all things to all people, so priorities must be set. This question has to be answered before any other decisions can be made. For example, in deciding on the direction of a laboratory during the planning process, managers might ask the following questions.

- Does the laboratory wish to continue providing the same level of service, or does the changing nature and mix of its patients and physicians require the development of new programs and services?
- Has there been an increase in request for certain procedures?
- Is there a rise in the number and types of reference tests?
- Do complaints continue to focus on specific areas of service?

These questions, and the resulting answers, come from feedback and information received from the hospital staff, laboratory personnel, physicians, and patients. From the answers and insight gained from the questioning process, the manager can identify problems and set the direction and goals for the laboratory.

Evaluating the Current Situation

Knowing where you are and how you got there is essential in determining where you are going. Understanding what resources are currently available and how they can be marshaled provides the base for any plan. Although a manager may feel that he or she has extensive knowledge of the department, taking the step of inventorying the assets of the laboratory in light of the desired goals can provide insights and guidance in the next steps of the planning process.

One point that should be emphasized at this stage because it is crucial to any management function is to include all personnel involved in the project in the decision-making process. This inclusion goes far beyond simple ego stroking; it is essential to the very success of any venture. To short-circuit this resource is to miss important information and advice and risk overlooking important obstacles that may later appear obvious.

Establishing a Time Frame

Once desirable goals and current capabilities have been identified, the potential of the laboratory to achieve these goals within an acceptable time period can be evaluated. The time factor is a key element in determining if a plan is realistic. Although most plans are severely limited by short-term constraints, steps can be taken to ensure that the situation improves over a longer period. Placing goals within the context of time frames enables managers to plan where they want their organization in 1, 2, or even 5 years.

Setting Objectives

At this stage of planning the manager must be clear in identify the target and select the best route to reach it. This is done by setting **objectives**, which allow the group to achieve the desired goal.

Understanding the distinction between goals and objectives is imperative at this stage: goals are the broad long-term ambitions of the organization; objectives are specific short-term standards that allow the manager to achieve the goal.

For example, the goal of the laboratory may be to improve the turnaround time for morning lab work. An objective that supports this goal could be to have all the fasting blood glucoses on the patients' charts by 7:00 AM. A goal is more philosophical, elusive, and admirable marker and it may be difficult to determine exactly when it has been achieved. By contrast an objective is a specific benchmark, for which there is not question as to whether the standard has been met.

There are four basic characteristics of a good objective.

1. It is clearly defined and understood.
2. It is obtainable and realistic.
3. It has a strict time period in which it is to be accomplished.
4. It is measurable.

Setting objectives is discussed more completely in the final section of this chapter.

Forecasting Resource Needs

An integral part of any design—and a major consideration during each step in the planning process—is the feasibility of the goal and each objective. Deliberation must be given to the availability of current resources and the possibility of obtaining the additional assets needed. To consider this factor, the manager may have to return to the first step and revise the goals accordingly. This issue further illustrates the ongoing cycle of the management process and the necessity of developing a sound and flexible strategy.

Within the time frame of the objectives established, arrangement must be made for the acquisition and use of appropriate equipment, instruments, supplies, work space, and personnel. The development of the laboratory's budget, both operational and capital (see Part 3: *Management of Financial Resources*), is the principle vehicle for accomplishing this task.

Implementing the Plan

Built into the design of a good plan is a strategy for anticipating and overcoming any obstacles or impediments. The manager has two basic avenues for implement a plan or obtaining the desired performance: (1) tools of persuasion, which focus on working with and through people; and, (2) tools of controls, which involve the allocation of resources. Selecting the proper mix of tools is a crucial decision in the success of the implementation strategy.

Tools of persuasion can best be described by listing key words associated with this method: communication, involvement, inclusion, education, training, cooperation, building confidence, support, consultation, feedback, sharing information and responsibility. These important people skill are covered in Part 2 of this book.

By virtue of their position and formal authority, managers have *two tools of control* that are crucial in obtaining and maintaining management control: (1) the allocation of financial resources (selection of equipment and supplies and number of employees) through the budgeting process; and, (2) the process of staffing and scheduling, or job assignments. Parts 2, 3 (*Management of Financial Resources*), and 4 (*Management of Laboratory Operations*) of this book all present information on these subjects.

The balancing of these two options determines the success of both the manager and the plan. Neglect or improper use of either tool results in a high likelihood of failure. By including the staff in the design of the project, managers ensure their support and refine the plan. Proper consideration of both material and personnel needs is a major factor in bring about a smooth operation.

Creating Feedback Mechanisms

Built into any plan must be provision for obtaining information on how the project is progressing so that needed revisions and corrections can be instituted. This stage, which completes the loop of the planning phase, requires collecting data for evaluation and continual incorporation into the management cycle. Information can be obtained and correction introduced through several avenues.

1. Monitored standards of performance can be set to measure the progress of the plan.
2. Informal meeting and conversation with staff and customers can reveal problems and recommendations for improvements.
3. Another suggestion, an analysis of the nature and types of problems that are encountered can be undertaken. Ideally, this should be accomplished through the organization's quality management program.
4. Formal meetings between managers and coworkers can be held to assess the current status and to make any necessary adjustments.

The nature of these and other information and feedback sources illustrates the continual nature of the management process. Upon completion of the planning process, the manager is ready to proceed with the next phase: *organizing the project.*

Organizing

After a plan has been designed, the first step is to gather together the necessary resources and people and develop a structure for putting the plan into action. Attention must be directed toward the efficient use of all resources, ensuring that the goals and objectives of the plan design are accomplished. As the organizational process advances, the need for continual modification of the master plan becomes evident, and may bring about updates in the way a group is organized.

The organizational process has two dimensions: (1) the formal hierarchy of work groups, job assignment, and lines of authority; and, (2) the network of informal relationships that forms in any organization—friendships, social groupings at lunch and after hours, and of course, the legendary, "grapevine." The smart manager takes advantage of both formal and informal relationships. Chapter 2 (*Organizations*) examines the nature of both formal and informal structures in organizations and the mechanisms for assembling these forces.

Directing

Directing is the most visible of all management functions. Directing includes seeing that the day-to-day tasks necessary to ensure a smooth running facility are done. This is the so-called human factor stage, in which both leadership and management skills come to the forefront. Planning and organizing have been completed, and the plan is now in progress. Because of the acute nature of the problems that must be addressed and the demands on the manager's attention, the manager can get trapped here and become a hostage of the system.

Faults overlooked in the planning and organizing phases become blatant as this point. Often the failure of a manager to take the time to plan contributes to the stress and frustration of "fire fighting;" that is, rushing from crisis to crisis, or simply "spinning their wheels," rather than making real progress toward their goals and objectives. Allocating time to each of the management functions enables the manager to avoid this "trap."

Controlling

Drucker has pointed out that there are two parts to giving instructions. The first part is to be sure that the instructions are clearly understood; the second part is to check to ensure that instructions have been followed. This is an important principle in all aspects of life. Imagine the outcome of the following scenarios.

- A teacher covers a topic completely and to great length, but the students do not expect the subject to be on the exam.
- A law is passed, but no provisions for enforcement are made.
- A company sends a bill but makes no effort to collect.
- A manager gives the staff 10 tasks, but the employees know that questions will be asked about only 2.
- A parent tells the child not to do something, but the child knows that the parent will not bother to check.

These examples emphasize the need for controlling, which is the process of checking up on the priorities established in the previous three management functions. The control function is the measurement and feedback mechanism of setting objectives. It completes the management function loop by comparing what has actually been accomplished with the original master plan in order to determine its success or identify need modifications.

The tools of persuasion and control are the primary mechanism for success in the controlling function. These should be matched with other approaches such as the quality management models present in the last part of the book, and management strategies (i.e., *MBO program*) in which standards are established, performance is measured, and corrective action is taken.

All this information is funnel backing into the planning phase, where the management process recycles and continues:

Planning →Organizing →Directing →Controlling →Planning →....

Management By Objectives

Management by Objectives (MBO) is a program that embodies all of the concepts in the management process. The idea, first introduced by Peter Drucker in the 1960s, incorporates the principles of planning, operating, directing and controlling and provides a mechanism to bring these concepts into everyday practice. Many textbooks correctly choose to discuss MBO with other leadership skills; however, it is included here as an illustration of the application of the functions of the management process.

One of the more interesting aspects of the latest quality management program sponsored by the Joint Commission on Accreditation of Healthcare Organizations (JCAHO) is a return to quality assessment and performance improvement standards that can be objectively measured which are an integral part of MBO programs.

At the core of MBO is communications. Its success or failure depends on how well employees comprehend the company's mission and objectives. Managers must understand where their staffs are headed and how individual employees perceive their jobs. Effective MBO programs require managers who are participatory in their leadership style; that is, managers who allow employees to share in the decision-making process. Chapter 7 (*Principles of Leadership*) covers these leadership styles in detail. In practice, MBO provides a formal mechanism for the most elementary principle of all human relations: Talking to each other.

Finally, to effectively design and implement an MBO program, the manager must understand and be skilled at writing and monitoring objectives.

Setting Objectives

Setting objectives, which is the heart of the MBO method, is in actuality an everyday occurrence. Diets, saving plans, vacation trips, and study time are all examples of setting objectives in everyday life.

To be effective, MBO objectives should aim to hit these targets.

1. **Follow well-thought-out plans and long-term goals**. Although objectives are short-term by nature, they should be an orderly part of the continuing management review cycle and should not be set according to arbitrary, aimless, and hastily made decisions.
2. **Be a collaborate agreement between supervisor and employee to provide for accountability and ownership of the objective by the employee**. The individual must identify with, and accept, the expected result.
3. **Be person-specific**. Although many objectives are the same for employees with similar jobs, objectives should be customized so that members understand their roles in meeting the mission of the organization.
4. **Be within the power of the individual to accomplish**. This means that objectives must be realistic and obtainable, yet at the same time encourage employees to reach toward their potential. This is a crucial factor. If an objective is unreachable, the employee will not take it seriously or will just give up. However, an objective that does not challenge the employee or that is too easy does not benefit either the organization or the individual.
5. **Be measurable**. There must be a way of knowing when the objective has, or has not been accomplished. The best measurements are quantitative. Number of tests performed, new tests implemented, employee turnover rate, amount of overtime, repeat tests, instrument downtime, phlebotomy redraws, variances from budget, and turnaround time ... are all factors that can be assigned a number and objectively measured. The more qualitative the objective, the more difficult it is to measure. For example, although good laboratory staff moral is an admirable ambition, it is best classified as a goal, broken into a subunit objective like turnover rate, and then assigned a quantitative unit such as a percentage of total staff.
6. **Have a designed time frame**. In addition to being purposeful, reachable, and measurable, objectives must be assigned a time period during which it is to be completed. Without this important benchmark, neither the workers nor their su-

pervisor know what is expected, the priority of the assignment, or when an evaluation is appropriate.

7. **Have built-in feedback mechanisms**. Employees must know how they are progressing so that they can make timely and independent adjustments. This feedback should be available on a continuous basis, not just at the time of the annual performance review. Also, it should be available first and foremost to the person who is responsible for carrying out the task. This is a major source of problems in MBO programs. If employees must depend on someone else for selected and prescreened information, or if they cannot be trusted with access to the necessary data, they are not truly empowered or responsible for the task. Under these circumstances the objective should not be assigned to them, because in reality it is the responsibility of someone higher up in the bureaucracy. Information may often be used as a means of power, control, and manipulation.

These points are summarized in Table 1 – 1.

Objectives should:

- Follow well-thought-out plans and long-term goals
- Be based on a collaborative agreement between supervisor and employee
- Be person-specific
- Be within the power of the individual to accomplish
- Be measurable
- Have a designated time frame
- Provide a feedback and information to responsible employees so they know how they are progressing and can make timely and independent adjustments

TABLE 1—1. Characteristics of Objectives in MBO

Table 1 – 2 show the MBO objectives of a Hematology supervisor who is making plans for installing a new instrument. This is a practical example of the management functions and planning process at work in the laboratory. When properly prepared, objectives become an effective tool for both the staff and the manager to plan the work of the department.

Implementing a MBO program

There are three phases in implementing an MBO program.

1. Managers must set the goals and objective for the organization in order to have a clear picture of what they wish to accomplish.
2. These objectives should be shared with the staff. Employees should be given the opportunity to develop their own priorities from the guidelines presented by the managers.
3. The manager and each employee must meet and come to a mutual agreement on the goals and objectives for the individual. This meeting should serve as part

of the foundation for the employee's periodic performance evaluation. From this session, both the manager and employee have a clear understanding of what is expected and how the employee's work will be evaluated.

Objective	**Measurement**	**Review**	**Evaluation**
Preliminary space and power needs assessment	Work order to Engineering	May 1, 2008	Work completed or outside contractor approved
Attendance at instrument training workshop	Attendance at program	May 15, 2008	Certificate of completion
Onsite installation of instrument and completion of procedure manuals	Instrument installed	May 30, 2008	Instrument installation accepted and procedures manual signed by director
Training and orientation of laboratory staff	In-service sessions completed	June 15, 2008	Signed in-service and and orientation sheets Quality-control database and preventative maintenance protocol established
Instrument operational	Report of test results	June 25, 2008	Parallel testing completed and signed by director

TABLE 1—2. Using an MBO Program to Install an Automated Cell counter

Implementing a MBO program finishes Chapter 1; the next chapter covers the topic of *Organizations* and how they work.

— Case Study —

Chapter One: Management

Bill and Ann, the chemistry and hematology supervisors, greet each other in the hall on their way to meet with Betty Harp, the laboratory director, and their fellow supervisors for the monthly manager's meeting.

"Well," Bill opened the conversation, "it's May and this is the time of year that administration always comes down hard on Betty to cut staff and eliminate overtime."

"How?" asked Ann. "I've only been here 3 months and all the supervisors complain about being understaffed. My section has been wiped out by long-term illnesses, and the only way we have made it is by overtime and with my working almost entirely at the bench, even working most weekends. I've had no time to get started toward my goals of upgrading the hematology section, and taking comp time has been out of the question. I don't know why I accepted this job without overtime, the workload has been unreasonable. At least the staff is getting paid for their extra time."

"I know," Bill nodded in agreement, "none of the supervisors like being on salary. In fact, our new tech, Sally, came here because we pay overtime. This year has been especially hard. It looks like every year is worse than the last, and they still push to reduce the number of labor hours."

"I agree," added Tammy, the microbiology supervisor. "Maybe if we all bring it up to Betty, something can get done. We need help so we can work reasonable hours, or they need to give us overtime."

The meeting went through the usual list of topics, and as Bill had predicted, the last item on the scheduled agenda was staffing levels for the coming summer months.

*****

After listening to the expected volume of complaints and arguments by the supervisors, Betty told the group that she had already expressed these concerns to administration and reviewed the laboratory's excellent productivity levels with the group. Administration had agreed with her that there were not to be any more cutbacks this year and that an aggressive recruitment campaign must be pursued to fill the open positions. Bill, Ann, and Tammy all exchanged looks of relief with each other and the rest of the supervisors in the room.

"However," Betty continued, "they are insisting that we eliminate our overtime problems. We are out of line with other departments; double that of most labs in our system. This must be reduced."

Holding up her hand to halt the outburst of comments, Betty explained. "To help in this area, all Technologists will be reclassified as professional staff and placed on salary. This alone will eliminate 50% of the overtime problem."

"It will also eliminate 100% of the fill-in help," responded Bill, as the others nodded in agreement. "Everyone in chemistry has had to work an extra day this past month just to meet minimal staffing requirements. I've only had one weekend off myself. It won't work."

"There will be a salary adjustment to make up for some of the loss in pay, just like when the supervisors went on salary," answered Betty. "I know we must carefully plan how to announce this to the staff, but administration expects us to support this plan. The corporate office bas especially targeted overtime reduction as a critical objective for each of the hospitals."

After listening to their objections, Betty reminded them of their responsibility as managers and asked them to keep the policy quiet, think about the best way to implement the change, and meet again next week to develop a plan.

"No way!" Bill commented to Tammy and Ann as they left the meeting. "I don't even like the salary status myself. We will lose all of our staff to other hospitals."

"Remember, we need to support management on this point," advised Sam, the blood bank supervisor. Look on the bright side; they are now formally recognizing us as professionals, rather than just hourly workers."

Each supervisor returned to his or her section contemplating the impact the policy would have on the staff members and how best to inform them of the new plan.

Chapter Sections for Review

- Roles of a Manager, particularly the manager's role as a servant and representative of the owners and employees
- The Management Process, especially the planning function ·
- Management-by-Objectives and Table 1-2

Questions for Discussion

1. Who do the supervisors represent in this situation?
2. What responsibility do the supervisors have in defending the employees' position? How far should they go in aligning themselves with the opinions of their employees, especially if the supervisors believe that their staff is right?
3. Should the supervisors be expected by management to support a policy with which they strongly disagree?
4. Using the functions of the Management Process, what would be the steps in developing a program to implement the new pay plan?
5. Did the hospital follow the process outlined in the MBO program?
6. How would a MBO approach have handled the concerns of administration about overtime in the laboratory?
7. Using an MBO program as a model, write the goal and objectives for reducing overtime in the laboratory; or, as an alternative, an MBO program for implementing the salary based program.

[2]

Organizations

— Chapter Two —

Organizations, those entities that result from people joining together in pursuit of a common cause, are examined in this chapter. The topics covered in this area complement the material in Part 2 of the text, in which the influence the organization has on people is explored, along with how its structure, social order, and policies affect the individual. This chapter looks at how an organization operates, functions, and interacts with itself and its environment. Organizations are examined through the following windows.

1. Business organizations as systems
2. Forces outside the control of the manager that influence both the organization and the manager's job
3. Formal and informal groups that structure organizations,
4. The role of authority within the organization
5. Organization charts, which serve as the formal presentation of the structural plan
6. A summary review of the principles of organizational structure and authority

Understanding the nature of organizations, their impact on society and individuals, and how they function as systems is crucial for managers who expect to be successful in directing organizations toward desired goals.

OBJECTIVES

After completion of this chapter, the reader will be able to demonstrate accomplishment of the following objectives.

1. Describe the characteristics of organizational systems.
2. Differentiate between those factors that managers can influence and those that are outside their control.
3. Explain how business entities, such as the medical laboratory, operate under the systems model.
4. Identify the characteristics, both shared and unshared, of formal and informal groups.
5. Design an organizational structure for a medical laboratory.
6. Compare and contrast the types and roles of authority that exist in a medical setting.
7. Prepare an organizational chart reflecting the structure and chain of command for a medical laboratory.

Chapter Highlights and Glossary of Key Terms

I. BUSINESS ORGANIZATIONS AS SYSTEMS

System: *A self-contained collection of interacting and interdependent components, working together toward a common purpose.*

A. Characteristics of Organizational Systems

Primary Tasks: *Defined duties that are necessary because of the nature of the system* 's *products or services.*

Hierarchy of Systems: *The process whereby self-contained subsystems develop within a parent organization, such as a laboratory within a hospital.*
Open Systems: *Systems that interact with their environment by both receiving and delivering products and services.*
Equilibrium: *A state of stability within and between the system and its environment.*
Self-Regulation: *The feedback process by which the system monitors performance and provides information to its members.*

B. Functions of Organizational Systems
   1. Input
      Input Mechanism: *The process through which needed resources are acquired and replaced.*
   2. Transformation
      Transformation: *The internal process whereby resources received through the input channels are converted into the products and services produced by the organization.*
   3. Output
      Output Mechanism: *The process of delivering the goods and services produced to the external environment.*

C. The Laboratory as a System

II. ORGANIZATIONAL FORCES SHAPING THE MANAGER'S JOB

III. STRUCTURE OF ORGANIZATIONS
Formal Bureaucracy: The *officially sanctioned lines of authority assigned by the owners of the organization.*
Informal Groups: *Alliances that form outside the boundaries of the formal bureaucracy from the interaction and allegiance of people with common interests.*

A. Formal Organizational Structure
   1. Design elements and factors
   2. Design strategies and models
      a. Bureaucratic models
      b. Situational models

B. Characteristics of Formal and Informal Groups
   1. Leaders
   2. Followers
   3. Group goals
   4. Shared opinions
   5. Performance and commitment expectations
   6. Sanctions

C. Group Management and Coordination

IV. AUTHORITY
Authority: The *empowerment by formal job classification of an individual to make commitments and act on behalf of the organization.*

A. Responsibility
B. Job-Related Authority
C. Types and Roles of Authority
   Line Authority: *Supervisory responsibility assigned through the formal delegation of authority.*
   Staff Authority: *Influence exerted through the control of support services, such as the business office and personnel, which provide recommendations to the line manager and set institution-wide policies.*
   Functional Authority: The *power to enforce directives, such as physician's medical orders, within the context and boundaries of a clearly defined specialty and span of control.*
D. Delegation of Authority

Delegation **[of authority]:** The *passing on to someone else the authority and responsibility to get a job done.*
1. Delegation routes
2. When to delegate
3. Fear of delegation

V. ORGANIZATION CHARTS

Organization Chart: The *formal written presentation of the structural plan of the organization.*

A. Traditional Organization Chart Format

B. Alternative Chart Formats

VI. PRINCIPLES OF ORGANIZATIONAL STRUCTURE AND AUTHORITY

A. Departmentalization

Departmentalization: The *grouping together of related activities to expedite the production process.*

Specialization: The *process of having an individual or group of people who are highly trained in a specific and limited area or task, with specialized work space and equipment, to effectively produce a product or service.*

B. Decentralization

Decentralization: The *process of assigning the decision-making process to those who are actually performing the work.*

C. Unity of Command

Unity of Command: The *process of ensuring that each individual reports to only one supervisor.*

D. Scalar Principle

Scalar Principle: *A linear system of authority providing a direct vertical link from the board of directors to the lowest-level worker.*

E. Span of Control

Span of Control: The *theory that there is a definable limit to the number of people one person can effectively supervise, within the boundary of specific work parameters and situations.*

F. Exception Principle

Exception Principle: The *principle of referring for resolution by a superior only those things that cannot be solved by the employees at their own level.*

Business Organizations as Systems

As mentioned frequently elsewhere in the text, human organizations by their very nature are social systems in the most classic sense. A system may be defined as a self-contained collection of interacting and interdependent components, working together toward a common purpose. Systems receive instructions and resources from external sources (input), process this internally (transformation), and deliver the finished goods or service to external users (output).

The medical laboratory is an excellent example of the systems principle. The laboratory receives an abundance of inputs, including supplies, staff, equipment, financing, and requests for tests, from many sources. The laboratory then uses these inputs to produce test results that are then delivered to the patient or physician. How the laboratory functions as a system is discussed later and is illustrated in Figure 2 – 1.

A social system, like a biological organism, can also be defined as a collection of interacting and interdependent components working together toward a common purpose. This description applies to systems ranging from the single-cell organism in microbiology to the complex business organizations of government and industry. They all function in close relation to both internal processes and their environment. In this chapter, organizations as systems are analyzed by examining their characteristics and functions. The chapter concludes with a brief look at the laboratory as a system.

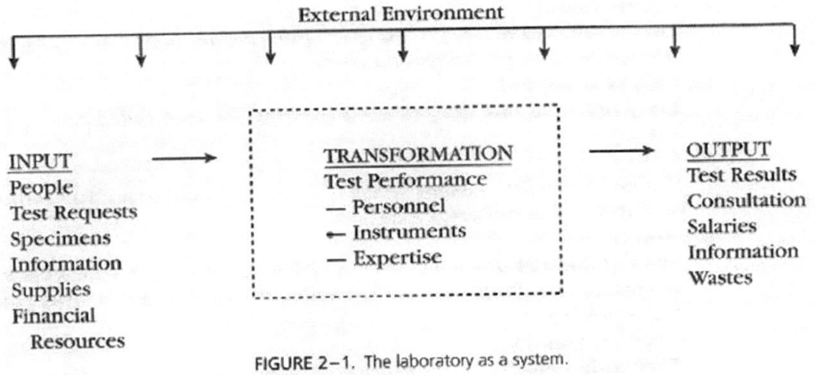

FIGURE 2–1. The laboratory as a system.

Characteristics of Organizational Systems

All organizations share the following six traits (see also Table 2 – 1):

1. They are made up of many interconnected parts that are both dependent on and supportive of each other; that is, they are **holistic** and **synergistic** with clearly defined boundaries. Each component acts on, and is acted upon, by the other members of the system, resulting in a cause-and-effect syndrome. Together the individual elements produce a holistic synergism that makes the system greater than its parts. In other words, by sticking together, the parts gain from the system much more than they could from being independent. There are also clearly defined boundaries to the system, which are identified by obvious landmarks or labels of ownership.

2. They have a purposeful activity or **primary task**. This trait is almost inseparable from the first. The system's reason for being is a commonly shared goal. The parts exist and are organized in such a manner as to achieve this purpose. Although the goals and objectives of an organization may temporarily change, the primary task must be accomplished if the enterprise is to survive. Laboratories, for example, are dedicated to the delivery of timely test results to their patients, even though they may have other functions, such as teaching students. The laboratory may be a poor teaching facility, but if it fails in the delivery of testing services it is either shut down or replaced. This primary mission obviously determines the distinct nature of the system.

3. The internal components change and become progressively more specialized as the organization increases in size and sophistication. This differentiation increases the interdependence and seeks to improve the efficiency of the entity. This process results in the development of distinct subsystems that develop their own character yet remain under the umbrella of the superior organization. This successive evolution develops into a **hierarchy of systems**, in which subsystems develop sub-subsystems as the need for specialization continues, each under the auspices of the parent. A hospital laboratory is an example of this specialization. Even though it is a distinct unit unto itself, it functions within the organization of the hospital by receiving and delivering specialized services. The laboratory, in turn, may have sections such as microbiology or the blood bank, which may function as self-contained subsystems.

4. Organizations operate as **open systems**, actively interacting with their environment by receiving and delivering products and services. This openness is an important concept because even the most comprehensive system must receive inputs from outside its boundaries to survive. Even a system as large as the earth must receive and exchange important support from other systems to maintain its dynamics.

5. Much like natural systems, organizations appear to seek a state of stability, or **equilibrium**. This characteristic can be both a strength and a source of frustration to managers, whose job is to influence the behavior or direction of the group. Because the mission of the organization defines its nature, the demands and tasks associated with this purpose create an inertia to develop around certain levels and tasks. Couple this with an inherent resistance to change, and a strong pressure to maintain the status quo coalesces.

1. Holistic and synergistic with clearly defined boundaries
2. Purposeful activity and a primary task
3. Hierarchy of systems
4. Operates as an open system
5. Seeks a state of stability and equilibrium
6. Self-regulating

TABLE 2—1. Characteristics of Organizational Systems

6. To meet each of the previous characteristics, the organization must have a mechanism for **self regulation**. To be successful, a system depends on specific behaviors occurring at exactly the right time. An effective feedback network must be in place, one that provides each of its parts with information about when and what services are needed. Biological organisms use various chemical and neurological methods to accomplish this. A business organization relies on the management process to monitor performance and provide information to its members.

Functions of Organizational Systems

Three activities must be conducted on a continuous basis if an organizational system is to continue to operate: input, transformation, and output. Inputs are transformed into products and services and are delivered as output. Each stage has specific needs and tasks. This cycle is illustrated in Figure 2 – 1.

Input

Through the **input mechanism**, needed resources are acquired and replaced. Supplies, knowledge, machinery, and labor are procured with the money received from the sale of the enterprise's products and services.

In social institutions such as governmental agencies, financial resources are provided in return for the expected delivery of services. Also received at this stage are requests for the products or services of the organization.

Transformation

Resources received through the input channels must be converted into the products and services offered by the organization. This **transformation** is achieved by the internal action of the organization performing the tasks established for these purposes. This process, which requires constant attention to the desires and needs of both the enterprise's customers and employees, is accomplished through a mechanism of continuous self-regulation.

Output

Through the **output mechanism**, products and services produced by the organization are delivered to its customers. In this export stage the enterprise satisfies its clients and receives the nourishment (payments or funds allocations) to renew itself through the input process. Failure to meet this goal results in challenges to the organization's legitimacy.

The Laboratory as a System

Laboratories are an excellent example of organizations as systems (Figure 2—1 above). As a system, laboratories take in reagents, supplies, and test requests; use the instruments and people in the department to perform the procedures necessary to obtain the results; and then deliver the results to their patients and other departments along with the wastes and by-products produced in the process. For this reason, the information and concepts presented in this chapter are highly applicable to laboratories, particularly as they function as subsystems of the hospital and health care systems.

Organizational Forces Shaping the Manager's Job

Many components affecting organizations are beyond the influence and control of a manager, yet they have a crucial impact on the manager's job. This important point should be clearly understood, and managers must be prepared to place these issues in their proper perspective if they are to be effective in leading an organization. Three main factors play such a role:

1. *The life cycle of the organization*. Organizations, like all systems, have a starting point, a stabilizing period, and a stage at which the enterprise must either terminate or begin anew. Each phase requires special consideration and exerts its own special effect on the manager.
2. *The external environment of the organization*. This factor, which is definitely outside the influence of the manager, shapes the character and capabilities of the institution. The external environment may include general economic conditions, laws and regulations, national and local customs, transportation routes, funding sources, available work force, and even weather conditions.
3. *The internal culture of the organization*. Many managers find this a point of frustration because they may think they control all aspects of their department but find themselves blocked by the history, lifestyle, and images of both the people and the organization itself. A new manager may dismiss comments such as "We've always done it this way" and attempt to make changes without a complete background investigation. However, this is a mistake. Although the explanation may seem irrational, there are usually valid reasons why a situation has developed in a certain manner. The manager, to his or her chagrin, may even find that things are done a certain way because of a pet peeve of one of the senior officers of the company, who may want to maintain the status quo for personal reasons. Respect and care must be given to these points as the topic of organizational structure is reviewed.

Structure of Organizations

It is difficult to separate leadership from the structure of the organization. They are in a mutually supportive relationship: *structure* is the result of leadership decisions, and leadership style is strongly influenced, if not determined, by the structure of the organization. For study purposes, we examine structural design in this chapter. Leadership styles are covered in Chapter 7.

In any enterprise two simultaneous organizational structures may complement, but often compete with, each other. The first is the **formal bureaucracy**, which is officially sanctioned by the owners of the institution and is given the authority and responsibility to carry out the organization's designated duties. Within the formal structure, members of the organization know whom they work for, whom they supervise, how their department relates to other groups, and even who supervises their boss. The formal bureaucracy consists of a specific organizational plan that can be drawn up formally in an organizational chart (*see figures. 2—2, 2—3, and 2—4 in the Principles of Organizational Structure and Authority section below*) so that the chain of command and chain of responsibility are clearly understood.

The second, less obvious structures are the **informal groups** that develop from the interaction and allegiance of people with common interests. These informal groups can arise from within the organization through the day-to-day activities of people working together or from social involvement with community, family, or recreational ties. The smart manager is aware of the potential of both structures and builds opportunities for groups and individuals to work creatively together by forming teams that develop from the natural flow of the work.

The formal aspects of organizational structure are discussed next, followed by a review of informal structural factors, including a comparison of the characteristics of the two types of groups.

Formal Organizational Structure

Managers need to consider four main factors in assessing the structural design of an organization.

- Design elements and factors
- Appropriate options, design models, and strategies
- Delegation of authority
- Formal organization charts

The information needed to design an effective and efficient organization structure should be readily available from the management plan. In practice the structural design is an important element of the management planning function, and the focus here is simply an in-depth exploration of one topic in the course of the planning process.

Design Elements and Factors

There are three paramount concerns in designing an organizational structure: the tasks to be performed, the people involved, and the workplace.

The tasks to be performed are the main object of attention in determining how a project should be organized. The types of equipment, the level of automation, and the nature of the product or service to be produced are all examples of factors that determine what work needs be performed and what is the best method for getting the job done.

The people needed and available to perform the work also exert a strong influence on how the manager organizes the enterprise. The existing skills and knowledge of the employees determine the extent and level of supervision necessary. The manager must know if a lot of close supervision and training are required. Can the staff perform independently with limited oversight from management? Motivation is an important consideration in deciding how the staff is organized (see Part 2 of book). The personal talents, educational levels, personality, and even cultural backgrounds of the members of the organization need to be taken into account in the organizational plan.

Where the work is performed is a third limiting factor. The total space available, the amount of storage room, the visibility and accessibility of workers and supervisors, and the proximity of rest areas are just a few examples of those physical elements that can influence how a company is organized. For example, cramped, isolated workplaces that make it difficult for the supervisor and the worker to communicate may hinder the performance of detailed work requiring extensive supervision. Instead, small work groups, each with its own supervisor, may be required. In large, wide-open spaces, where the workers can summon assistance quickly, less personal supervision is needed.

With these three factors in mind, the manager can look at different options for streamlining the organizational efficiency of the department. One way to gather information is to examine facilities with similar work traits. Following is a discussion of several broad models for organizations. This presentation is not meant to limit the ingenuity of the manager but to generate ideas from what researchers have found in analyzing the structures of different organizations.

Design Strategies and Models

The essence of any structural organizational plan is the relationship between people within a group and between the groups themselves. From this premise, structural strategies and models fall into two broad groups: bureaucratic models and situational models.

Bureaucratic Models

Bureaucratic models focus entirely on the relationship between people and rely on the hierarchy's formal chain of command. The advantage of this approach is that there is a clear understanding of who is in charge and who is responsible for specific areas of work.

Bureaucratic models can be divided into two types, depending on the level of control exercised by the top echelon of managers. Models that maintain tight reporting ties with each subunit and require that all decisions be checked with "headquarters" before action can be taken are part of a centralized system. A decentralized management structure attempts to bring the decision-making process as close to the work site as possible.

Max Weber, a social scientist who worked in the early part of the 20th century, identified the following five basic features of a bureaucratic model.

1. Each job has a formally established set of official duties (the modern job description).
2. There is a hierarchy-based chain of command.
3. Rules and regulations are consistently applied.
4. The system works as its own "formalistic personality" without the attachment of human emotions.
5. Hiring and firing are based on qualifications and performance, and the worker is protected from the arbitrary and unpredictable whims of any one particular manager. This feature is often cited as the reason for the "lifetime employment" or "one-company career" characteristic of the 1950s and 1960s, which is now being challenged in today's rapidly changing world economy.

Situational Models

Situational models attempt to tailor the organizational structure to the specific job needs dictated by the work situation. This is accomplished by looking at both the type of work to be performed and the ability of the staff to work independently.

Joan Woodward and associates have developed a *technological model* based on the company's type of production process: (1) small-batch production; (2) large-batch and assembly-line production; and (3) production processes that have a long-run and continuous output, for example, chemical and petroleum companies. Woodward found that successful organizations with small-batch and long-run production processes tended toward similar structures—more loosely defined job descriptions and more delegation of authority to those actually performing the work. Those successful enterprises involved in mass—production techniques, such as automotive and assembly-line plants, seemed to exert tighter supervision of the workers and maintain a dominating administration that required strict reporting and control of the manufacturing system.

Another situational approach uses a matrix scheme to identify the need for different structural arrangements in an organization. This plan grades crucial variables in each unit by grouping them according to the task to be performed, the types of personnel needed, and the history of each section. These variables are tallied, and each work group is placed in a cell of the matrix, which then matches the group to one of the following structural strategies.

1. Work that consists of repetitive tasks and needs a minimally trained work force falls into a routine strategy.
2. Non-repetitive work that requires independent judgment and is performed by a professionally prepared staff requires an engineering strategy.
3. A craft strategy is best when the products are unique and workers are extremely skilled but the basic production process for each item is similar.
4. For work that allows a wide latitude in investigation and for more abstract products, as in research and development, a heuristic (discovery) strategy is recommended.

Companies and institutions that use situational models are more likely to have organizational charts and structures that reflect a team concept (Fig. 2 – 4 below), rather than the traditional hierarchical format illustrated in Figures 2 – 2 and 2-3 below in the *Principles of Organizational Structure and Authority* section.

Characteristics of Formal and Informal Groups

All organizations consist of both formal and informal structures. Formal structures are designed around the mission plan; informal structures result from the relationships that are formed by the interaction of people. These two forces exert simultaneous, and continuous, pressure on the direction and success of the enterprise. Formal and informal groups have many things in common because both depend on how people function in groups. They both have leaders, followers, purpose or mission, shared opinions on how things should be done, performance and commitment expectations, and sanctions for those who do not meet these expectations (Table 2 – 2).

Leaders

Leaders of formal groups are appointed by the owners or their designates. Informal leaders emerge from within the group itself, either because of a perceived need or personal charisma. Both types of leaders may have the talent for attracting followers, but informal leaders must depend on their personal attributes, whereas the supervisor's authority is upheld by the bureaucracy. It is not unusual for a manager to play both roles, as we discuss in Chapter 7.

Group Traits	Formal	Informal
Leaders	Appointed	Charisma
Followers	Recruitment incentives	Personal attraction
Purpose	Profit or social goals	Peer motives
Shared opinion of how things should be done	Organizationally driven	Social norms and mores
Performance and commitment expectations	Job and task standards	Issue-focuses
Sanctions	Organizational rewards and punishment policies	Peer pressure

TABLE 2—2. Formal and Informal Group Characteristics

Followers

Followers join groups because of perceived mutual benefit. They are attracted to business companies by the financial incentives offered for their services. Informal groups offer shared values, communal concerns, common interests, and the fellowship of friends as rewards for membership. Organizations provide opportunities for the fulfillment of all of these human attributes..

Group Goals

Groups exist so that individuals can accomplish something that is beyond the ability of one person. The aim of the formal group is to support the mission of the company. The informal group's objectives center around meeting the needs of individual members according to the group's perception of those needs. When individual members and the group as a whole believe that their interests match those of the institution, both benefit tremendously. When their interests conflict, serious harm can result. The manager's role is to bring these two potent forces together so they can work toward a common goal.

Shared Opinions

A frequent cause of breakdown in communications and team spirit revolves around the issue of how things should be done. Disagreement over a company policy or a manager's decision is a strong stimulus for the formation of informal alliances, particularly if the point of contention appears to be unfair or arbitrary.

Although managers cannot be expected to please their employees all the time, they can prevent problems concerning differences in opinion by sharing information with the staff and, most important, including employees in the decision-making process. This strategy accomplishes two things: first, it helps the staff to understand the reasons for the decision; and secondly, it enables them to buy into the plan by feeling that they are part of the organization.

Performance and Commitment Expectations

Both formal and informal groups have very specific performance and commitment expectations. The formal organization dictates its wishes through job descriptions, written policies, and product standards. Informal cliques make compliance demands on their members through the social and

personal behavior mores of the circle in which they function. Informal groups also have very strict issue-related norms tied closely to the rules of etiquette, civility, and manners.
By definition, for a group to form, the individuals must share common beliefs about some issue; be it religious, social, recreational, or economic.

Sanctions

Formal business organizations impose sanctions through the financial reward system and its disciplinary procedures. Other groups enforce compliance by using tactics that rely on the personal and social needs of their members. These can include the positive benefits of belonging, praise, camaraderie, recognition, and friendship of peers. Negative sanctions in informal groups can range from temporary rejection, with verbal and emotional shows of displeasure, to expulsion and ostracism.

Group Management and Coordination

Managers should not view the presence of informal groups in the workplace as bad or see them as natural enemies of the "system." Informal groups frequently play only recreational roles for their members or respond to specific stimuli within the organizational environment.

Many of the informal groups that form in response to internal factors offer the alert manager the opportunity to take advantage of spontaneously developed improvements. These may have been initiated by the group in order to adapt to work situations. The goal of a manager is to build these two forces—formal and informal groups—into a confluence of energy directed toward support for the mission of the organization.

Authority

The concept of authority and how it is exercised and delegated is an important factor in the operation and structure of an organization. In organizations, **authority** is the empowerment, by formal job classification, of an individual to make commitments and act on behalf of the firm and to decide how resources, rewards, and penalties are used to ensure that designated goals and responsibilities are achieved. In short, authority is the power to act. The term "authority" is often used synonymously with words such as "power," "influence," "knowledge," and "control." Coupled with two other concepts, appointment and responsibility, a good picture of authority begins to emerge.

The extent to which the manager has to check with a superior before proceeding with a decision describes the measure of the individual's authority. This is an important defining factor. Managers may be told that they have the authority to do a job, but if they must check with another person before proceeding, their power is limited, and the real authority lies somewhere else.

This point is a major cause of breakdowns in communication and smooth organizational functioning. Progress on a project may cease because of the organizational logjams that develop when everyone has to wait for clearance before continuing. For this reason, sufficient authority must accompany responsibility for a particular work situation or job.

Responsibility

Responsibility and authority are, or should be, coterminous. When responsibility is assigned without the authority to act, the situation can quickly deteriorate into one of blaming and buck-passing, with everyone trying to avoid becoming the scapegoat rather than working together to get the job done. When work assignments and job descriptions are accompanied by the correct amount of both authority and responsibility, there is a harmonious flow of organizational energy toward completion of its tasks and mission. Everyone has an understanding of what he or she has to do in performing his or her duties.

Job-Related Authority

An illustration of the authority-responsibility match is in the writing of job descriptions. A good job description details the extent of authority a worker has when assigned a job. One way to accomplish this is to match each duty or work assignment with a rating that designates the level of authority. For example, the degree of authority can be ranked from highest to lowest on a scale of 1 to 4.

1. Part of regular duties. No prior checking required. Report any problems through routine communication channels.
2. Take any action necessary, but let the supervisor know as soon as possible during the normal work schedule.
3. Must attempt to check with supervisor before intervening, but can take emergency action if needed before a supervisor can be contacted.
4. Must clear any decision before proceeding.

Job Description Abstract 15:00—23:00 Shift Supervisor

Task	**Authority Level**
Perform testing services according to procedure manual	1
Change testing protocol and policies in special cases	3
Reject unacceptable specimens	1
Perform instrument maintenance	1
Request service assistance from outside vendors	2
Call in additional (overtime) staffing	2
Order routine supplies	1
Approve special supplies or authorize rush shipment charges	3
Discipline staff	3

Key:
1 = no prior checking or special notification required
2 = notify supervisor ASAP, during normal working schedule
3 = must attempt to consult supervisor before, but may take action as necessary
4 = not authorized to act without consulting supervisor

TABLE 2—3. Laboratory Task and Authority Level Scale

Table 2-3 gives a sample of laboratory tasks, with the corresponding authority level. Note the predominance of authority assignment at level 1; levels 2, 3, and 4 are relatively rare. This is an important feature of the authority-responsibility match. There should be few, if any, authority level assignments of 3 and 4, or this is not a description of that person's particular job, but of someone else's. Authority levels 3 or 4 should be on the job description only to help clarify the limits and boundaries of the duties for which the worker is responsible.

Types and Roles of Authority

Formal authority can be grouped according to the role of the manager and the department within the organizational structure. Line managers exert direct authority through the bureaucratic hierarchy of the organization. Staff and functional managers exercise their influence through the services they provide or their relationships to other managers.

Line authority takes two forms in a hospital-based laboratory. First, within the confines of the department itself, authority takes the straight-line route from administration to department head to supervisor to the staff. However, in its bureaucratic relationship, the laboratory serves a supportive role to the nursing department by providing services that augment their duties.
Within the hospital, straight-line authority flows from administration through nursing to other departments. This is illustrated by the fact that, when administration is not present, as on the evening shift and holidays, the house supervisor assumes administrative responsibility for the institution.

Staff authority is exercised through such staff departments as the business and personnel departments —those areas that provide supportive services in a more indirect fashion. These staff departments exercise their influence by making recommendations, providing specific support services, giving assistance and advice in technical areas, facilitating paperwork and other procedures, and developing general hospital policies. Their power may be subtle and ambiguous, but a manager ignores their advice at great peril.

There are also numerous examples within the laboratory of staff functions. These include such positions as the safety officer or quality assurance coordinator, whose ability to implement change depends on the action of the section supervisors; however, their recommendations carry great weight in the policies of the department and in the ability of the supervisors to perform their jobs effectively.

Functional authority is best illustrated by the relationship of physicians with the laboratory and hospital. Despite being outside the formal organizational structure of the hospital and having no direct supervisory control over its employees, doctors have the power to enforce their directives within the context of a clearly defined span of authority. Functional authority allows specialists (accountants, physicians, engineers) with expertise in a particular area to exercise control within the boundaries of their specialty.

All three types of authority may be present in one individual or department. Within the laboratory, for example, supervisors have line authority over those below them in the bureaucratic structure, yet the department itself provides testing services (staff authority) to the hospital. The laboratory also has functional authority for setting testing parameters in such matters as patient preparation or specimen collection criteria and in establishing reference ranges.

Delegation of Authority

Delegation [*NOTE: this section relates to the delegation of **authority** and not delegation of **work**, as the term is often used. Although there are some common or similar themes and issues, they are different topics. Work assignments are covered in the chapter on Job Design and Job Description. Delegation of work (e.g., giving one person's work to someone else) is an entirely different focus than is discussed in this section in the context of assignment of authority*] is passing on to someone else the authority and responsibility to get a job done. This definition, as simple as it may seem, is really fraught with danger.

It implies trust of the other person, as well as the risk associated with the loss or giving up of control. This task can reveal the confidence that managers have in themselves and in their people. No matter how talented, no manager can do everything. Sooner or later out of necessity he or she must ask for assistance or assign some duties to other people.

Delegation Routes

In essence, all authority is delegated from the owners of the organization to the board of directors to the chief executive officer; this is the organizational structure. Delegation can be permanent or temporary. Temporary delegation is the short-term or single-project assignment of authority and responsibility that are normally a superior's.

For example, a laboratory supervisor may delegate to a staff technologist the job of writing a procedure or evaluating an instrument for possible purchase. These tasks would normally be part of the duties of the supervisor, but they are assigned to the technologist on an individual basis. Insecure supervisors, or those who do not trust the ability of their staff, may be reluctant to delegate. However, this inaction causes managers to miss the opportunity for staff development, fail to tap the staff's knowledge and expertise, and lose the obvious time-saving advantage.

When to Delegate

There are several important factors in deciding when, how, and to whom to delegate. Foremost is the ability of the employee to handle the assignment. The employee need not currently be experienced in the area but must have the potential to perform the task with little additional training or under minimum guidance from the supervisor. This is an excellent opportunity for a manager to develop staff, provide a job enrichment experience, and allow a person and the laboratory to grow professionally.

Other delegation factors center on the time management skills of the manager and the nature of the tasks. Managers should not view delegation as something that is forced on them by their own time constraints or because of the frustration of the workload. Delegation should be a positive aspect of the total management plan, one that takes advantages of the abilities and talents of all the staff.

The task itself may dictate who can perform certain duties. For example, if the institution refuses to disclose certain sensitive information, such as financial or quality assurance statistics, to employees other than designated managers, the ability of the manager to delegate a task requiring such information is limited.
Also, if it takes longer to train or provide the necessary instructions to perform the assignment than to actually perform the task, delegation can become a catch-22 situation for managers. To avoid this dilemma, delegation should be part of an overall long-term staff development plan, through programs such as continuing education, so that the manager develops faith in the ability of the staff to tackle challenging projects.

Fear of Delegation

Letting go can be difficult for some managers. Because of a lack of confidence in either themselves or their staffs, managers may fear delegation and see it as a personal threat to their position or even use it as a way of punishing their staffs. As we will discuss in Chapter 7, the leadership style of managers depends on how they perceive their workers. Managers who feel that their people are inherently lazy, dislike work, generally shirk responsibility, and lack initiative are not willing to delegate. In contrast, managers who view their employees as responsible, desirous of doing a good job, naturally talented, and creative encourage their workers to grow and to expand their horizons.

Organization Charts

The **organization chart** is the formal written map of the structural plan and authority delegation. It attempts to clarify the bureaucratic relationships between both individuals and work groups.

One point that needs emphasizing: the organization chart is not an end in itself but only the visual presentation of the structural plan. Anyone can draw up a schematic in a few minutes. However, to design an effective system involves the analysis of work flow, an understanding of the nature of the work, and a definitive plan on how best to fit groups together to achieve a smooth working relationship between the various parts. Organization charts are a technique for planning and fitting the parts together, not the end result. Most organization charts are filed in the personnel manual after completion, never to be seen or consulted again. This cannot be allowed to happen to a management plan; otherwise, the institution muddles along without any direction or guidance.

Analysis of an organization chart reveals important personality traits of a company. First, it shows the relationship of the members to each other and how they interact and communicate with one another. It may also yield clues about the management philosophy of the company's leaders.

Traditional Organization Chart Format

Figures 2 – 2 and 2 – 3 show examples of traditional organization charts for a laboratory. Note how many management layers there are between the top manager and the bench worker. An organization chart that has many management layers is referred to as a tall structure (Figure 2 –2), whereas one that has few management layers is called flat (Figure 2 – 3). In drawing up the actual diagrams, note how the lines show direct line authority relationships. The chart may be either position-specific or simply show the relationships of various departments to each other. Departments that are high in the pyramid are superior in corporate rank and show who reports to whom. Those horizontal to each other on the chart have similar rank and position. Horizontal relationships also establish the boundaries of responsibility and span of control for each department.

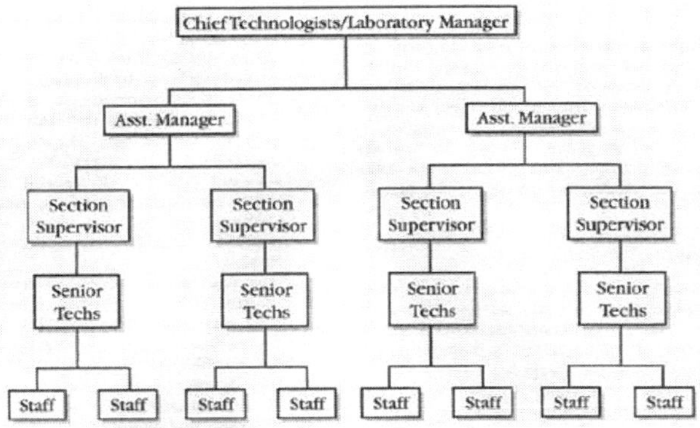

Figure 2—2 Laboratory Organization Chart (Tall-Structure Design)

Alternative Chart Formats

Some attempts have been made to get away from the bureaucratic pyramid-style organization charts, which sometimes serve to build fences between sections. Figure 2 – 4 shows a different structure, one that focuses on the organizational interdependence, rather than on the segregation and division of each department.

[note: Figures 2 – 3 and 2 – 4, are on the following page]

- *Departmentalization*: Related activities are grouped together to expedite the production process, that is specialization.
- *Decentralization*: The decision-making process is brought as close to those who are actually performing the work as possible.
- *Unity of command*: Each individual must have only one boss.
- *Scalar principle*: Supervision should be a linear system providing a direct vertical link from the board of directors to the lowest-level worker.
- *Span of control*: There is a definable limit to the number of people one person can effectively supervise, with the boundaries of specific work conditions.
- *Exception principle*: The manager and staff are able to do their jobs without having to check with a supervisor about every detail.

TABLE 2—4. Principles of Organizational Structure and Authority

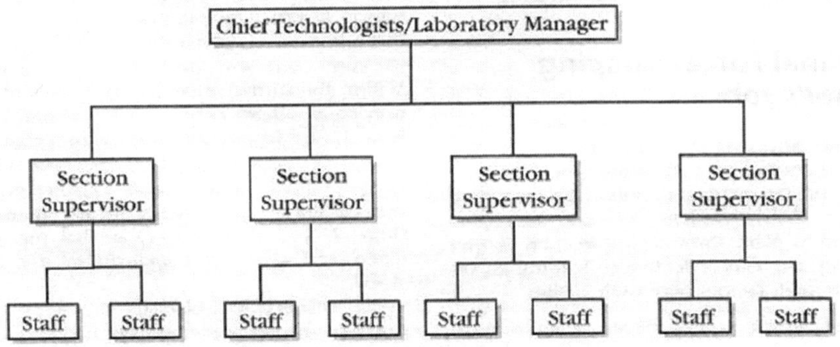

FIGURE 2—3. Laboratory Organizational Chart (Flat—Structure Design)

Principles of Organizational Structure and Authority

With this conceptualization of organizational structure and authority, several design principles become evident. The following points are considered elementary to any organizational plan: departmentalization, decentralization, unity of command, scalar principle, span of control, and the exception principle. Part 4 of the book contains detailed information on how these factors apply in a laboratory setting, and applicable comments are noted later with each principle, as well as summarized in Table 2 – 4.

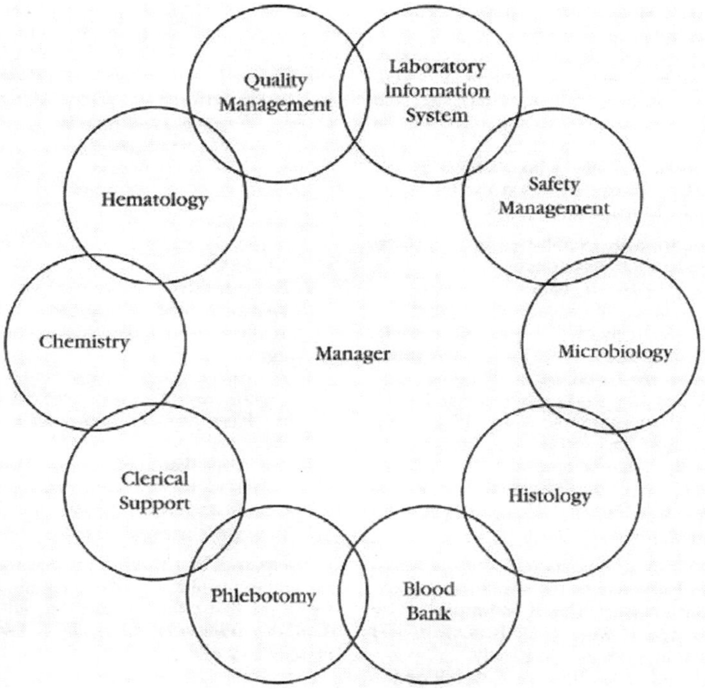

FIGURE 2—4. Laboratory Organizational Chart (Team—Structure Design)

Departmentalization

Departmentalization, the grouping together of related activities to expedite the production process, is a key management decision. Units are usually formed to take advantage of the efficiency that comes from having a group of people who are highly trained in a specific area, with the specialized work space and equipment, to effectively produce a product or service. This process is called specialization and is one of the oldest industrial principles, first described by Adam Smith in 1776 in The Wealth of Nations. Departmentalization and specialization usually continue from the highest to the lowest level of an organization. The production line of car manufacturers is a good example of this principle.

In the laboratory, specialization can be based on such factors as the type of specimen received (hematology, urology, microbiology) or the function performed (quality assurance, safety). Units can also be grouped by geographical location or project, or because close coordination of certain activities is required.

Decentralization

There are two main advantages to **decentralization,** the process of having the decision-making process close to those who are actually performing the work. First, it ensures that the people who are responsible for the task and who know the most about everyday operations are familiar with and share the objectives of the firm. Secondly, it frees upper—level managers to focus on broader issues, which only they can deal with.

In determining the extent of decentralization and the types of decisions to be delegated, managers have to consider the ability of staff and the well-being of the whole organization. The level of contacts with outside parties, the potential for commitment of company assets, the competence of the staff, and the consistency in the policies of the company are factors that limit the extent of decentralization.

Unity of Command

Unity of command states that each individual must have only one boss. This is an important principle, especially in health care institutions, where there are several strong, and often conflicting, lines of authority coming from staff and functional parties as well as immediate line supervisors. In reality, laboratory technologists receive instructions and orders from many sources during the course of a normal day. These sources include nurses, patients, physicians, and their own supervisor. They must, however, always have a clear understanding of who they report to for directions and consultation when problems arise.

Unity of command, also referred to as *unity of direction,* can best be implemented by assuring a parity of authority and responsibility. A single manager should control and coordinate the people and resources needed to carry out an assignment, and that manager should report only to a single superior.

Scalar Principle

According to the **scalar principle,** there should be a linear system of authority that provides a direct vertical link from the board of directors to the lowest-level worker. This hierarchical structural format is designed to ensure clear communication channels and management controls throughout the organization and to prevent confusion in the work force, operational breakdowns, and the sabotage of authority by competing interests. Terms such as "chain of command" and "career ladder" reflect this principle.

Span of Control

Span of control hold that there is a definable limit to the number of people one person can effectively supervise within the boundary of specific work conditions. For example, the U. S. Army has set a goal of one squad leader for every four soldiers, with a maximum allowable number of nine people.

When the work consists of routine and repetitive tasks, errors and problems can be readily traced, and when work areas are open, a large number of employees can be viewed simultaneously. In such a situation, as along a production line, many companies have found that very few supervisors per employee are needed. In the medical laboratory, however, where highly technical work is being performed on sophisticated instruments and a great deal of attention by the supervisor is essential, a large ratio of supervisors to employees is required. How a company deals with this principle determines to a great extent the number of management layers that are necessary.

Exception Principle

The **exception principle** allows the manager and staff to do their job without having to check with a supervisor about every detail. Only those problems unresolvable at the employee level, or those issues concerning company policy, are referred to a superior. This rule frees both employees and managers to get the job done rather than write reports and attend unnecessary meetings.

This chapter on Organization concludes with this review of the principle of organizational structure and authority. The next chapter will deal with the issues of *communications*, an absolutely necessary process if the laboratory is to be successful.

— Case Study —

Chapter Two: Organizations

"The chemistry instrument is down again, and I can't reach the laboratory manager to authorize calling in the service tech!" exclaimed the frustrated evening supervisor.

Because of budget cuts, the laboratory had opted for Monday through Friday only business hours service contracts on their major instruments, and the manufacturer would send a service person after these hours only if they received a purchase order number authorizing the service. According to hospital policy, only department managers could request a purchase order

Chapter Sections for Review

- Design Strategies and Models
- Delegation of Authority
- Decentralization

Questions for Discussion

1. Look at the organizational charts in Figures 2 – 2, 2 – 3, and 2 – 4 in the book. What kind of structural design do you think this hospital has?
2. What type of job-related authority does this supervisor have in this situation? Is this an appropriate match?
3. What kind of structural design and authority assignment action would you recommend to remedy the situation?

[3]

Communications

— Chapter Three —

No matter how great the plan or how talented the person, if managers cannot communicate effectively with other members of the team, their ideas and inputs are doomed. Although it is not listed as a separate management process, communication is an integral part of each management function. It is embedded in every action taken. This chapter reviews the process through which messages are formatted, transmitted, and received. The obstacles to effective communication are discussed, along with the development of a strategy for overcoming these obstacles and improving the process.

OBJECTIVES

After completion of this chapter, the reader will be able to demonstrate accomplishment of the following objectives.

1. Describe the six phases of the communication process.
2. Discuss the channels through which organizational members receive information and transmit messages.
3. Identify barriers to effective communications.
4. Develop a strategy for overcoming communication obstacles and improving the process.

Chapter Highlights and Glossary of Key Terms

I. THE COMMUNICATION PROCESS

Communication*: The act or process of receiving and transmitting messages.*

Sender*: Person wishing to transmit a message.*

Message*: The actual format of the communication effort, including verbal and nonverbal signals, symbols and language transmitted.*

Mode of Transmission*: The vehicle by which a message is sent: oral, written, nonverbal, recorded, or third party.*

Receiver*: The target of the message, either an individual or group.*

Decoding*: How a receiver translates the message.*

II. COMMUNICATION NETWORKS AND CHANNELS

A. Communication Directions

Formal Communication: *The official communication messages (e.g., memos, directives, work orders) generated by the business activities of organizations.*

Vertical Communication: *Formal messages that are channeled through the hierarchical network of the organization (top ~ bottom).*

Horizontal Communication: *Communication activity that occurs during the normal conduct of business, including the exchange of services, information, and work orders between departments, managers, and staff.*

B. Means and Methods of Communication

Dynamic Communication: *Live discourse in which all parties can simultaneously exchange ideas and information and receive spontaneous feedback.*
Canned or Packaged Messages: *Messages that are delivered in formats that prevents the recipient and sender from responding to each other instantaneously.*

1. Communication routes
2. Communication formats
   Written Messages: *Messages such as memos and video programs that are prepared and transmitted by mechanisms other than a face- to- face encounter.*
   Verbal Messages: *The actual delivery of the message.*
   Nonverbal Messages: *The associated signals, body language, facial expressions, voice tone, context, and connotation of the words that are transmitted with the verbal components of the message.*
3. Nonverbal language

III. PERSONAL AND ORGANIZATION COMMUNICATION LINKS

IV. BARRIERS TO COMMUNICATIONS

A. Structural Barriers
   Spatial Constraints: *Barriers, such as geography and job duties, that isolate people from the normal communication channels of an organization.*
B. Problems of Semantics
   Semantics: *The branch of communication science that studies the denotation and connotation of words and messages.*
   Denotation: *The exact dictionary meaning of a word or phrase.*
   Connotation: *The context and nonverbal messages associated with a word or phrase.*
C. Technical Problems
D. People Barriers
   1. Perception factors
      Perception: *How a message is viewed from the standpoint of the receiver*
   2. *Interpersonal factors.*
      Credibility: *Worthiness of a person as perceived by another individual within the context of trust, honesty, and competence.*
E. Outcome Problems.

V. IMPROVING THE COMMUNICATION PROCESS

The Communication Process

Communication requires both the delivery of a message to another person and the assurance that the message was correctly received and understood. This two part process must clear the six distinct hurdles listed next and summarized in Figure 3 – 1 for the **communication process** to be successful.

1. The **sender** or person transmitting the message has a particular understanding of its meaning, why it is being dispatched, the designated target, and the desired response. All of these factors are **encoded** into the formulation of the message.
2. The **message** itself —how it is worded and presented— is an important variable. In addition to the words selected; voice tone, gestures, and verbal images all have associated connotations that imply meaning or even hidden messages. Words and signals are heavi-

ly dependent on the language of the group (shoptalk, dialect, vernacular) and the shared level of knowledge.

→	<u>SENDER</u>
	Motives
	Action Expected
	Context
	Credibility
	Empathy
		→	<u>MESSAGE</u>
			Semantics
			  Denotations
			  Connotation
			Format
			  Written
			  Verbal
			  Nonverbal
				→

→	<u>TRANSMISSION</u> Route Dynamic Canned/Packaged Technical Problems	→	<u>RECEIVER</u> Perception Credibility Context Decoding Personal Agenda	→
→	<u>FEEDBACK</u>	→	<u>SENDER</u> → Message → Transmission → Receiver → Feedback → Sender → ...	

FIGURE 3—1. The Communication Process

3. The **mode of transmission** selected — oral, written, nonverbal or through a third party — influences how a message is interpreted and acted upon. The channel through which it is received (organization structure or grapevine) and the stature of the messenger (friend or foe) all influence the effectiveness of the delivery. The level of activity — or "noise," to use communication jargon — that is going on at the same time, combined with the competing rivals for the attention of the audience, affects the likelihood of the information to reach its target unaltered.
4. The **receiver,** the person or group receiving the message, brings to the relationship a background and perceptions that may be quite different from those of the sender. In addition, the emotional state and social status of the receiver in relation to the sender may affect receptiveness. Demographics (audience size, age, sex, job position, education, and so on) also play a key role in the dissemination process.
5. How the receiver translates the communication determines the response. This **decoding** is dependent on both the previous four factors and the receiver's understanding of the message within the historical context of previous communiqués and exchanges.
6. Feedback and clarification of the message must be included in the communication effort; otherwise, the whole effort simply collapses. This can be accomplished by an active interchange between the sender and receiver to help avoid confusion or by observation of

the response of the receiver to the message. In any event, the sender must follow through and ascertain that the message was received and understood and that appropriate action was taken.

This chapter addresses the issues surrounding each of these steps. First, the network of formal and informal communication channels is reviewed. Second, the barriers that block effective communication are discussed. Finally, methods for overcoming and improving communications are presented.

Communication Networks and Channels

Members of organizations receive communications from two sources: (1) the formal communications network of the organization, which exchanges information through work orders, memos, meetings, policy manuals, job descriptions, performance reviews, newsletters, and the normal interactions of the members in pursuit of their duties; and (2) informal sources, including the news media (newspapers, journals, magazines, television, and radio), professional colleagues, salespersons, and, of course, the gossip grapevine, which is always active in any group. Communication networks and channels are discussed here according to the means and methods by which the communications arrive.

Communication Directions

Formal communication comes from two directions in a company — from above or below within the organization. These **vertical communications** take the form of memos and other directives that come down through the bureaucratic hierarchy and the responses and other information that make their way back up through the same network. **Horizontal communication** occurs in the course of the normal exchange of services, information, and work orders, when managers and staff talk to each other as peers.

Every person is familiar with the characteristics of the informal communications network — the so-called grapevine. The informal network is a valuable source of information, important to both managers and staff.

Although the grapevine can be constructive and informative if used properly, it has a reputation for exerting detrimental effects on its victims. Most workers have either experienced the sting of the gossip grapevine personally or seen its effect on others. Yet, despite its destructive nature and reputation for error, the grapevine's future appears secure. Managers cannot destroy the grapevine, but they must be cognizant of its existence and effects. The best antidote appears to be a management style that encourages a spirit of inclusion, openness, and involvement, along with the timely sharing of information that may affect employees and their jobs.

Means and Methods of Communication

The number of methods by which we receive information is increasing rapidly. The latest additions include fax machines, video monitors, electronic mail, and computer networks, and even more timely and comprehensive information sources are being developed. These innovations notwithstanding, communication still breaks down into two groups, depending on the amount of live interaction between the parties: (1) **dynamic communications,** whereby both parties can simultaneously exchange ideas and information and receive spontaneous feedback, and (2) **canned or packaged** messages, which are delivered in formats that do not allow the recipient and the sender to respond instantaneously to each other. Communication routes (dynamic or canned) and formats (verbal or nonverbal) are reviewed next.

Communication Routes

The most vivid example of *dynamic* communication is the personal meeting, in which the parties can sit together and discuss a topic face to face. With modern technology, such conversations can also be conducted via the telephone, computer networks, and videoconferences.

Canned or *packaged* messages can also be transmitted in a variety of forms, including written memorandums, short notes on Post-Its attached to reports, taped video or audio programs, and third-party messengers.

Communication Formats

Communications can take several forms, and each has its advantages and disadvantages. The message can be presented in written or verbal form. For definition purposes and to simplify discussion, if a message is not verbal (that is, oral), it is written. For example, computer data and recorded visual presentations are considered written messages. This distinction is important when the manager is considering the tools and techniques available for preparing a message and selecting the best route for delivery. *Writing* has the advantage of being easy to document. It allows readers to study the message without worrying about whether they have mistranscribed some point when taking notes. **Verbal messages** enable the manager to be seen or heard as a person and overcome some of the formality that often accompanies a written notice.

Equally important is the hidden message that accompanies all communications. In written communication this message involves "reading between the lines"; in oral communication it is referred to as the nonverbal message. If this issue is not addressed by the manager in planning a presentation or communiqué, the target audience may become more concerned about the hidden message — what was not said or the manner in which it was said — than in the actual wording of the message itself.

Nonverbal Language

Nonverbal communication has received a lot of attention. Such communications are the signals transmitted by the demeanor or behavior of the sender. How the managers dress, the tone of voice, extent of eye contact, office furniture and arrangement, and the timing or place of the visit all give the receiver hints as to the seriousness or importance of the message. The old adage that "*actions speak louder than words*" points to the importance of placing the message in the proper context.

Nonverbal messages and signals are transmitted through every aspect of the communication. *Tone of voice* is an important amplifier of the signal. For example, a substantial pay raise may be perceived in a negative light if the supervisor's tone of voice implies that the raise was not altogether deserved.

Body and facial expressions such as frowns, slouched body, crossed arms, or an inattentive or faraway look may be interpreted by the receiver as signs that the sender is in a hurry or has more pressing things to think about. How a person is dressed also transmits messages about priority and respect for the receiver.

Personal distance and movement also send messages. One of the more pronounced actions that a sender or a receiver can take to demonstrate a keen interest in the other party's message is to make a *direct physical movement* toward the other person. To experience the effect of this strategy, do this maneuver the next time you are talking to a family member, friend, or colleague.

> Specifically, when talking with someone, make eye contact, move a couple of inches toward the person, or purposefully turn your ear in a direction that shows the individual that you very much would like to hear what they are saying, that it is interesting and important to you.

Of course, the movement should be positive and nonaggressive. Notice the impact it has on the recipient, their reaction/expression.

Physical environment, including choice of furniture and the layout of an office, convey power issues. Whether meetings are held in the boss's or employee's office, how luxurious or spartan the accommodations are, how much space is allowed to the visitor, and the types of furniture in reception and conference rooms have all been identified as factors in the message. Even such subtle or inadvertent factors as *room temperature and lighting* may demonstrate the sender's concern for the receiver's comfort and importance.

The connotation of *time* can be strong. One story circulating among the sales staff of a laboratory supply company stated that if the boss invited you to breakfast, you were going to fired; if you were invited to lunch, it would be a business meeting; and if you were invited to dinner, you were getting a bonus.

These factors point out the importance of consistency, clarity, and attention to detail in selecting both the message and its delivery medium.

Personal and Organization Communication Links

Managers, like all employees, receive messages from both inside and outside the organization by maintaining personal contacts with other individuals as well as receiving information through formal news sources. This is done out of both wisdom and necessity. Managers who depend solely on formal sources of information can lose touch with the pulse of the company, risk being unprepared for sudden changes, and miss crucial clues to what is behind the actions of executives and staff. Managers must also cultivate ties with colleagues, fellow professionals, and community sources that can provide insights into messages that are circulating through both the formal and informal communications channels.

Barriers to Communications

There are five types of barriers to effective communication. These barriers, which are reviewed in the next section and summarized in Table 3 – 1 are: structural, semantic, technical, relate to human factors, and outcome objectives.

Barrier	**Action**
Structural	Remove or find alternative routes
Semantic	Pay attention to both content and context of message
Technical	Find alternative routes or times
People	Provide training, groundwork, feedback, explanations, reassurance, credibility, and trust
Outcome	Ensure that the outcome is within the ability of the receiver to Perform

TABLE 3—1. Communication Barriers and Improvement Strategies

Structural Barriers

The organization itself, its design and bureaucratic patterns, can present major obstacles as well as advantages. Even though the design is meant to streamline the exchange of information and feedback, the size of the organization may present an obvious difficulty. The number of managers and supervisory layers, the number of employees, and the size of the physical plant all complicate efforts to "get the word out" to interested parties.

Because of its dynamic nature, an enterprise is continuously adapting to change. By the time a message reaches the intended users, the data may be irrelevant and obsolete. The continuous modifications in bureaucracy and personal relationships, matched with the hazy and often overlapping responsibilities inherent in such an environment, complicate correspondence further. Messages may be delivered to one place but not the other; out of sheer confusion, they may even be diverted to a group with similar duties or title.

People may be isolated from the communication channels by both distance and job position. Grouped together, these are referred to as **spatial constraints.** Geographic separation is an obvious impediment to communication. Employees may be bound to specific work locations or be unable to engage in everyday interaction with fellow workers because of a job that requires constant monitoring of instruments or equipment. If the communication network is heavily dependent on one person passing along documents or directives to another, the system can become clogged or simply break down when one link in the chain fails to continue the process.

Problems of Semantics

Attention must be given to both the *content* **(denotation)** and the *context* **(connotation))** during the formulation of messages. **Semantics** is the branch of communication science that studies these aspects of words and messages.

We have all found ourselves in extremely awkward situations when we didn't know what to say but stood groping for the right words. Perhaps we wished to express our condolences or ask the boss for a raise or request a favor of someone. Perhaps we were trying to decide how to give advice or respond to criticism or ask someone to stop an annoying habit. These and other circumstances emphasize the effect language has on how a message is given and received. Senders must consider not only the message they want to deliver but also how it will be received. Will the receiver be grateful and appreciative, take offense, become defensive or even turn hostile?

Semantic problems revolve around words and their meanings. Meaning is much more than what is covered in a dictionary; it includes ancillary issues such as tone of voice, place and setting, and the spirit in which the words are spoken and written. Besides the obvious differences presented by slang, job talk, and regional and local customs, *how* a particular word or phrase is said creates certain perceptions in both the sender and the receiver.

There can be a great disparity between the verbal and nonverbal signals transmitted. A person can say one thing but mean something else, be sarcastic, or convey other hidden meanings. This equation also includes the receiver who may "hear" one thing, even though the speaker said something entirely different. For these reasons, problems of semantics must be addressed in every communication effort.

Technical Problems)

Technical problems can occur during the transmission and reception of a message. They may include defects in the equipment (static, poor image, and so on), the environment (background noise, distracting activity), or the medium (torn paper, lost messages). Additionally, there are numerous rivals for the attention of the audience — in other words, information overload. These problems can result in the message being distorted, delayed, or even blocked entirely. For these reasons, the sender must ensure that the correspondence arrives at the target in the manner and format intended. Technical problems may be overcome or avoided by selecting an alternative route and communicating at times when there is less interference.

People Barriers)

"Say what you mean — and mean what you say!" This adage embodies the essence of people talking to each other. Barriers can exist because of individual differences in background and perception, or they can be thrown up intentionally in an effort to hide ulterior motives.

People bring to every exchange the sum of their educational, life, and work experiences and their previous interactions with the other person. The person across the table may be not only different in makeup and personality but also preoccupied with other matters — in other words, not on the same wave length. People barriers to communication generally involve problems with perception or interpersonal relationships.

Perception Factors)

This broad group covers personal issues ranging from the emotional to the attitudinal to the functional preparation and skills of the individual. Many studies on **perception** have demonstrated that we see what we are looking for and usually completely ignore or block out what we do not recognize or have not been trained to understand. Puzzles or brainteasers illustrate this point. When the solution is revealed, we are astonished that we did not see something so obvious. This principle carries over to all of our interactions, in both our personal and professional lives: The sender of a message may have said one thing, but the receiver may have heard or perceived something entirely different.

Emotions, attitudes, and physical and mental fatigue also color our perceptions. Problems sometimes seem insurmountable — until after a break, a little distance, a good night's sleep — the solution may suddenly appears crystal clear.

Perception is also strongly influenced by the individual parties' perspectives, particularly if one person outranks or is seen as a threat to the other — that is, there are real or perceived differences in personal, social, and business status.

Studies have shown that subordinates, like all people, hear what they want to hear or simply ignore conflicting information and gray areas. This phenomenon is called *selective perception* or the *halo effect* and is closely tied to the emotional and attitudinal state of the participants. To overcome perception problems, managers must invest time and attention in training and laying the groundwork for communications, as well as providing extensive opportunities for feedback, explanations, and reassurance.

Interpersonal Factors)

Differences in background and communication skills, as well as relative social and personal differences between the parties may impede communication. At the core of personal relationships is the issue of **credibility** between the participants. Credibility encompasses many other broad concepts: *trust* in purpose and character, *honesty* and dependability of the information provided, *competence* in objectivity in judgment, and, of utmost importance, the *empathy* and enthusiasm shown for the other person and the project.

Artificial barriers usually center around issues of self interest and hidden agendas. These barriers are expected and considered proper when negotiating business deals and contracts, but they are extremely destructive in the workplace, where teamwork and dependability are crucial. If someone begins to suspect that a person is hiding something or trying to "put something over," the breakdown in net communication accelerates as each person begins to build safety nets and defensive barriers.

Authority (job and social status) is often cited as being a natural hindrance to communications, but this criticism is unjust. People expect someone to be in charge. But when personal ambition, jealousy, and insecurity are added to the boss mentality, authority becomes a barrier. People start to protect their turf, exhibit attitudes of negativism and indifference, or simply tune out.

Outcome Problems)

No matter how skilled the sender is at communicating the message, if the receiver cannot perform the requested task, the communication has not been entirely successful. Outcome is also closely tied to the acceptance of the message by the receiver. The receiver may perceive that the task or project requested has a low priority. Obtaining results is the purpose of management, and communication skills are an integral part of that purpose.

Improving the Communication Process)

A vital part of communication skills is the ability to be a *good listener*). This is true on the receiving end, but is absolutely essential to the sender. Listening involves not only hearing or seeing the overt sounds or images transmitted but also correctly interpreting the message sent or received. Listening is a two-way partnership. Poor listening results in a person's not hearing or hearing incorrectly what was said or missing part of the message. Good listening involves asking questions, seeking feedback, showing interest in the speaker and subject, and looking for clues and signals that may reveal the need for further clarification or repetition.

Effective communication also involves *empathy*) with the person on the other end of the communication line. Empathy allows the sender to prepare the message with the needs of the audience in mind. There is no substitute for genuine concern and interest; this sentiment always comes through loud and clear. Unfortunately, *apathy*) or negative feelings and misplaced emotions are also just as easily detected and in most cases drown out any other portion of the message.

Sending a message through several different routes) is a highly effective way to gain attention. Repetition allows the recipient to properly interpret the missive, place it in context, and develop an appropriate response. Familiarity may produce boredom, but it also increases the comfort level.

As a review, to improve the communication process (also see Table 3—1):

- Be a good listener
- Be empathy toward other participants
- Send messages through several different routes

The next chapter with deal with techniques for Decision Making and Problem Solving.

— Case Study —

Chapter Three: Communications

"Where did you get this information?" the laboratory manager asked the supervisor.

"One of the evening techs told me about the plan last night when I was checking to see if anyone needed time off during the next month schedule," responded the supervisor.

"It's amazing how accurate what you told me is; however, the plan to move additional techs and phlebotomists to the night shift in order to support our new reference lab programs is only one of the many options that were discussed yesterday. But maybe there's a lesson here. Since the grapevine works faster than management, and since any changes will directly affect the evening and night shifts, I think it would be a good idea if you take responsibility for this part of the program. You must work closely with me, the director, and administration. We will try to hold all meetings in the afternoon after you come to work. Again, most important: While most of the work at this stage is confidential and only in the very early planning stages, you will be responsible for keeping your staff informed, and try to stomp out these wild rumors before they get started."

Chapter Section for Review

- The Communication Process
- Communication Directions
- Interpersonal Factors
- Improving the Communication Process

Questions for Discussion

1. Which communication direction channel appears to be the most active in this laboratory?
2. What link in the communication process seems to be the weakest in this situation?
3. How would you respond to the laboratory manager if you were the supervisor?
4. What advice would you give to the supervisor in handling the communication problems concerning the project and the staff ... particularly, possibly competing issues between ... confidentiality and leaking of management planning and discussions ... and keeping the staff "informed?"

[4]

Decision Making and Problem Solving

— Chapter Four —

Decision making and problem solving are such integral parts of daily life, encompassing every aspect of management and personal action that discussing them as separate subjects may seem impossible. Because of their importance, however, decision-making and problem-solving skills must be given top priority. Without proper training and attention in this area, the manager and the laboratory simply muddle through, postponing everyday decisions until they become acute. Such laboratories then find themselves engulfed in crisis management, running from fire to fire without making any discernible progress. This chapter describes the decision-making process as a series of eight steps and provides a selection of analytic tools that may improve the ability of the manager to make wise decisions.

OBJECTIVES

After completion of this chapter, the reader will be able to demonstrate accomplishment of the following objectives.

1. Recognize the features of a good decision.
2. Identify the role that human behavior plays and its influence in the decision-making process.
3. Explain the steps to making a sound decision.
4. Select from the available qualitative and quantitative techniques to resolve the problems and decisions faced by a laboratory manager.

Chapter Highlights and Glossary of Key Terms

I. CHARACTERISTICS OF A GOOD DECISION

Decision: *A conscious choice made after evaluating the available alternatives, for the purpose of achieving a specific result.*

II. THE HUMAN ELEMENT

III. STEPS IN MAKING A SOUND DECISION

A. Recognition
B. Investigation
C. Definition

Deviation: *A one-time, random human error.*

Effectual Problem: *The symptom or surface sign that may hide the real cause of a problem.*

Causal Problem: *The root cause of the problem.*

D. Identification of Alternatives
E. Solution Evaluation and Selection
F. Implementation and Follow-up

IV. DECISION-MAKING TECHNIQUES

A. Qualitative Tools

1. Personal judgment
2. Solicitation of advice

   Brainstorming: *A technique used in groups whereby everyone freely and spontaneously throws out ideas and solutions for later evaluation without regard for validity.*

   Synectics: *A group whose members are brought together as a problem-solving team.*

   Nominal Grouping: *A highly structured meeting in which individuals write their original ideas in private, with the alternative solutions anonymously presented to the group for discussion and then voted on and tallied in secret.*
3. Systematic Option Review

   T Chart: *A technique for evaluating alternative solutions by writing down the advantages and disadvantages of each option.*

B. Quantitative Tools

Operations Research: *A branch of management science that specializes in quantitative tools.*

Probability Analysis: *A procedure for measuring risk by assigning a value, expressed as a percentage, to the likelihood of a specific event occurring.*

Queuing Theory: *A decision-making technique that recommends the number of servers needed to handle an unpredictable workload.*

Linear Programming: *A tool for allocating limited resources among competing needs by applying mathematical values to each solution variable.*

Simulation: *The use of computer-designed models to imitate real-life conditions and test different intervention strategies.*

1. Probability analysis

   A Priori Probability: *Predictions obtained by deductions based on assumed conditions.*

   Empirical Probability: *Probability factors determined from the recording of actual events over a specific period of time.*

   Subjective Probability: *A prediction based on the knowledge and experience of the decision maker.*

   Payoff Matrix: *A matrix, or chart, that compares the probability potential of the alternatives identified.*

   Decision Trees: *A schematic presentation that demonstrates the probability potential of selecting a particular course of action at specific decision option points.*
2. Queuing theory
3. Linear programming
4. Simulation

Characteristics of a Good Decision

Good decisions require both careful thought and thorough planning. A well made **decision** should have the following features.

1. It should be based on a complete investigation of the root causes and potential problems, as well as the obvious symptoms.
2. It should identify and evaluate alternative solutions.
3. It should involve the selection of the best solution by in-depth analysis of the available information.
4. It should encompass an effective strategy for implementing the solution.

Timing and the setting of priorities are also crucial in making decisions. This chapter examines the decision making and problem-solving processes within the framework of organizations and discusses both a step-by-step decision making model and the tools and techniques available to the laboratory manager.

The Human Element

The human element can quickly cloud the decision making process. Emotions, prejudices, peer pressure, and personal interest can exert tremendous influence on the choices made. These factors can never be completely eliminated, but they must be controlled. This can be accomplished through sound management and decision-making procedures.

Human factors are not always bad. However, they should be recognized for what they are and given appropriate consideration. *Disclosure* is often proposed as an effective control method and balancing action — providing the participants have the *power* and *independence* to consider its impact and to act accordingly.

The most effective way to deal with the human element is to turn it into an asset by using objective analytical tools to evaluate the situation and allowing the human touch to provide the perspective and context for selection and implementation. A model for problem solving and associated analytic tools are presented in the following sections. The manager must consider each stage carefully and apply the available analytical techniques to the deliberations.

Steps in Making a Sound Decision

A model for making a decision or solving a problem can be broken down into eight steps, as shown in Table 4 – 1 and reviewed in the next section. Each phase offers the decision maker both a challenge and an opportunity. By paying attention to the details of each stage, the laboratory manager can build the framework for choosing the correct course of action.

Step 1:	Recognition that there is a problem or need for the manager's intervention
Step 2:	Investigation and analysis of the cause and extent of the problem
Step 3:	Definition of the nature and boundaries of the problem
Step 4:	Identification of alternative solutions
Step 5:	Evaluation of each option, within the context of the management plan and objectives of the laboratory
Step 6:	Selection of the best alternative
Step 7:	Implementation of the solution
Step 8:	Follow-up on the success and progress of the decision, and institution of needed modifications

TABLE 4—1. Decision-Making and Problem-Solving Process

Recognition

Step 1 in making any decision or solving a problem is to become aware that something is wrong and needs the attention of the manager. This message may arrive from many different sources — as a complaint from a physician or employee or as a flag in the quality control data, for instance.

Recognizing a problem is not as simple as it may appear. What appears to be a problem may be only a random occurrence, and the manager can waste a lot of time and energy tracking down something that will fix itself. The earlier the problem is recognized, the sooner priorities can be set for resolving it.

Investigation

After the laboratory manager becomes aware of a problem, the situation must be investigated. Step 2 includes collecting data, interviewing staff, and gathering information that may shed light on the nature and seriousness of the problem. During this fact-gathering stage, the manager should be alert to ancillary issues that may have contributed to the problem but were not at first readily apparent.

Definition

Step 3 in the decision-making process is to define the problem. President Lyndon Johnson once pointed out that when a problem has been defined, the solution often becomes obvious to all. Other authors have found that formulating the correct question is 80 percent of the solution. Determining the exact extent and boundaries of the problem enables the laboratory manager to target the investigation toward specific objectives.

Defining the problem means determining all the issues and aspects of the question, including people, equipment, communication, supplies, and the work flow itself. At this point, attention should be given to ascertaining the depth of the trouble and questioning the boundaries of the definition. Here are some questions to assist in this process.

- Is this only a symptom of a more serious or wide spread problem?
- Is it a one-time **deviation** from the standards or a random human error?
- Is the problem as it initially appears, only an **effectual** (surface) **problem**; or should it be investigated further to uncover the root or **causal problem?**

The answers to these inquiries help define the nature and urgency of the problem being researched. The laboratory manager can note the similarity between this step and troubleshooting procedures common in quality control and instrument malfunction investigations.

Identification of Alternatives

Determining what solutions are available to remedy the situation is step 4 of the decision-making process. At this stage the manager may wish to solicit advice from other members of the staff or even assign the problem to a committee to recommend solutions. Although the committee system is often criticized as being too slow and ineffective, it is one of the best sources for ideas to resolve organizational problems.

The key at this stage is to be aware of as many alternative solutions as possible; the manager then has a range of options from which to choose. The manager should avoid the temptation to examine each alternative in depth as it is discovered and instead wait until a number of solutions are collected. Although some proposals can be rejected outright, considering each alternative as it becomes known is time-consuming, and the manager may settle on a poor choice simply because of time constraints.

Solution Evaluation and Selection

After the pool of feasible solutions has been compiled, a thorough evaluation should be conducted (step 5), and the best alternative selected (step 6). Some suggestions can be ruled out immediately. For those deserving serious consideration, a variety of tools can be used to select the most suitable alternative. Both qualitative and quantitative techniques are discussed in the next section.

Implementation and Follow-up

Steps 7 (implementation) and 8 (follow-up) should be fully integrated into the management functions and process of the laboratory. Developing a plan to implement the final decision and devising a mechanism to monitor compliance are part of the management functions (see Chapter 1) and illustrate the central role of decision making in the overall operations of the laboratory.

The seven steps are synthesized into four by Roger Martin, in the article *How Successful Leaders Think* (HBR June 2007):

- First, determine which features of a problem are salient, then look beyond to find other relevant factors (i.e., what's important, pertinent to defining and investigation the situation).
- "Second, consider multidirectional and nonlinear relationships, not just linear ones."

  This is to not just assume a single direct causal relations between a problem and a single happening [i.e., (cause — effect) this happen, then so did this]. For example, the morning collections may *not* be late solely because the third shift phlebotomists decided to arbitrarily start printing out a list and labels of patients to be drawn in the morning collection at 3:00am instead of 1:00am, as they were supposed to; however, it may be found that the ward clerks begin to put AM orders in the computer after Midnight, because someone in the Hospital Information System department thought the screen would be more streamlined, if only the currents days tests where displayed (i.e., *if* the ward clerks put order in the evening before, they could not see or check until after midnight to review that days requests).
- "Third, they see the whole problem and the parts fit together.
- Forth, they creatively resolve the pensions between opposing ideas and generate new alternatives." p. 139.

Decision-Making Techniques

Techniques for evaluating decision options can be divided into qualitative and quantitative methods.

Qualitative Tools

Qualitative decision-making tools involve personal judgment, solicitation of advice, and systematic option review.

Personal Judgment

People begin at birth to develop skills in choosing between competing options. These skills grow with maturity and experience. In addition to the judgment gained through life experience, the specific duties and demands of the workplace and profession become familiar through formal training and career advancements. This personal knowledge is a vital resource in evaluating alternatives and making decisions.

Solicitation of Advice

Asking for opinions, organizing a committee, seeking a consensus from colleagues and coworkers, and delegating the task to staff members are all examples of soliciting advice and using the experience and insight of other members of the laboratory.

Forming a group or committee to focus on a problem is one of the most common approaches to decision making. Listed next are several successful techniques for collecting suggestions from a group.

- **Brainstorming**. Everyone freely throws out ideas for later evaluation without regard for initial validity or criticism: *idea popping*.
- **Synectics.** People with a variety of backgrounds are brought together as a troubleshooting team.
- **Nominal grouping.** In a highly structured meeting, individuals write down their original ideas and then present them to the group. Group members then vote on and rank-order each suggestion secretly to discourage peer pressure and encourage creativity. This technique is similar to brainstorm; however the anonymity is intended to allow suggestions and input to flow without possible fear or intimidation from other members of the group.
- **Delphi method.** In a modification of nominal grouping, the input and opinions of experts are solicited on questionnaires before the meeting. The results are then discussed and voted on anonymously. The Delphi method is more commonly used in making decisions in which forecasting future events or trends are important.

Systematic Option Review

Systematic option review involves prioritizing each option according to its apparent attractiveness. A **T chart** is one popular format for evaluating facts and information. This technique has been borrowed from accounting. The problem and proposed solution are written down at the top of the page, a line is drawn down the middle (hence the name T), and the advantages and disadvantages are listed on either side of the T. This visual presentation of the proposal often clarifies the opportunities and risks associated with each option and make the selection process more objective. Table 4 – 2 shows a T chart for making the quantitative beta human chorionic gonadotropin a STAT test, available on all shifts.

Problem: Request by ER Medical Staff for STAT BHCG
Proposed Solution: Train staff on evening and night shifts to perform test

Advantages	**Disadvantages**
Satisfy patient service needs	Training time
Spread of workload and productivity	Lack of trained staff
Improved turnaround time	Shortage of personnel
Additional trained staff	$2 increase in cost of test
Educational opportunities	Disruption of work flow
	Increased workload of shifts

TABLE 4—2. T-Chart Analysis

Quantitative Tools

Quantitative tools include both quality control (QC) measures and financial data. One branch of management science that specializes in providing quantitative tools for decision making is called **operations research (OR).** The four main areas of OR are as follows.

- **Probability analysis**, which measures risk by assigning a value, expressed as a percentage, to the likelihood of a specific event occurring.
- **Queuing theory**, which provides recommendations for the number of staff (phlebotomists, clerks, technical personnel, and so on) needed to handle an unpredictable, or randomly accessible workload (i.e., any one, or number, of patients could request service at a particular time; like "business hours," of a retail store — one customer or twenty could walk through the door at any moment).
- **Linear programming**, a tool for allocating limited resources among competing needs.
- **Simulation**, which designs models to imitate real life conditions so the different intervention scenarios can be compared

OR management is the application of these quantitative techniques to business situations.

Probability Analysis

Probability analysis is most useful when the manager is faced with choosing between several different options under conditions with significant risk or uncertainty. An estimate of probability *(P)* of a certain outcome or event happening is calculated numerically so that it can be compared with other options.

An **a priori probability** is obtained by deductions based on assumed conditions. For example, a flip of a coin has a 50 percent probability (P = .5) of coming up heads. However, the outcome of a single toss cannot be predicted with absolute certainty. Similarly, the laboratory goes to great lengths to establish normal (or reference) ranges for its procedures and patient population, but it cannot predict with certainty where a particular patient's results will fall before the test is run. Delta checks, a type of statistical quality control procedure, depend on comparing current results with previous tests to detect possible errors.

Empirical probability is determined by recording actual events over a specific period of time and calculating the number of times each event occurs. This technique is used when the laboratory establishes QC ranges for a new lot of reagents or controls. It may also be used to predict turnaround time for a test, STAT response times, and absenteeism.

Subjective probability is just that — subjective. Based on the knowledge and experience of the individual or group, a prediction is made of the likelihood of an event occurring. This technique, like decision making, is a common process. When technologists are asked how soon a result will be ready or how much longer a reagent will last on an instrument, they can usually predict the answer with fairly good accuracy, even though no formal study has been conducted.

Two techniques have proved helpful in applying probability analysis to business situations: the **payoff matrix** and **decision trees**. These procedures are especially useful for cost-benefit analysis of different alternatives. In addition, the decision tree can be modified for use as a *flow chart* (see the chapter on *Laboratory Information Systems*) .

> **Here is an example of probability analysis: Financial impact of performing tests in-house**
>
> Laboratories must frequently decide whether to perform a test in-house or send it to a reference lab. A payoff matrix (Table 4 – 3) and decision tree (Figure 4--1) are used to determine the financial impact of performing protein electrophoresis in the lab. Here are the known data:

- *Empirical data:* An average of 75 protein electrophoresis tests is sent to reference laboratories per month.
- *Subjective potential:* There is a 70 percent probability *(P* = .7) of doing 125 tests a month, as determined from conversations with physicians and complaints about turnaround times.
- Net profit per test
  - Send to reference lab: $5 per test
  - Perform in-house: first 75 = $2 per test;

		Send Test Out		*Bring Test In-House*	
Volume (Tests per Month)	*P*	Potential Income ($)	Expected Income ($) (Potential Income × Probability)	Potential Income ($)	Expected Income ($) (Potential Income × Probability)
75	1.0	375	375	150	150
100	.8	500	400	525	420
125	.7	625	438	900	630
150	.3	750	225	1,275	383

TABLE 4—3. Payoff Matrix Analysis

each additional test = $15 per test

Analysis (see also Table 4—3 and Figure 4—1): The *potential* for profit goes up as the volume of tests increases; however, when *probability (P)* is included in the equation the options become more realistic — $900 versus $630 at 125 tests/month. The manager must obviously include other factors, such as turnaround time and patient service needs, in making a decision, but the tools of probability shed significant light on the impact of a course of action on the total operations of the laboratory.

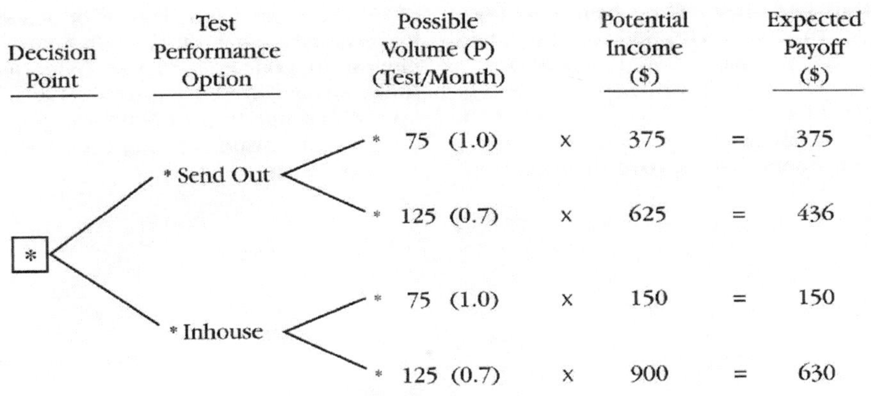

FIGURE 4—1. Decision-Tree Analysis

Queuing Theory

Computer programs for queuing, linear programming, and simulation are widely available. The manager, however, should know how and when to use these tools, which are ideally suited to the fluctuating and unpredictable work flow of the medical laboratory. Queuing theory was originally designed to determine the number of airline reservation clerks needed for a given time period and is designed to determine the staffing requirements of a workstation with the following operational needs:

1. Need for prompt service
2. Need for an adequate number of servers to meet an urgent demand
3. Unpredictable timing of service requests
4. Unpredictable duration of service time

The input variables used by most queuing programs to determine the appropriate staffing level of servers (e.g., phlebotomist, technologists, instruments) include:

1. Average number of units (e.g. specimens, patients, clients) requesting or arriving for service during a designated period of time (hour, shift, day, test run)
2. Average number of units waiting for service
3. Average waiting time until service begins
4. Average time to process a unit
5. Maximum time acceptable to wait for results or service

Once these parameters have been determined, they can be entered into a queuing program for staffing level calculations.

[below are two web sites from *EventHelix.com*[tm] with additional information on Queueing(sic) Theory Basics, including Little's Theorum and several equations used in staffing level projections] [connected June 1, 2007]
http://www.eventhelix.com/RealtimeMantra/CongestionControl/queueing_theory.htm
http://www.eventhelix.com/RealtimeMantra/CongestionControl/m_m_1_queue.htm

Linear Programming

Linear programming was designed to resolve the following types of problems.

- Limits and restraints on the availability of resources (staff, time, expenses)
- Constant need for decisions as to allocation of these limited resources among competing needs
- Pressure to maximize income and minimize losses

Managers may not be aware that they use linear programming techniques subconsciously in everyday decisions; however, you will easily recognize that linear programming is a normal thought process in life.

The process of elimination and selection illustrates the procedure. Here are some questions and variables associated with this type of decision.

- Does the instrument perform all the tests required, or is additional equipment necessary?
- Are the throughput and turnaround time acceptable?
- Is the price within the laboratory budget?

Linear programming then applies a mathematical value to each variable to solve the problem.

Linear Programming example: Requirements for the main chemistry analyzer

- Turnaround time (routine processing time)
  $\leq$ 20 minutes for all tests including enzymes
  $\leq$ 10 minutes for STAT CHEM 6 (glucose, BUN, lytes)
- Specimen Requirement:
  $\leq$ 50 *u*L per test

- Throughput (tests per hour)
  $\geq$ 60 samples per hours

- Test available:
  $\geq$ all routine tests
- Price:
  Instrument = < $100,000
  Cost per test = $\leq$ $1.20

<u>Analysis</u>: By solving for each of these variables, an informed decision can be made when these criteria are applied to each instrument being considered.

Simulation

The computer has made possible the development of models that closely duplicate the conditions found in real-life settings. These models attempt to identify important variables, which the manager can then manipulate to test the impact of different options on the system. An example of simulation might be a computer projection of the impact on length of patient stay in the hospital if CPK isoenzymes are batched and run at different times (e.g., every 2, 4, or 8 hours) instead of on a STAT basis.

Critics point out the difficulty of isolating all possible variables and accurately measuring their influence. However, as computers and computer simulation become more sophisticated, they will be even more useful to the manager. Used in conjunction with the other decision-making tools, the possibilities are limitless.

By applying the tools discussed in this chapter to the decisions and problems encountered in the medical laboratory, managers can improve their chances of selecting the wisest course of action and increasing the efficiency of the laboratory. These techniques, in concert with the other techniques and skills covered in Part 1, provide the laboratory manager with a significant amount of knowledge that can be directed toward assuring both personal and institutional success.

The next chapter covers the *Management of Change*.

— Case Study —

Chapter Four: Decision Making and Problem Solving

The hospital administrator has suggested to the laboratory manager that she consider opening a satellite specimen collection and service center in the new medical office complex that is being built next door to the hospital. Several reference laboratories have approached the building manager about renting such space already, and the administrator is concerned about the possible loss of outpatient business to these reference labs.

Upon investigation the laboratory manager obtained the following information.

1. The laboratory is now receiving an average of 12,250 tests a year from the doctors who will be moving into the new office complex.
2. The laboratory has a net profit from these tests of $10 each. This is expected to drop to $5 a test in the satellite station because of costs associated with rent, salaries, and other expenses.
3. From market research conducted by the hospital, the number of tests received from the new satellite station would at least remain the same and has an 80% possibility of increasing to 20,000 tests a year because of new physicians who will occupy the building and convenience for current patients.
4. From the same studies, it was found that there is only a 70% chance of maintaining the current volume of tests from these sources, and that there is a high probability (100%) that the test volume will drop to only 9,000 a year if a satellite station is not opened.

Chapter Sections for Review

- Steps in Making a Sound Decision
- Qualitative Tools
- Probability Analysis
- Decision-Tree Analysis (Figure 4—1) and Payoff Matrix Analysis (Table 4 – 3)

Questions for Discussion

1. Prepare a decision tree analysis of the problem.
2. From this analysis, what appears to be the best solution?
3. Are there other factors that need to be considered in making a decision (e.g., maintaining market and patient base, service needs of the community)?
4. What qualitative tools may be helpful in the decision-making process?

		Possible Volume(*P*)	Potential Income	Expected Payoff
Satellite station:	Open	20,000(0.8)	$100,000 (@$5/test)	= $80,000 [$100,000 **x** 0.8]
	Not Open	- 12,250(0.7)	$122,500 (@$10/test)	= $85,750 [$122,500 **x** 0.7]
		- 9,000(1.0)	$ 90,000 (@$10/test)	= $90,000 [$90,000 **x** 1.0]

Management of Change

—Chapter Five—

The management of change is a reflection of the management process. Planning for change must be an inclusive and integral part of the four management functions. For practical purposes, and to avoid repeating the management functions already discussed, this topic is divided into two parts: the nature of change and management of the change process. The change process is further broken down into four stages: diagnosis, planning, implementation, and follow-up. Note the similarity between these phases and the phases of the management process (planning, organizing, directing, and controlling) described in Chapter 1. This similarity is intended.

OBJECTIVES

After completion of this chapter, the reader will be able to demonstrate accomplishment of the following objectives.

1. Explain the role of change in the life of an organization and the manager's responsibility for both controlling and initiating change.
2. Identify the sources of conflict and resistance to change.
3. Discuss the change process, including the incorporation of the change process into the overall management plan of the laboratory.
4. Design a plan for intervening and implementing a change strategy.
5. Track the progress of a change program.

Chapter Highlights and Glossary of Key Terms

I. CHANGE: A NATURAL PROCESS

Change: *To become different, usually in response to a stimulus requiring an action or adjustment.*

II. MANAGEMENT RESPONSIBILITY FOR CHANGE

Change Agent: *The person initiating the change effort.*

Client System: *The target of the change agent's intervention effort; the entity that may need or desire a change.*

III. THE NATURE OF CHANGE

A. Sources of Change
B. Sources of Conflicts and Resistance to Change

IV. MANAGEMENT OF THE CHANGE PROCESS

A. Diagnosing and Analyzing Change
B. Change Strategies
   1. Participation and involvement strategy
   2. Informed strategy
C. Implementation
   1. Job functions
   2. Organizational structure
   3. People changes
D. Follow-up Cycle: Continuous Change Management

Change: A Natural Process

It is an undisputed fact that **change** is inevitable. In actuality, if the elements of our life (physical and mental maturation, family, job, social ties, and so on) did not change (i.e., grow), this would be a source of great concern. Given the acceptance of, and desire for change, it may seem puzzling that this issue should require a separate section in management textbooks and receive the extensive attention it does in business literature and research. This attention results from one additional force generated by change, namely, *resistance!*

Resistance is part of the natural flow of the change process. Diet, health, retirement, reconstruction, and reconciliation plans are everyday examples of the extent that individuals go to in order to ward off and prepare for the inevitable. Given this fact, resistance to change should come as no surprise to the laboratory manager. Just as obvious are the reasons for resistance: loss of personal control, fear of the unknown, and apprehension about the "real" objectives of management- in a word, insecurity.

The antidotes for resistance to change are also just as apparent: openness, inclusion, and participation in the decision-making process — in a word, communication. This common understanding of the continuous process of change, resistance, and antidote lays the groundwork for a review of change in the laboratory and the role of the supervisor in managing the process.

Management Responsibility for Change

As the representative of both the owners and employees of the institution, the manager is responsible for adjusting to, and initiating change. Too little change results in a department that is stagnant and ineffective; too much unmanaged change leads to confusion and chaos. The manager's role as a **change agent** in this balancing act is closely tied to the target of intervention. In change management terminology, the individual or unit that needs or desires the change is called the **client system**.

Viewing the design of a change strategy in a consultant-to-client (change agent-to-client system) relationship helps the manager gain perspective on the inherent conflicts that accompany such decisions. It also enables the manager to achieve the measure of objectivity that allows the change process to be incorporated into the overall management plan of the laboratory.

The Nature of Change

Consistent with the organizational systems theory reviewed in Chapter 2, change exerts constant pressure on the organization's tendency toward stasis. The laboratory receives and delivers the forces of change through the input-output mechanisms by which it and its members interact with the social and economic environment. Researchers who study group dynamics have found that this stress drives the organizational system from the steady (or frozen) state through a process of thawing and regeneration and on to a new plateau by refreezing in a new steady state. This process is illustrated in Figure 5 – 1.

The forces of change bombarding the organization come from many sources, both internal and external; they are shaped by the resulting resistance that arises to these challenges. Sources of change, conflict, and resistance are reviewed in the following sections, as are strategies for managing change. Understanding the origins of these change impetuses and resistance is important in developing a plan to lead the organization as it continues to adapt and grow.

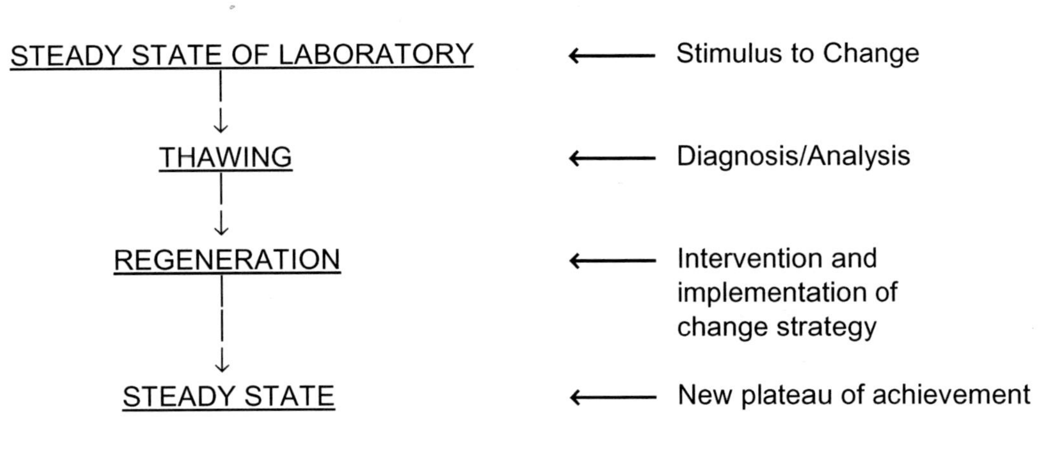

FIGURE 5—1. The Change Process

Sources of Change

In all institutions, change is generated through movement, growth, and advancement. These stimuli may arise from changes in the following areas.

- The *knowledge base,* both the broad advances in the arts and sciences in general and the specific technology of laboratory instrumentation and methodology.
- The *scope of management* duties and responsibilities and the application of specialized business skills and concepts to nonprofit and social organizations.
- The *issues and problems* facing managers, society, and individuals as their needs and desires progress into the future.
- The *environment,* as physical resources are depleted and must be renewed.
- The *increasing rate of change* in all these areas and resulting decrease in the response time allowed for the manager to make and implement needed adjustments.

The energy created by these tensions precipitates conflicts and resistance as the old, familiar, and seemingly secure positions are motivated to move on to a new level.

Sources of Conflicts and Resistance to Change

Another part of the manager's job is making decisions about the allocation of scarce resources (money, schedules, time, and work priorities) among competing demands. This duty can also be considered the wellspring for the conflicts and resistance resulting from members who may perceive themselves as "losers" when required to change and adjust to decisions imposed on them.

Insecurity, cited earlier as the reason for resistance to change, can be a genuine concern based on the reality of the situation or a function of an erroneous evaluation based on poor communications and misinterpretation of the impact the change will have. Whether justified or misplaced, the resulting responses of the people involved can cause havoc in the workplace if not properly managed. The conflict and resistance arising from insecurity may come from a variety of sources and assume several different forms. They all, however, center around the workers as individuals and their relationship with the organization.

Self-interest, be it social position, status, or economic well-being, is an important factor. If people perceive that they have something to gain or lose from changes in the system, whether real or imaginary, they can be expected to take advantage of the opportunity or try to protect themselves from harm.

Assessment differences are another impetus for conflict and resistance. Such differences can arise because of a disagreement over interpretation and judgment, limited information, or a lack of understanding of the situation. These differences can be particularly potent if individuals assess the potential impact on their wellbeing in a way that is markedly different from the projections of management — in other words, if there is a lack of trust.

A perceived *loss of control,* whether real or not, can result in a strong attempt to maintain the status quo. Fear can develop through a perceived reduction of autonomy or a challenge to the person's comfort zone. Apprehension about hidden agendas or the "real" objectives of the decision maker can contribute to this fear. This fear may also be a factor in the *low tolerance for change* of staff members who have held a particular position or operated a specialized piece of equipment for a long time. When faced with a change in job duties or equipment, they become defensive and uncooperative in order to reinforce and emphasize their worth to both themselves and the organization.

Finding ways to overcome the normal conflicts and resistance to change is an important challenge for all managers. The best approach lies in the effective use of the tools and skills discussed in preceding chapters.

Management of the Change Process

The kinship between the change process and management has already been established. Whereas management seeks to guide the overall progress of the organization toward specific goals, the change process focuses on identifying needed modifications and developing a strategy for adjustment. Four stages enable the manager to incorporate new ideas and innovations into the overall management plan of the laboratory: diagnosis, strategy development, implementation of plan, and follow-up. These steps are outlined next and in Table 5 – 1.

1. Diagnosing and analyzing the need for change
   - Management planning function
   - Decision-making skills
2. Designing a change strategy
   - Situational changes
   - Organizational development
3. Implementing the change plan
   - Job functions
   - Organizational structure
   - People changes
4. Follow-up cycle: Continuous change management

Table 5—1. Change Management Process Model

Diagnosing and Analyzing Change

The need for change may become evident from many sources, including the quality control process. For example, there may be a drift in the QC data or an increased turnaround time for STATS. It may come from increased complaints about service from physicians, patients, or staff. There may be excess overtime or work hours. Change may also develop from diverse external sources, such as the information received from seminars, literature reviews, or contact with sales people and colleagues from other laboratories. Whatever the source of the revelations, a systematic investigation should be conducted to identify exactly what kind of change needs to be pursued. Suggested guidelines for diagnosing and analyzing change and other organizational problems can be found in the management planning function (see Chapter 1, and specifically Table 4—1 in Chapter 4 listing the steps in making a sound decision).

Change Strategies

A review of the management planning function shows that a manager can use two primary means of intervention: tools of persuasion and tools of control. These intervention tools can be placed on a continuum ranging from a participatory strategy of education, discussion, and fact presentation (in which the manager attempts to gain support by convincing the workers that the change is in their own, and the institution's, best interest) to an approach of explicit orders (in which the staff is informed of the change and coerced by threats of disciplinary action if they do not accept or adjust to the new policy). What tools managers select are determined by their leadership style (participatory or dictatorial; see Chapter 7), the implementation route selected, and the particular circumstances surrounding the event.

A change strategy built on a participatory leadership style centers on providing information about any impending change at the very first stage of the decision making process and on soliciting the advice of those who will be affected.
The following example illustrates the expected effect of two change strategies, persuasion and control, on a tech who learns about the acquisition of a new instrument that will automate tasks this person has spent most of his or her career performing.

Scenario 1

Participatory and involvement strategy (persuasion). The tech is called into the manager's office for a discussion of the problems (increased workload and requests for faster turnaround) of the current methodology. The tech is asked to investigate and make recommendations about available instruments that might be useful in updating the department.

Scenario 2

Informed strategy (control). The manager walks into the department with the service representative and asks the tech to help with the measurements for the new instrument that will be arriving in 2 months. (Of course, the tech has already heard about the change through the grapevine. The manager fully intends to have the tech trained in the operation of the new instruments but forgot to let the tech know and to find out which training session the tech would like to attend.)

If you were the tech, which scenario would you prefer? Your answer suggests which change strategy is most appropriate and most likely to result in a smooth transition to an automated department.

Implementation

The laboratory manager has three avenues through which to implement change: *job functions, organizational structure,* and *people.*

Job Functions

Job functions, or *tasks,* can change because of the adoption of revised policies and procedures or the introduction of different *technology* (new instruments and equipment). The redesign of job responsibilities is an ongoing process in the laboratory and is the most frequent method for introducing change. Almost all changes involve modifications in jobs; the increasing pace of specialization and technological change makes this an excellent intervention point for the manager. Change, like medicine, is easier to accept if it is part of the job enrichment, training, and professional growth that should accompany the incorporation of new technology and procedures into the laboratory.

Organizational Structure

Changing the bureaucracy by reorganizing the management hierarchy is a popular strategy for big corporations and top administration. The news media are full of reports of companies announcing such changes in efforts to renew and improve the corporation. "New blood," "top-heavy," "streamlined decision making," "eliminating middle-management waste," "cost cuts and reduction of overhead," "restructuring," and "downsizing" are all reasons cited for reorganization.

At the department level, structural changes can be introduced through changes in supervisory and management styles. In particular, a move to a more participatory decision-making style that includes changes in the delegation of authority, span of supervisory control, coordination, and communication channels has been successful in implementing change.

People Changes

A manager can implement changes through people, either by replacement or by changing the attitudes and behavior of the current staff. Change is normally expected when a new supervisor is promoted or brought on board, a technologist with specialized skills is hired, or an educational program is completed.

Managers may feel it is easier and quicker to bring in new talent rather than develop an existing staff member. There is, however, considerable risk involved in this decision. Possible mistakes revolve around selection, compatibility, orientation, learning and adjustment time, and recruitment expenses. In addition, the current staff may feel rejected, resentful, and disappointed. This policy may also be a sign of a failure on the part of the manager to encourage an environment of trust and loyalty. There is no question that there are situations in which only a new person can satisfy special needs, but a major part of any ongoing management plan must be the development of new leaders from among existing staff.

Follow-up Cycle: Continuous Change Management

After the need for change has been identified and a plan developed and implemented, the progress of the program must be monitored to make needed modifications and ensure success. The feedback mechanism should be built into the management controlling function and make use of the monitors established during that phase of the management process.

In anticipation of the types of standards and performance criteria that will be needed to keep track of progress in the change program, the manager should be aware that there are three possible responses on the part of the staff to the changes:

1. They can accept and provide active support for the program.
2. They can passively comply with the new requirements.
3. They can resist the new plan with varying degrees of aggression.

Whereas the first action is highly desirable, no manager can expect enthusiastic support for every decision. It is often a welcome relief just to find that the staff is willing to "give it a try." However, active resistance must be dealt with and overcome. As pointed out in the first part of this chapter, resistance can be avoided and overcome by including in the decision making process the people who will be affected by the change. If this step is not attended to at the beginning of the change cycle, the manager may have to stop the process and deal with this issue when it is most inconvenient. When resistance or lack of support is encountered, an analysis of both the source and objection must be conducted and appropriate steps taken using the tools of persuasion and control available to the manager.

This concludes the chapter on the *Management of Change*, and the first part of the book; <u>Management of Organizations</u>. The next chapter, *Motivation to Work*, begin the second part of the course dealing with the <u>Management of Human Resources</u>, or working with people, a vital skill for any manager, especially in the medical laboratory.

— Case Study —

Chapter Five: Management of Change

"Well, I agree," responded the chief technologist to the information presented by the chemistry supervisor, "both routine and special chemistry have grown too large and complex for one supervisor to handle. I spoke to the pathologists and they agree it's time to make special chemistry its own section with a supervisor and staff. We thought it would be a good idea, however, if you oversaw the transition and recommended a plan along with staff assignments and who we should consider for the new special chemistry supervisor."

"I don't know," answered the chemistry supervisor. "There shouldn't be any problems with the equipment, but I'm not sure how the staff will like it, and I certainly don't want anyone to get mad at me about choosing a new supervisor. You know both Tom and Mary are still disappointed about not being promoted last time."

"Welcome to management," commented the manager, nodding in agreement. "We would like to promote someone from within, and there are a lot of excellent techs in your section. Think about it, and get back with me about a possible plan."

Chapter Sections for Review

- Sources of Conflict and Resistance to Change
- Management of the Change Process (Table 5—1)
- Change Strategies
- Implementation

Questions for Discussion

1. What type of reception do you think the staff will give the impending change?
2. What kinds of resistance might the supervisor expect to encounter when implementing the plan, and why? How can the supervisor best deal with the resistance?
3. What are the best avenues through which to implement the change in this situation?

PART 1: BIBLIOGRAPHY

This book is presented as a 2nd edition, revision, update, additional text content, and sequential of: Varnadoe, Lionel A; Medical Laboratory Management and Supervision: *Operations, Review, and Study Guide*; F. A. Davis Company, Philadelphia; 1996. Following is the initial bibliography (p.54) plus additional current citations.

Adler, RB: Communicating at Work. McGraw-Hill, New York, 1992.

Bennett, AC, and Tibbitts, SJ: Maximizing Quality Performance in Health Care Facilities. Aspen Publishers, Rockville, MD, 1989.

Drucker, PF: Management: Tasks, Responsibilities, Practices. Harper & Row, New York, 1974.

Drucker, PF: Managing the Nonprofit Organization. HarperCollins, New York, 1990.

Gupta, SK, and Cozzolino, JM: Fundamentals of Operations Research for Management. Holden-Day, San Francisco, 1975.

Haimann, T: Supervisory Management for Healthcare Organizations, ed 4. The Catholic Health Association of the United States, St. Louis, 1989

Hillier, FS: Introduction to Operations Research. McGraw-Hill, New York, 1990.

Litterer, JA (ed): Organizations: Structure and Behavior, ed 3. John Wiley & Sons, New York, 1980.

Lyles, RI, and Joiner, C: Supervision in Health Care Organizations. Delmar, Albany, NY 1986.

Martin, Roger; *How Successful Leaders Think*; Harvard Business Review, vol. 85, no. 6, June 2007; pp. 60-67, 139

Mintzberg, H: Mintzberg on Management. The Free Press, New York, 1989.

Resnik, MD: Choices: An Introduction to Decision Theory. University of Minnesota Press, Minneapolis 1987.

Schulz, R, and Johnson, AC: Management of Hospitals and Health Services, ed 3. CV Mosby, St Louis, 1990.

Varnadoe, LA: Designing a mission-oriented laboratory. American Journal of Medical Technology, 44(12): 1145, 1978.

Woodward, J: Industrial Organization: Theory and Practice. Oxford University Press, New York, 1965.

Internet reference, referrals, and suggested citations

[below are two web sites from *EventHelix.com*tm with additional information on Queueing(sic) Theory Basics, including Little's Theorum and several equations used in staffing level projections]

http://www.eventhelix.com/RealtimeMantra/CongestionControl/queueing_theory.htm
http://www.eventhelix.com/RealtimeMantra/CongestionControl/m_m_1_queue.htm
[connected July 3, 2007]

Medical Laboratory Management and Supervision

Part 2: Management of Human Resources

[6]

Motivation to Work

— Chapter Six —

> "But, interestingly, our research show that the most important managerial behaviors don't involve giving people daily pats on the back or attempting to inject lighthearted fun into the workplace. Rather, they involve two fundamental things: enabling people to move forward in their work and treating them decently as human beings."
>
> Amabile, Teresa M., and Steven J. Kramer; *Inner Work Life*; Harvard Business Review Vol 85 No 5, May 2007; p. 81

Leadership, motivation, management—those words are so often used as synonyms that they are frequently seen as one and the same. In fact, many one-line definitions describe management as the "process of getting thing done through people." This approach is correct but incomplete. Leadership and motivation are essential elements of the management process; however, management goes further and includes the coordination of other factors, such as financial and material recourses, as well as people. In the same vein, motivation is a crucial part of leadership but not the entire picture. Leadership focuses on directing a *group* of people toward a designated goal. Motivation, by contrast, deals with what makes *individuals* act the way they do.

Objectives

After completion of this chapter, the reader will be able to demonstrate accomplishment of the following objectives.

1. Define motivation in the context of the workplace;
2. Describe the major theories of motivation;
3. Distinguish between content and process models; and,
4. Relate motivational theories to managing professionals in the medical laboratory.

Chapter Highlights and Glossary of Key Terms

I. DEFINITION OF MOTIVATION

Motivation: *The reason people do the things they do.*

A. Motive

Motive: *A desire or need that acts as a stimulus for action.*

B. Definitional Limitations

C. Attitude

Attitude: *People's outward disposition toward their job tasks and coworkers.*

II. MAJOR THEORIES OF MOTIVATION

A. Content Motivational Theories

Content Motivational Theories: *Theories that examine the internal forces that drive the individual toward specific actions.*

1. Maslow's Hierarchy of Needs Theory
2. Herzberg's Two-Factor Theory
3. McClelland's Achievement Model
4. Alderfer's ERG Theory

B. Process Motivational Theories

Process Motivational Theories: *Theories that seek to understand "how" people are motivation.*

1. Vroom's Expectancy Theory
2. Adam's Equity Theory
3. Skinner's Reinforcement Theory

C. Other Motivational Theories

III. APPLICATION OF MOTIVATION THEORIES TO THE WORKPLACE

A. Leadership, Work, and Job Satisfaction

Job Satisfaction: *The degree to which employees feel their jobs meet their needs and wants.*

B. Goal Setting

C. Pay

Material Pay: *The tangible or monetary part of the paycheck.*

Psychic Pay: *The intrinsic rewards that give us a good feeling about ourselves and work.*

Definition of Motivation

The term **motivation** encompasses many images. It implies the existence of incentives, motives, and purpose. It also incorporates ideas about the drive, desires, and needs of an individual. Motivation can be cited as the reason someone behaves in a certain manner or is blamed for failure; for example, although they were obviously the better team, they were just not motivated enough to win." It is also a source of hope; for example, "If only I could motivate my child to get better grades," or "I know we have the talent, if we could just motivate the staff to pull together as a team."

"Motivation" can be defined concisely as the reason people do the thing they do. This simplification addresses question such as "why do we act in the way we do? And "what will cause us to change or do thing differently?' In this definition, motive is the key component'

Motive

"Motive" is not only the root word for motivation but also the essence. Discovering the motive for an action such as murder or robbery has provided both suspense and solution to real-life and fictional mysteries. Once the motive has been revealed, most of the other clues begin to fall in place. This also applies to the workplace. By identifying and understanding the motives and reason people work, and what they are looking for in a job, we can develop a plan that matches the motivation goals of the individual with those of the organization.

Definitional Limitations

It is tempting but erroneous to conclude that a causal relationship exists between motive and reaction. Taken to its extreme, this definition of "motive" implies a cause-effect model. However, human beings are much more complicated than this simple explanation implies. Certainly we react in an immediate and very predictable manner to a harsh stimulus such as pain. In the complex area of people, with their often competing personal, physical, emotional, social, and family priorities, predicting a specific reaction to an isolated stimulus is extremely difficult, if not impossible. This point is illustrated by the fact hat a person may view a situation or comment as humorous at one time, yet take it as an insult at another time under very similar circumstances.

Attitude

What a manager wants most from a motivational plan is to understand what causes people to behave in a certain manner and how to get staff member to perform consistently according to the standards of the institution out of their own desire and not because they are afraid or forced to do so. A word that embodies these objectives is attitude: "*That technologist has a bad attitude.*" "*They certainly have an attitude problem.*" "*There is nothing like a willing worker*" .... These statements all encompass this management wish.

Attitude in the workplace is a person's outward disposition toward his or her job and coworkers. A primary goal of the manager is to help the staff develop and maintain positive attitudes toward the laboratory and its mission. The next section reviews the major theories about achieving this goal in the workplace.

Major Theories of Motivation

Motivational theories can be divided into tow broad groups: (1) content theories, which examine the internal forces that drive the individual to specific action; and, (2) process models, which attempt to explain the person's reaction to external stimuli. Both approaches try to explain why people act the way they do. Each concept also recognizes that specific action is dependent on both the personality of the individual and their interaction with the external environment. By focusing on the topic from different vantage points, manager may gain insights that enable them to reach an understanding of the needs and expectation of their employees and to develop an incentive plan that incorporates the goals and objective so the staff into those of the laboratory.

A simple example of the difference between **content** and **process** models may be:

> **You are attending a meeting, and suddenly the speaker asks everyone to stand up, and everybody does.**
>
> **The question is, who is motivated, you or the speaker? *If* you had felt the urge to stand on your own, understanding why you had this motivation (internal) would be a content process; *if* the only reason you stood up was that the speaker instructed you to (*they wanted you to stand up*) this would be a process model (external).**

Content Motivation Theories

Four content theories have gained wide respect in the business community: Maslow's hierarchy of needs theory; Herzberg's two-factor theory; McClelland's achievement model; and, most recently Alderfer's ERG theory. Two of these, Maslow's and Alderfer's, emphasize the satisfaction of needs to explain the motivational process. Herzberg, while still citing the importance of needs satisfaction, proposes that some workplace-related factors can generate dissatisfaction in the employees, whereas others offer promise as motivators. McClelland's achievement model ties the strength of behavioral motives to the individual's assessment of the likelihood of achieving a specific goal. An overview of each of these approaches is presented next.

Maslow's Hierarchy of Needs

Abraham H. Maslow in 1954 offered a theory that prioritized basic human needs into five categories ranging from the most fundamental physiological needs to the most fulfilling, self-actualization. The primary needs take priority and must be satisfied before the secondary needs can be pursued.

Designed originally to explain human motivation in pursuit of life goals and for use by psychologists in the treatment of their patients, Maslow's model is widely applied in the workplace. Table 6 – 1 shows the relationship between the workplace and the role work plays in the satisfaction of basic human needs. The nature of the work and the tasks performed are themes that are repeated in all motivational models. In Maslow's theory, needs are ranked according to their urgency.

Need	**Job Function**
Self-actualization	Challenging work that allows for creativity, autonomy in decisions, continual learning, and opportunity for professional growth
Esteem (ego)	Position in company and associated privileges, such as prestige of job title; location, size, and furnishing of office; respect, recognition, and admiration of colleagues and fellow employees and comparative salary level Personal worth reinforcement and feeling of competence and pride in work
Social	Identification with and membership in a group Opportunity to participate in social relationships with peers
Safety	Benefits such as health insurance and retirement plans Safe working conditions Fair personnel policies, including job security and protection from arbitrary dismissal
Physiological	Level of income, particularly amount of discretionary (take-home) pay

Table 6 – 1. Role of Job Functions in Fulfilling Maslow's Hierarchy of Needs Theory

Primary or lower-level needs include:

- **Physiological needs**: The most basic biological survival needs such as food, water, air, rest, and sex.
- **Safety needs**: Physical and psychological security and stability, and freedom from deprivation, fear, or threats.

Secondary or higher-level needs include:

- **Social needs**: Affiliation, affection, friendships, a sense of belonging, acceptance, and being part of a group of peers.
- **Esteem (ego) needs**: Personal respect and independence, recognition for achievement, and appreciation from other.
- **Need for self-actualization**: The highest-level need. Need for fulfillment and realization of potential, both as a creative person and as a member of society.

Maslow emphasized one point that the manager should keep in mind when applying the needs model to the workplace: *Satisfaction of any one level is not enough.* It just drives the individual to seek a higher plane of accomplishment. As the employee moves to a higher level in the needs hierarchy, these new needs gain even more urgency than the previous level. Two examples illustrating this factor are that top managers appear much more restless and dissatisfied than workers employed at the lowest rungs of the organizations; and also, pay raises usually have only a short-term (*about 3 months*) positive effect on an employee's performance. This point often frustrates managers, who, after addressing staff complains and granting pay increase and privileges, soon find themselves facing even bigger challenges. Managers should seize this opportunity and tap into this new level of motivation energy as employees look to the job help them reach their newfound aspirations.

For laboratory managers, needs satisfaction is especially relevant. The laboratory offers many intellectually challenging and fulfilling opportunities; however, if the need for security and stability is not satisfied through the pay scale and benefit programs and the technologists are worried about how they are going to pay their bills and feed their families, these primary concerns assume disruptive priority over the higher needs satisfaction potential offered by the laboratory. For these reasons, more than just labor competition (e.g., salary surveys) factors must be incorporated into the compensation packages of workers. (See the discussion of the pay model at the end of the chapter).

Alderfer's ERG Needs Theory

Although similar to Maslow's hierarchy of needs, Clayton P. Alderfer's ERG model condenses the number of categories to three;

- **Existence (E) needs**: physiological, safety, and other elements necessary to support existence (Maslow's physiological and safety needs).
- **Relatedness (R) needs**: interpersonal relationships, acceptance, and belonging (Maslow's social, and part of esteem needs).
- **Growth (G) needs**: creativity, challenge, and personal growth on the job (Maslow's self-esteem and self-actualization).

The ERG model contains several additional differences from Maslow's needs hierarchy. One of the main variations allows a person to be operating at different levels at the same time and includes a frustration-regression process when an individual is frustrated in satisfying higher-level needs such as the need for personal growth, lower-levels needs (regression) grow in intensity.

Alderfer's ERG theory builds on several presuppositions:

1. **Needs frustration**: The less a need is satisfied, the more the desire for it increases.
2. **Frustration regression**: The less successful an individual is in satisfying a higher-level (relatedness or growth) need, the greater the importance of fulfilling the previous level. For example, for a person who is frustrated in achieving personal growth, maximizing friendships and personal relationships (relatedness need) becomes the major emphasis.
3. **Satisfaction progression**: As a person satisfies one level of needs, the desire for higher-level needs increases proportionately.
4. **Growth progression**: The more growth level needs are fulfilled, the more intense the desire for additional growth.

Herzberg's Two-Factor Theory

This theory, like many other practical models, has generated considerable criticism from behavioral scientists because of its research methodology; however, it still enjoys tremendous success in the workplace. Criticism has mainly centered on the use of critical-incidents format research methods, which may have influenced the responses of the participants. Also, study populations were all male engineers and accountants. Nevertheless, many successful motivational programs tailored to professional workers are based on Herzberg's study.

Motivators	Hygiene Factors
Achievement	Policies and administration
Recognition	Competence of supervision
Work itself	Relationship with supervisors, subordinates, and peers
Responsibility	Working conditions
Advancement	Working conditions
Personal growth	Salary
	Status
	Personal life factors

Table 6 – 2. Herzberg's Two-Factor Model of Motivation

Frederick Herzberg identified two groups of factors that play roles in job performance. Each is essentially independent of the other and affects behavior in different ways. One groups called **hygiene factors** (also referred to as "maintenance factors" or "dissatisfiers") because they prevent job dissatisfaction; the other is called **motivation factors** ("motivators" or "satisfiers") because they seem to stimulate employees to strive for superior performance. Table 6 – 2 list job determinants that are considered either motivators or hygiene factors under the Herzberg model.

The most basic illustration of the difference between hygienic and motivational factors is the example of whether a person takes a bath or not. If a person comes to work without washing for several days, fellow employees will notice and this condition will have an impact on the staff; however, if you are properly groomed (i.e., hygienic) no one will notice or give you special credit for this action. Hygiene factors are negative and tend to stir up problems when present; while motivational factors have the positive effect toward influencing the employee toward productive goals. You must be well groomed (*i.e., hygiene factors in the workplace must be clean*), but no one is going to give you an award for taking a bath (i.e., sound management practices), *except perhaps comments right after the problem has been remedied.*

Hygiene factors appear to be related more to the workplace (context, or where work is performed); they are *extrinsic* in character (Table 6 – 2). Motivators appear to be intrinsic in nature, arising out of the content of the work that the employee performs (i.e., the work itself). The two types of factors are independent in the sense that if one group is satisfied, the other may remain unfulfilled. For example technologists may love their work (motivational elements present), yet be extremely unhappy about their paycheck or supervision (i.e., poor hygiene). If hygiene factors are not properly attended addressed (e.g., poor working conditions or insecurity), workers may become dissatisfied and irritated and the motivational aspects of work will not be functional. A good hygiene climate brings about a satisfied or contended worker but may provide no motive to excel. To allow motivational forces to flow within the laboratory, the manager must properly attend to both elements of the work process.

McClelland's Achievement Motivation

David C. McClelland hypothesized that even though there are definite needs that provide explanation for behavior, the strength of a specific motive is directly linked to the opportunities offered by the situation. This theory holds that individuals have three work related needs.

1. The need for achievement (job and career success)
2. The need for power (control and influence)
3. The need for affiliation (warm, friendly relationships)

Each person has the potential to act with a variety of options depending on the relative strength of a motive (i.e., degree of "aroused motivation") matched against the possibilities provided. This concept has been quantified in the model below to show the relationships between these factors.

Aroused Motivation	=	Strength of the motive	x	Perceived possibility of achieving the objective	x	Expected value of the objective

---

Managers want their staffs to be highly motivated. Although individuals may have personal motives for reaching the productivity and quality objectives of the laboratory, if these goals are unrealistic or the personal benefits of achieving the goals are limited, the staff may become discouraged.

Motive is a major component of laboratory j ob descriptions and performance reviews. IF objectives and rewards involve Herculean efforts or are unfeasible, the technologist may simple give up, no matter how attractive the potential rewards (money, promotions, and so on). An important point of the achievement equation is that if the individual scores a minimal or negative value on any of the factors, a low level of aroused motivation results.

Process Motivational Theories

The process approach, as noted earlier, seeks to understand how people are motivated, in contrast to the content theories, which are concerned with the internal motivational forces. Three primary process theories have achieved popularity: Vroom's expectancy theory, Adam's equity theory, and Skinner's reinforcement theory.

Vroom's Expectancy Theory (VIE)

Victor H. Vroom proposed a theory of motivation that explains behavior as a process of making choices in direct response to the expected potential for reward. This concept developed from the opinion that humans are rational and thinking beings who act in anticipation of their own best interest. The resulting motivational theory suggests that people believe two things.

1. Effort will bring reward
2. The effort expended will be related to the perceived value of the reward to the person.

Based on these assumptions, this theory concludes that people make a choice between alternative courses of actions according to how they perceive the resulting benefits. Five variables have been identified that influence the selection decision.

- **Expectancy**: the belief that effort brings performance and performance leads to rewards.
- **Outcome**: the perceived expectancy that the outcome from the effort (reward) will actually be realized.

- **Instrumentality**: the degree of faith in the belief that current efforts may make possible *(i.e., be instrumental)* achieving even larger or moiré long-term rewards. For example, although efforts on the job are directed toward the immediate reward of money, this money may be instrumental in obtaining another item, such as a new car.
- **Valence**: the value place on the available rewards. The more highly valued the prize, the more motivated the individual; the less desirable, the less motivation.
- **Choices**: a quantified mode, called the VIE equation (***VIE** is another label that is sometimes used for this theory*), has been develop to demonstrate the relationship between these factors and the likelihood of a person's choosing to behave in a certain manner:

M = V **x** I **x** E

Motivation (or effort extended) **=**
Valence **x**
Instrumentality **x**
Expectancy

Adam's Equity Theory

Imagine the outcome from a conversation between two technologists, Bill and Tom, who have just received their annual reviews and found that they had been graded alike and received the same pay raise.

> Bill perceives himself as a hard worker, particularly in relationship to Tom, who has a reputation for disappearing, taking long breaks, having sloppy work habits, and not being helpful to coworkers.
>
> The other tech, Tom, views himself as being more productive than the rest of the crew, specifically in the ability to do more work in half the time, and feels that once his work is done, it is all right to disappear, while everyone else moseys along, taking his or her own good time to get things done.

Given this illustration, which tech do you think will adjust his efforts based on the performance review and sense of equity?

This scenario provides the bases of the *equity theory* propounded by J. Stacy Adams. Equity theory holds that employees are motivated by the degree of equity that they *perceive* in their work situation, especially compared with people in similar positions. If employees feel they are paid less than the job demands or less than others performing the same duties, they adjust their efforts accordingly.

The key concepts in the equity theory are *comparison* and *perception*. Comparison can be inside the organizations, as in the salaries of coworkers, or external, as in the wage rates of other laboratories. The workers, according to this theory, have several options to correct perceived inequity.

1. Alter their efforts, or inputs, by either increasing or reducing production.
2. Alter the outcomes, or rewards, by seeking more pay or benefits.
3. Cognitively distort the relevance of the inputs and outputs, that is, rationalize or rethink the importance of the differences.
4. Leave the company or look for another field of employment.
5. Influence others to change their efforts.
6. Change the target of comparison.

Skinner's Reinforcement Theory

B. F. Skinner's theory of motivation is based on the observation that we tend to behave according to the way we are treated. In principle it states that we repeat performances for which we are positively rewarded, or we avoid actins that bring about undesirable consequences. It differs from most other models in that it focuses on the environment, rather that on needs, motives, and personality as an explanation of motivation and behavior.

This theory has been the recipient of some sharp criticism because its theoretical databases are drawn from the work of B. F. Skinner, a behavior psychologist who studies are mainly based on the response of animals to harsh, often painful stimuli. For example, a mouse or chicken would receive either food or an electric shock depending on which button it hit. The animal eventually either figured out the system, become psychopathic, or starved to death. This theory has proven extremely useful, however, in designing most performance evaluation systems because of our cultural belief that rewards should be tied to performance: *A good worker should receive more money or privileges than one who is less proficient and, as a result pay increases are directly linked to the performance evaluation.*

Other examples of the application of this theory to the workplace are goal-related management models such as the Management by objectives (MBO) and total-quality management (TQM). These programs point out that employees and organizations work best when all the members understand their duties and the related expectation, and when rewards are tied directly to the achievement of the goals and objectives.

Following are listed the components of reinforcement theory.

- **The law of effect**: This law proposed by E. L. Thorndike, states that we act in response to expected consequences. Behavior that provides pleasurable or desirable rewarded most likely reoccurs; behavior that results in discomfort is avoided.
- **Stimulus**: an event that influences or leads to a response.
- **Response**: Behavior that results from a stimulus.
- **Reinforcement**: the consequence of an action or response. Reinforcement may be positive in nature and meant to bring about or encourage desirable behavior, or it may be negative, designed to cause the individual to avoid undesirable behavior. Negative reinforcement can take the form of punishment or withholding of desirable consequences. The timing and scheduling of the reinforcement messages are important aspects of this theory.
- **Behavior modification**: The application or practice of reinforcement theory, as expressed in the law of effect:

  Stimulus → response → reinforcement → stimulus .... →

Other Motivational Theories

Books on motivation, both personal (self-help) and business are usually at the top of any best-seller list. Our appetite for this material appears insatiable, and we seem to be willing to pay a good price for a book that offers new hope or promise. Most, if not all, of these publications attempt to apply the theories presented here or a least provide anecdotal evident of new motivational ideas. Noted hare are several important authors who have made contribution to our understanding of the topic.

Among authors making contributions are Douglas M. McGregor (theory X and theory Y) and W. Ouchi (theory Z). Thee authors and their theories are covered in Module (lesson) seven because they suggest that worker performance arise from the way managers view their subordinates (i.e., leadership), not from within the employees themselves.

Researchers such as E.E. Lawler have explored the role of money in worker satisfaction of needs. Lawler pointed out the important link between performance appraisals, compensation, and achievement of organizational goals.

Many authors have built on the theoretic work of Erick Erikson and Chris Argyris about the relationship between maturity (age and life-stage development) and motivation. These researchers have documented that, as we progress along life's path, what we want and expect from our work changes in priority and perspective. A summary of these and other findings about the life cycle of workers is presented in the following job-maturity matrix, which ties life goals and developmental stages to job expectations.

- 20 to 30 years of age: *a time of searching and exploring work and life alternatives*
- 30 to 40 years of age; *high commitment to career advancement goals.*
- 40 to 45 years of age: *a period of questioning career and life choices; frequently evolving into a midlife crisis*
- 45 to 65+ years of age: *a time of increasing stability, acceptance, and commitment to job, family, and retirement.*

Application of Motivation Theories to the Workplace

The participant may ask, "What do all of these theories about motivation mean to me, and how do they apply in the real world of laboratories and medical technologists?" The answer to these and similar questions are found in module (lesson) seven, which is devoted to leadership skills, and the topics that follow.

Leadership, Work, and Job Satisfaction

In essence, leadership is the application of motivational principles to the workplace. Leadership relates directly to the role that work itself plays in the motivational process. Managers control the assets and operations of the organization from which workers receive their pay and other benefit programs, hire-fire decisions, career advancement opportunities, work and job assignments, job security, and to a large extent, reassurance of their personal worth. The factors all combine to determine the degree of **job satisfaction** realized by the individual from the work performed in the laboratory.

Job satisfaction is the degree to which employees feel their jobs meet their needs and wants. Job satisfaction is directly reflected in absenteeism and turnover rates, as well as the attitude and functional performance level maintained by the worker. The age of the employee, occupational level, and organization size all contribute to the perception of job satisfaction.

Although any single laboratory manager may not have complete control of all these factors, every manager, by definition, has tremendous influence on some aspect of the job that directly affects the staff. Even first-level section supervisors (e.g., hematology, chemistry, second shift) control aspects of the work that are crucial to satisfying the motivational needs of the employees: *job assignments, work schedules, performance evaluations, and, most important, the day-to-day personal connection between the individual and the sometimes faceless organization within which the laboratory functions.*

Goal Setting

Goal setting incorporates the themes contained in several motivational proposals, including expectancy, reinforcement, and achievement theories. The most widespread example of these techniques are management by objectives (MBO) (Module 1) and total-quality management (TQM) Module 20). Other examples include job description preparation and performance appraisals conducted as part of the management process of laboratories. In goal setting the manager and the employee come to an agreement about what to expect from each other and develop a plan to reach mutually shared goals.

Pay

The pay model focuses on the definition of pay. Two types of pay are awarded to employees. The first type, **material pay**, is the tangible, or monetary, part of the paycheck. The second, **psychic pay**, consist of the intrinsic rewards that give us a good feeling about ourselves and our work. Material pay includes salary, fringe benefits, holidays, vacation, insurance, as well as the "perks" of the position such as a corner office with a view or company furnished automobile. Psychic pay is psychological in nature and includes pride in work; the feeling of acceptance by and belonging to a team, and the positive feedback we receive from our boss and coworkers. This model is closely tied to both content and process motivational theories, particularly the needs-satisfying models of Maslow and Herzberg. Material pay takes care of the lower-level needs; psychic pay addresses the higher, or motivational, needs.

Although first-level section supervisors (e.g., Hematology, evening shift, or Phlebotomy supervisors) may have limited influence on the amount of pay workers receive, the play a significant, if not overriding role in the amount of psychic pay their staffs take home. Psychic pay accounts for the starving artist and Mother Teresa phenomena, whereby the person may receive only subsistence pay but devotes his or her life to a cause in return for a huge psychic paycheck. A large amount of one type of pay can make up for a deficiency in the other.

Figure 6 – 1 presents the pay model within the context of staff recruitment and retention as well as motivation. This graph demonstrates that to achieve these two goals of staffing and motivation, any gap in "total pay" must be eliminated. It also answers the question, "How do you motivate your staff?" **Easy —your pay them well.**

Like the VIE and McClelland's achievement equations, the pay model formula summarizes the application of the theories presented in this unit. The degree of aroused motivation or extended effort that laboratory managers get from their staff is directly tied to the total motivational paycheck issued, including both material and psychic pay.

Material Pay + Psychic Pay = Total Motivational Paycheck

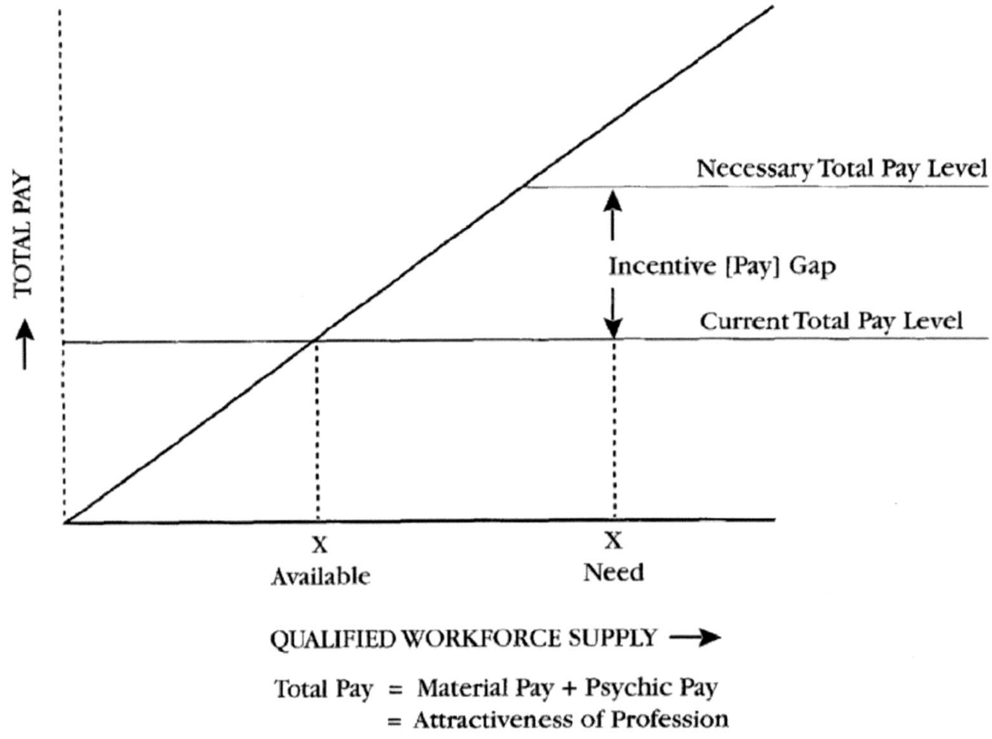

Figure 6 – 1. Total pay model. (from Varnadoe, LA: Keeping medical technologists in the workforce: Recruitment, retention, and motivation under CLIA'88. ASCP Teleconference Series 4985:6, 19993, with permission)

"How do you motivate your staff?" **Easy —your pay them well**. This insight concludes *Motivation to Work*. The following chapter: *Principles of Leadership*.

— Case Study —

Chapter Six: Motivation to Work

"What's the matter with George now," exclaimed the laboratory manager? "What do you make of this request to transfer to blood bank? He loves hematology and is the best tech we have here."

"I don't know," answered the assistant chief tech, "maybe he is upset about not being promoted. He doesn't seem to be willing to work with the new supervisor, although everyone has spoken well of her. Se is certainly sharp on doing diffs on bone marrow slides, almost as good as George, Dr. Smith told me."

"I don't think that can be the reason. We went to great lengths trying to convince him to accept the position before we even considered looking for someone else. Keep your ears open. I certainly don't want to lose such a talented person in hematology, especially since we are short of help now."

Shortly after the meeting with the assistant chief tech, the laboratory manager came across Dr. Smith talking to George, and overheard her asking him: "Why don't you bring in any more bone marrow slides? I know you enjoyed going over them, and the diffs you performed were very helpful and saved me a lot of time."

"I don't know," was the response given by George. "The new supervisor is really good, and I like her. However, she said that it would save a lot of time if we left the bone marrows for her. She could then do them and bring them in to you when there was time. You know, we have been extremely busy since we were cut back one tech, and she is only trying to make things work better, by letting us do the more routine things and not having to worry about all the special tests we had to do before."

Chapter Section for Review

- Content Motivational Theories, especially Maslow's hierarchy of needs and Alderfer's ERG needs theory
- Pay model

Questions for Discussions

1. From a motivational perspective, what is George's problem?
2. In Maslow's hierarchy of needs model, which need is not being satisfied (Table 6 – 1)?
3. What level of management (i.e., administration/laboratory management/supervisor) is responsible for this motivational problem?
4. Using the Pay model as an application strategy, what steps can the hematology supervisor take on her own to improve motivation of techs like George?

[7]

Principles of Leadership

— Chapter Seven —

Leadership has been partially defined in the previous module in order to distinguish ii from motivation. Often these two concepts have been used interchangeably; however, in practice they are quite different. Motivation deals with the *reason* people act the way they do, whereas leadership attempts to use motivational principles in an effort to achieve organizational goals. It is the *matching* of the goals and the objectives of these two entities, the individual and the institution that is the essence of leadership.

Leadership, like management, has been given about as many meanings and explanations as there are people discussing the topic. Several popular definitions follow:

- Some proponents have suggested that leadership is tied to the personality and persuasive talents (i.e., charisma) of the person, as demonstrated by the great leaders of history.
- Others point out that the situation or special circumstances enable a person to rise to the occasion. In another setting, the person may have simply remained anonymous, or someone else may have been just as successful in meeting the challenges.
- Still another common belief is that it is the power, either the formal authority or money that makes the leader. With the same resources and the right job, we can all succeed.

These opinions of leadership and how it develops all have elements of truth. They raise the salient question: *are leaders born, or can they be trained*? All of us have weakness, special talents, and strengths. Some people make friends and influence others easily, but they may have trouble organizing or lack the necessary analytical skills. There are those who are natural organizers, but they may have difficulty dealing with people and need direction in selecting goals and solving problems. Other may be talented in analytical and troubleshooting situations, but deficient in organizing and people skills. We each, however, can build on our strengths and tackle our weaknesses through training, education, and experience. The answer to the leadership question is that leaders are made, not born!

Within the context of motivation, **leadership** can be defined as the process of influencing the efforts of other to achieve designated organizational goals. This is the *directing function* in the management process model: to persuade, direct, inspire, guide, and bring about a commitment to a common cause on the part of the participants.

This module reviews the organization factors that influence and stimulate leadership, discusses popular leadership models, and provides several examples of leadership techniques.

OBJECTIVES

After completion of this chapter, the reader will be able to demonstrate accomplishment of the following objectives.

1. Define leadership within the context of the functions of management.
2. Recognize the three factors that determine leadership success.
3. Compare and contrast the concepts and advantages of major leadership models.

4. Apply leadership principles to the management of organizations such as the medical laboratory.

Chapter Highlights and Glossary of Key Terms

I. ORGANIZATIONAL FACTORS THAT INFLUENCE LEADERSHIP SUCCESS

Leadership*: The process of influencing others to achieve designated organizational goals.*

- A. Corporate Culture and Delegation of Authority

  Corporate Culture*: The way things are done in an organization: the habits, traditions, customs, processes, and social mores of the institution.*

- B. Management Style

  Management Style*: The general behavior and philosophy of a manager or an organization toward the employees, particularly the degree of participation allowed in the decision-making process.*

II. LEADERSHIP MODELS

- A. Personal Traits of Leaders
- B. Leadership Behavior
  1. Employee-oriented versus production-oriented leadership styles
  2. Structure versus consideration leadership styles
  3. The Managerial Grid®

     Managerial Grid®*: A graphic depiction of leadership styles in relation to concerns for people and production.*
  4. Theory X and Theory Y

     Pygmalion effect*: A theory that holds that people (students, employees) tend to act in the way they are expected to act by their leaders (parents, teachers, supervisors, etc.)*
- C. Situational Leadership Models
  1. Contingency models
  2. Continuum of leadership
  3. Normative theory

III. APPLICATION OF LEADERSHIP PRINCIPLES

- A. The management process
- B. Path-goal theory

Organizational Factors that Influence Leadership Success

The institution's bureaucratic structure, or management style, and culture provide the ground rules whereby leadership either flourishes or falters. Within the boundaries set by an organization lies not only the opportunity for development but also the restraints on growth. Corporate culture and management style encompass both the nature of the enterprise (its product, services, and social and business charter) and the management systems that allocate formal power and authority.

Corporate Culture and Delegation of Authority

Leadership is tied to both social (community, culture) and organizational expectation place on managers. The **corporate culture** establishes the climate and rules under which management operates. These cultural factors are then reflected in the management style of the organization and the way that it delegates authority to its managers.

Authority, with was discussed in a previous model, briefly refers to the authorization (i.e., empowerment) to act in the name of the organization. The associated power implies the ability to sanction others to ensure compliance with established rules, directives, or objectives. Sources of power range from the allocation of rewards and punishment to the control of vital information. The framework for the cultivation of leadership skills depends on how an institution deals with these issues in its administrative systems; the role of managers as the link between the organization, its members, and the outside community; and, the individual proficiency of its managers.

Management Styles

Rensis Liker suggests that organizations have four discrete leadership systems or management styles.

1. **Exploitative and authoritative**: Managers view workers only as tools and means of production and feel no further obligation to them.
2. **Benevolent and authoritative**: In this *paternalistic* approach, managers feel they know what is best for their employees and need only inform and direct their actions, without seeking any feedback.
3. **Consultative**: The manager feels the opinions and advice of the staff are useful, but all decisions remain the exclusive purview of the manager.
4. **Participative**: Input and responsibility for decision making and performance are placed directly on the staff, or as close to the production process as possible, with only general guidance and oversight from management. This is an inclusion team approach, in which the worth of all members is recognized.

Lower-level managers have a greater opportunity to learn and practice new leadership skills in an organization that has a participative management style. Companies with an authoritative culture not only stifle creativity but also encourage their managers to adopt this style as their own. Leadership models are reviewed in the next section.

Leadership Models

Three factors that are involved in leadership are the leader, the followers, and the situation. The motivation of followers, which was covered in a previous module, shows that leadership is not a one-way relationship. Models depicting the other tow parts of the equation center on the personal traits and behavior of leaders and the impending circumstances of the situation.

Personal Traits of Leaders

Some managers excel in leadership positions; other fail miserable. The question is: *what skills, temperaments, talents, or special training do successful managers possess that others lack*? Are some people born leaders, or do they pick up these attributes through experience and interaction with other successful leaders?

Early studies made detailed analyses on the intellectual, physical, social, and psychological qualities of “successful leaders” in both formal and informal settings. However, this research failed to develop a list of characteristics that applied in all situations. Although “charisma” (an especially elusive term with many meanings and contexts) appeared to be a common trait of informal leaders, investigators discovered that sometimes irascible and amicable leaders were equally successful in business settings. Traits of effective leaders found in one survey differed from those of another. This result did not discourage researchers, however, as is evident in the popular biographies and news stories of business and political leaders.

When common personal traits proved elusive, attention turned to how leaders treat their coworkers. Perhaps the clue to successful leadership was in the work environment or support network. This line of thinking opened the way to the next phase of research: *leadership behavior.*

Leadership Behavior

The next wave of research focused on the behavior of leaders instead on their personal traits. This research has proven more productive and resulted in several widely accepted leadership models.

- the employee-oriented versus production-oriented leadership styles.
- the structure-consideration leadership style.
- the Managerial Grid®.
- theory X – theory Y model and the associated theory Z model.

Employee-Oriented Versus Production-Oriented Leadership Styles

In the late 1940s the Survey Research Center a the University of Michigan conducted research to determine which types of supervisory behavior led to the highest level of productivity and individual satisfaction in small work groups. This study compared supervisors from work groups that had a high-level of productivity with those with low levels of output.

The initial surprise was the finding that the supervisors with the best productivity levels had strong ties to their employees, spent more of their time in actual supervision rather than in production work, supervised less closely while allowing workers more latitude in performing their duties, and demonstrated concern for their people both on and off the job. These managers were called *employee-oriented.*

The low-level production groups, in contrast, were dominated by *production-orient* supervisors, who tended to emphasize high productivity at the expense of all other factors. They viewed their workers as only tools for use by the company in the manufacturing process and spent the majority of their time on production-related problems.

Other investigations by researchers such as Liker have supported the theory that employee-oriented managers tend to outperform production-oriented managers. However, this model was not supported in all situations.

Structure versus Consideration Leadership Styles

Ralph M. Stogdill and later researchers such as Paul Hersey and Kenneth Blanchard found two principal dimensions to leadership behavior: initiating structure and consideration.

Leadership behavior associated with *initiating structure* is marked by emphasis on actively directing the staff toward getting the work done: paying attention to assigning particular tasks; specifying and clarifying what is expected of subordinates and the uniformity of the procedures to be followed; and, personally deciding what and how work will be done.

Consideration behavior is typified by managers' efforts to explain their action, treat workers as equals, listen to subordinates' concerns, look out for their personal welfare, give advance notice of changes, and be generally friendly and approachable.

The behavior of an individual leader is, in practice, a mix between the two patterns. The relationship between these two dimensions has been graphically illustrated in the Ohio State Leadership Quadrants Matrix (Fig. 2-1). Studies have shown that groups with leaders who score high in both dimensions usually demonstrate the best overall performance. The complementary nature of these two dimensions led to the development of models that demonstrated this connection. The most notable, and the one most widely used for training managers in leadership skills, is the Managerial Grid®. Hersey and Blanchard further expanded this model to include the life cycle of the workers (see Chapter 1 also) as an important factor in determining situational leadership styles.

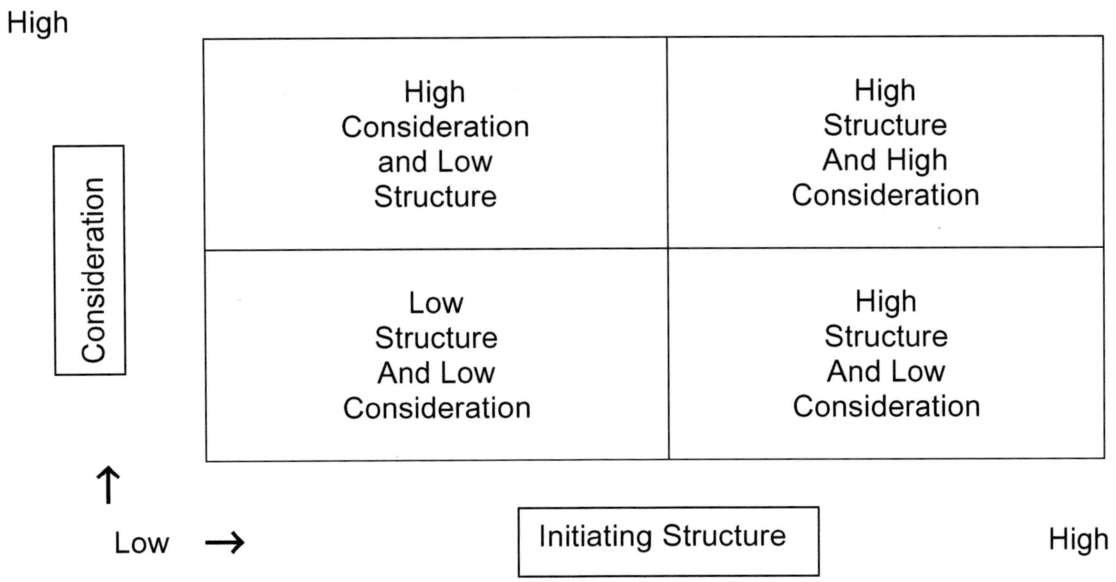

Figure 7 – 1. The Ohio State Leadership Quadrants (Illustration developed by Ralph M. Stogdill)

The Managerial Grid®

The **Managerial Grid®** shows the relationship between a concern for people (consideration orientation) and concern for production (structure orientation). The Grid®, which was developed by Robert R. Blake and Jane S. Mouton, shows that high concern for both factors is crucial to the successful manager.

In developing the Managerial Grid®, Blake and Mouton proposed that management style is influenced by five factors,

1. The aptitudes and assumptions of the manager.
2. The policies and procedures of the organization.
3. The day-to-day operational situation.
4. The social and personal values of the manager.
5. Chance.

From the research database and the listed assumptions, a grid was prepared that ranked concern for people on the vertical axis and concern for production on the horizontal (Fig. 7 – 2). Using a scale of **1** (for low concern) to **9** (for maximum concern), the attitudes and work attributes of managers can be plotted on the matrix to reveal their leadership style. Once known, managers can then take appropriate action to improve their leadership abilities.

The 81 possible points on the Grid® have been synopsized as seven basic leadership styles, as shown in Figures 1- 2.

According to Blake and Mouton, the **9,9** team leader approach is the most effective leadership style. To use the Managerial Grid® to improve and strengthen leadership ability, the leader should go through the following steps.

1. Identify their current style.
2. Decide for themselves the best style for a given situation.
3. Determine what attitudes and behavior changes are required to reach their goal.
4. Encourage management to develop the organizational culture necessary for the preferred style to flourish.

Remember this techniques ranks concern for people on a scale of 1→ 9; on a graph with Concern for Production with a corresponding ranking. The resulting leadership styles can be grouped into the following descriptions:

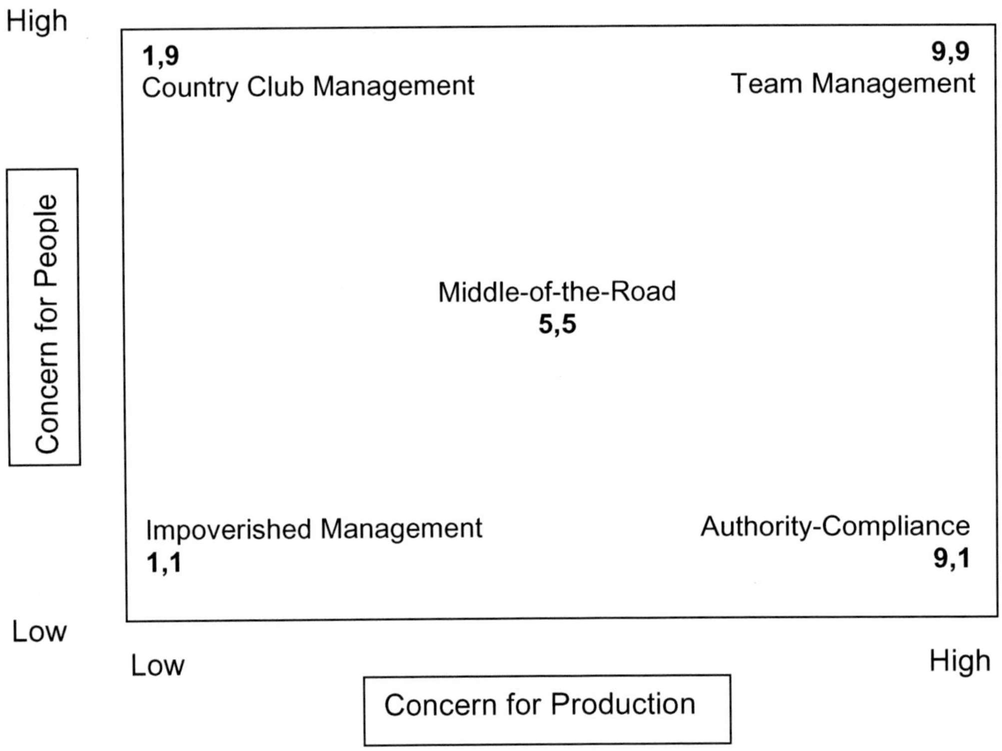

Figure 7 – 1. The Managerial Grid® [illustration resource — Blake, RR, and Adams McCanse (formerly Blake, RR, and Mouton, JS: Gulf Publishing, Houston, TX, 1991)]

1,1 Impoverished Management (low concern for both people and production) *Exertion of minimum effort to get required work done and to just sustain organization membership (i.e., keep their job).*

1,9 Country Club Management (high concern people, low emphasis on production) *Thoughtful attention to the needs of people for satisfying relationships leads to a comfortable, friendly organization atmosphere and work tempo (i.e., keep the people happen, and produce enough to get by).*

5,5 Middle-of-the-Road Management (equal concern for people and production, but not high focus on either) *Adequate origination performance is possible through balancing the necessity to get out the work with maintaining morale of people at a satisfactory level*

9,1 Authority-Compliance (high concern on production, to the neglect of people issues) *Efficiency in operation results from arranging conditions for work in such a way that human elements interfere to a minimum degree.*

9,9 Team Management (high concern for both people and production) *Work accomplishment is from committed people; interdependence through a "common stake" in organization purpose leads to relationships of trust and respect.*

Theory X and Theory Y

Another popular approach to identifying the behavior that makes good leaders is the *theory X, theory Y* model proposed by Douglas McGregor in 1960. This concept is a close simulation of the widely observed **Pygmalion effect** so adamantly propounded in education circles. This principle, named for George Bernard Shaw's play **Pygmalion**, states that students tend to learn and perform in the manner anticipated by their teachers. If students perceive that teachers expect them to do well, they do. If they pick up signals that they are expected to perform poorly, the prophecy becomes self-filling. Some teachers have countered that their expectations are based on the past performance of the students; however, numerous studies have verified the influence on this phenomenon.

McGregor proposes that leadership behavior is based on the manager's assumption about the nature of people, which in turn, translate into the level of performance achieved by their employees. *Expectancy* and *reinforcement* motivational theories also support this approach.

According to this model, *theory X* managers believe that people:

- Are inherently lazy and dislike work
- Must be coerced into performing their duties by constant supervision and maintenance of tight operational control
- Have no ambition and little interest in improving their efficiency on their own and must be prodded to produce.

Managers who hold theory X philosophies tend to be autocratic and dictatorial and allow for little input from their staff.

Theory Y managers, by contrast, believe that:

- Work is a natural part of life
- People have a high degree of ingenuity and creativity that they are eager to apply to the job
- Worker potential is only partially tapped by the company
- Workers are self-learners and seek responsibility for their performance
- Workers exercise self-control and self-discipline if they are committed to a goal, and the strength of this commitment depends on the reward associated with the achievement.

Theory Y managers are participatory in their leadership style, actively seek advice and counsel from their coworkers, and allow employees to share in the decision-making processes.

More recent work on the theory Y assumptions of successful leadership behavior has led writers such as Ouchi to propose a slightly modified *theory Z*. This concept developed from attempts to combine Japanese management techniques with American mores. Managers holding theory Z assumptions believe that the self-controlled and self-regulated characteristic of workers contained in theory Y is cultural and, as a result, changing societal goals must be included in today's workplace. For example, according to theory Z, productivity and rewards are not the only objectives of people; issues such as the quality of their work lives are also crucial to their motivation.

Situational Leadership Models

Many researchers have noted that forces other than behavior contribute to the success of a manager as a leader. The most notable of these are the circumstances in which the manager must operate. Three models have been proposed to identify and deal with this variable; *contingency theory*, *continuum of leadership*, and *normative theory*.

Contingency Model

Fred E. Fielder's theory takes into account the suitability of certain types of behavior in certain settings. This contingency theory of leadership applies the same standards to leadership as to management: *the effective leader must be able to analyze the situation and develop a satisfactory strategy for intervention.*
The contingency model proposes that the success of a manager as a leader is contingent on two factors: *the leadership style of the manager and the favorableness of the leadership situation.*

Leadership style, according to Fielder's theory, can be either *relationship-oriented* or *task-oriented*. These terms are largely self-explanatory. Relationship-oriented people emphasize good interpersonal relationships as an important means of accomplishing work-related goals. Task-oriented supervisors focus on completing a job first and taking care of people as secondary to accomplishing their primary mission.

Favorableness
is defined by Fielder as the amount of power, control, and influence wielded by a manager in a particular set of circumstances. Three components establish the favorableness dimensions of a situation.

1. **Leader-member relations**: the level of confidence and trust between the leader and members of the staff. This is the most important factor, according to the contingency model.
2. **Task structure**: the amount of formal structure imposed on work assignments. Assembly line jobs, which are highly structured, present the manager with the most control over the action of workers. Unstructured task settings, such as the work performed in the medical laboratory and other technical positions in which the employees may be as knowledgeable as the supervisor, provide the leader with considerably less control.
3. **Position power**: the degree of influence that the manager exerts on the reward and punishment system of the institution.

Fielder and associates have suggested that situations that are either very favorable or very unfavorable are usually handled best by a task-oriented leader. Relationship-oriented leaders appear to be most effective in situations that are considered moderately favorable or only moderately unfavorable.

One additional point is pertinent for the application of the contingency model. The selection of the right person for a leadership position is extremely important to the success of both the leader and the enterprise. Matching the right person who has the right leadership style for the situation is a crucial management responsibility.

Continuum of Leadership

The leadership models presented so far represent an either-or, polar approach to leadership. Robert Tannenbaum and Warren H. Schmidt recognized that leaders are usually somewhere between the two extremes. They developed a model based on the relationship between managers and staffs and the level of participation allowed in the decision-making process. They proposed a *continuum of leadership* model ranging from completely autocratic to democratic. According to this theory, managers could move along this continuous line, adjusting their leadership style to fit the situation.

The continuum of leadership recognizes seven degrees of freedom*:* *boss-centered* leadership occupy the first three degrees of the continuum*; equilibrium*
, is the center of the scale (position 4); and *subordinate-centered* leadership is described in 5 – 7 range of the scale.

Illustration: Continuum of Leadership

(1) Autocratic style — Democratic style (7)

↓ ↓ ↓ ↓ ↓ ↓ ↓

Boss-centered (1 – 3)	Equilibrium (4)	Subordinate-centered (5 – 7)

Boss – centered leadership can be identified in positions 1,2, and 3 of the scale.

1. Total use of authority by the supervisor: supervisor makes all decision and merely announces the decision to the workers.
2. The manager makes all decisions but attempts to sell and persuade the staff on the validly of his or her viewpoint.
3. The boss makes all decision but invites input, suggestions, and questions for the staff.

Equilibrium — shared boss-subordinate leadership — is at the midpoint of the scale.

4. Managers make the decision but seek support and approval for the subordinates.

Subordinate – centered leadership falls in the 5 to 7 range.

5. Supervisor gathers the data and defines the problems, then seeks suggestions and recommendations for solutions before making a decision.
6. Manager provides information, supervision, and guidance but requests that the staff make the decision.
7. Managers focus on setting general policies and procedures for the department but allow total freedom, and responsibility to the employees to function and make decisions within these broadly defined boundaries.

Some authors have extended this scale beyond 7 (democratic) to include a *laissez faire* style, closely aligned with the **1,1** *impoverished management* and **1,9** *country club* positions on the Managerial Grid® (Table 7 – 1). This leadership type has, for all practical purposes, deserted all responsibilities for productivity, allowing the workers absolute freedom in setting their own performance standards.

Normative Theory

Victor H. Vroom and Phillip W. Yetton suggest a leadership model that also depicts the extent of participation allowed in the decision-making process. This approach, which is similar to the continuum theory, proposes that managers are capable of adjusting their leadership style to meet the particular circumstances of a given situation. The *normative theory*, also referred to as the *Vroom-Yetton decision mode*
l, provides normative guidelines and recommendations for the way a leader should make decision in a specific set of workplace conditions.

The nomenclature of the normative theory classifies each decision-making method as **A**utocratic (**I & II**), **C**onsultative (**I & II**), or **G**roup-oriented.

The five possible behavior styles identified by Vroom and Yetton are as follows.

- **A-I**: Manager makes decision based on the current information available.
- **A-II**: Manager seeks necessary information from subordinates before making a decision.
- **C-I**: Managers shares the problem with selected individuals before making a decision.
- **C-II**: Manager shares the problem with all the members of the group but makes the final decision.
- **G**: Manager shares the problem with the group and a decision is reached by consensus.

Application of Leadership Principles

What do all these theories mean to a manager at work, and how can they be used in the laboratory to provide leadership?

The answer lies in the topics reviewed in the management and motivation sections of the text. People who work in medical labs must constantly guard against making the focus of their work a tube of blood or a lab specimen rather than the needs of the whole patient and the worker's role in the delivery of health care. Likewise, the total management process of planning, organizing, directing, and controlling must be kept in mind as a manager studies the individual components of each stage.

The Management Process

Leadership is the most active part of the *directing* function: however, directing can be effective only if it is preceded by a well-designed strategy, developed in the planning and organizing stages of the management process, and if it is followed through with a strong controlling phase. Neglect in any of these areas will sabotage the entire program.

Good leadership is reflected in several areas, including the confidence of the manager in delegating authority and power and the design and implementation of sound job descriptions and work assignments. The importance of work in filling the motivational needs of workers was emphasized in the previous chapter, and the effectiveness of the manager in tapping the people resource through programs of job enrichment and professional growth is a measure of leadership skills. These topics are explored in Chapter 9 and 10, devoted to job descriptions and performance appraisals.

Path-Goal Theory

One approach, which brings together both leadership and motivational principles in an application model, is the *path-goal theory* proposed by Robert J. House. This theory emphasizes the *role* of the leader in providing and streamlining a path by which subordinates can achieve their own and the institution's goals. The path-goal theory is essentially a contingency leadership behavior model in that it recognizes that leadership success is tied to both the behavior of the leader and the situation. House list two crucial factors that the leader must consider in designing a strategy to deal with the work environment.

1. The characteristics of the workers — their training, individual traits, personal needs, social backgrounds, etc.
2. The nature of the tasks to be performed — such as the complexity, degree of organizational structure, stress, danger, and monotony.

The leader then addresses two elements:

1. The *goal* component, in which the managers enhance the number and types of rewards (or pay) that subordinates can receive for achieving work-related goals; and,
2. The *path* facet, in which the leader clarifies the routes for obtaining these goals and removes obstacles that may impede employees from realizing their potential.

The concepts contained the path-goal theory are reflected in many management systems. The elementary principles of informing people of what is expected of them, showing them how to accomplish their tasks, and aligning the achievement of work-related goals with the rewards program are crucial components of such management techniques as management–by-objectives, quality circles, and total-quality-management. The concept of leaders providing guidance, coaching, counseling, and instructions to their staff is also an excellent example of the *service* role of managers.

Although an integral part of the function of management, as explained in the first part of the chapter, leadership is the process of bring together the goals and objectives of both the organization and its members.

In summary, <u>leadership</u> is dependent not only on the personal talents of managers but also on the characteristics of their followers and the circumstances of the situation. We address issues involved the <u>Management</u> <u>of</u> <u>Work</u> <u>Groups</u> in the next chapter.

— Case Study —

Chapter Seven: Principles of Leadership

"What are we going to do about Betty and Larry?" asked the laboratory manager. "We need them badly, but the chemistry supervisor said that they just don't seem to get it."

"I know," responded the blood bank supervisor. "I wasn't looking forward to training them in my section, either. They're OK, but just barely. I don't know how they will do on the second shift with a new supervisor coming and everything."

"That's what everyone is saying. Tom in hematology was especially critical, and that was their first department! However, we do need them badly," answered the laboratory manager. "I'll have to make sure the new supervisor lets me know immediately if there is a problem, and I will just have to keep a close eye on the situation until we can find more help."

(Six months later, during a meeting between the second shift supervisor and the laboratory manager)

"I must say you have done a fine job on the shift, especially having to work with Betty and Larry," remarked the laboratory manager to the section shift supervisor.

"Aren't they great techs!" answered the supervisor. "I've never seen two young persons catch on so fast. They were just what I expected, after I ran into the Med Tech program director at the local college when I first came to town. He told me that I was going to be getting two of his best students."

Chapter Section for Review

- Management Styles
- Theory X and Theory Y, and the Pygmalion Effect
- The Management Process

Questions for Discussions

1. Why do you think Betty and Larry did so poorly during their orientation?
2. Why do you think they excelled under the leadership of the new second shift supervisor? What made the difference?
3. Look at the managerial grid in Figure 7 – 2. What do you suspect is the leadership style of the second shift supervisor?

[8]

Management of Work Groups

— Chapter Eight —

In any organization two groups simultaneously exert pressure on the direction and success of the enterprise. One is the formal structure designed around the mission of the laboratory. The other is the informal structure — the relationship that are formed by the interaction of people. These two structures share many characteristics in their makeup and in the manner in which they operate.

This chapter focuses on the functions and management of work groups as they relate to the organization's formal structure; how individuals relate to the group; behaves as a unit; how the group interacts with other work groups; informal groups and the organization itself; and, techniques for the management of groups.

OBJECTIVES

After completion of this chapter, the reader will be able to demonstrate accomplishment of the following objectives.

1. Define motivation in the context of the workplace.
2. Identify the common characteristics of both informal and formal work groups.
3. Describe how individuals relate to and are affected by their interaction with work groups.
4. Explain the functioning of the group as a common unit.
5. Discuss the factors that influence inter-group transactions.
6. Recognize how management and leadership principles can be applied to the supervisor of work groups.

Chapter Highlights and Glossary of Key Terms

I. WORK GROUP CHARACTERISTICS

***Group**: A collection of individual persons consisting of a leader, followers, a purpose or mission (profit or social), shared opinions on how things should be done, performance and commitment expectations, and sanctions for those who do not meet expectations.*

A. Work Groups versus Informal Groups

B. Definition of a Work Group

***Work Group**: A collection of individuals who share the characteristics of all groups and are gathered together to perform specific functions that benefit the whole organization.*

II. INDIVIDUAL GROUP INTERFACE

A. Interpersonal Relationships

1. Personal image

***Personal Image**: The combined effect of how we see ourselves and how we think other see us.*

2. Behavior expectation
3. Personal benefits

B. Role Expectations

***Role**: Our behavior (personal or work) in response to group and individual expectations.*

III. WORK GROUP BEHAVIOR

***Synergism**: The process whereby the whole (group or organization) becomes greater (i.e., more productive and effective) than the sum of its individual parts.*

A. Work Group Functional Factors

***Emergent Behavior**: A term assigned to the efforts of the group as a whole, their behavior that "emerges" from the internal interaction of the group members.*

B. Work Group Dysfunctional Factors

IV. GROUP INTERACTION

***Ownership**: Communal (or group) identification or possession of a goal, workspace, cause, image, or item as one's own.*

A. Factors Influencing Inter-group Relationships
B. Union-Management Interaction
   1. Group formation: Why do employees join unions?
   2. Management-union relationships

V. MANAGEMENT OF GROUPS

A. Group Building and Teamwork
B. Leadership Strategies
   1. Structural techniques
   2. Team building: Organizational development strategy

   ***Teamwork**: The focusing of the group's united and shared energy on a common goal.*

C. Inter-group Management

Work Group Characteristics

The common features of **groups** are summarized in Table 8 – 1. All groups, either formal or informal, include:

- A leader
- Followers
- Purpose or mission, be it profit or social
- Shared opinions on how things should be done
- Performance and commitment expectations
- Sanctions for those who do not meet expectations

Work groups are organized to meet the needs of the organizations. Although unique in their mission, work, groups must be placed within the context of the shared characteristics of all groups to provide an understanding of how they coalesce and function as a single entity.

Group Traits	**Formal**	**Informal**
Leaders	Appointed	Charisma
Followers	Recruitment incentives	Personal attraction
Purpose	Profit or social goals	Peer motives
Shared opinion of how things are to be done	Organizationally driven	Social norms and mores
Performance and commitment expectations	Job and task standards	Issue-focused
Sanctions	Organizational rewards and punishments polices	Peer pressure

Work Groups versus Informal Groups

Leaders of formal work groups are appointed by the owners, whereas informal leaders emerge from within the group itself because of either a communal need or personal charisma. Followers join both types of groups because of perceived natural benefits such as financial incentives, shared values, and fellowship.

Groups exist to enable individuals to accomplish something together that is beyond the abilities of one person. The purpose of work groups is to support the mission of the company, whereas informal group objectives center around meeting the needs of its individual members. Agreement on how things should be done to accomplish group goals is an important cement for all groups.

Work groups dictate performance and commitment expectation through job descriptions, company policies and procedures, and production standards. Informal groups make compliance demands on their members through the shared mores of the group. Sanctions for failing to meet expectations are imposed on work groups by the financial reward and disciplinary system of the organization. Informal groups use sanctions that rely on personal and social needs of their members (i.e., peer pressure).

Definition of a Work Group

A **work group**, by definition, shares the characteristics of all groups. It is a collection of individual persons gathered together to perform specific functions for the benefit of the whole organization. Its management justification lies in the principle of specialization of work, in which the total output of the organization is greatly enhanced by allowing individual persons or groups to become highly proficient in a special part of the production process.

The laboratory is an excellent example of this concept. Already a highly specialized entity, the lab requires an even greater level of specialization to effectively deliver services. The night shift may be generalists in meting the STAT needs of the hospital; however, they must be specialist in the coordination and organizational skills necessary to function across a broad range of disciplines and deal with the competing demands for their attention. These skills can be contrasted against the enormous depth (hence limited scope) of knowledge necessary to perform many of the highly technical procedure in the modern laboratory. The laboratory cannot function without both types of work groups.

Individual-Group Interface

Groups and individuals maintain a push-pull relationship. Each puts pressure on the other to change and adapt. The character and performance of each is molded by this dynamic interaction. Individuals are the substance of a group and provide the source of its energy. In return, the group enables individuals to achieve goals far beyond what they could accomplish by themselves.

The importance of members to the group must be kept in perspective throughout this review. If the people desert the group, it disappears. If the group disbands, the individuals simply seek other alliances. However, the group has a tremendous impact on it members in both shaping their daily work lives and providing boundaries for their futures, which are accomplished through the interaction of the individuals with members of the group and from contact with other groups.

Interpersonal Relationships

People have definite goals and expectation for their interactions with other individuals. How they respond to fellow members of the group is guided by several factors, including how they view themselves (personal image), how they believe others will behave (behavior expectations), and what they expect to receive for the relationship (personal benefits).

Personal Image

How we see ourselves and how we think others see us combine to form our self-concept or **personal image**. The importance of this self-image to our well-being and success in social intercourse is demonstrated by the attention psychologists give to identifying its parameters and developing techniques for improving and healing this fragile entity. Sell-concepts include our personal goals, belief systems, assumptions about ourselves and others, social and moral values, confidence in our ability to perform in the workplace, and amount of control we exercise over our affairs.

Behavior Expectations

If personal image matches our expectations of how fellow humans are supposed to behave, harmony is achieved. If it does not, the conflict must be resolved. **Behavior expectations** are derived from the experiences and feedback we have received from our daily encounters. Our personal image and the behavior expectations we hold for others are an extremely complex montage of family, genetic, cultural, and religious factors that science is only beginning to understand. The resulting emotional and personality package defines the nature of the person who comes to the group and the type of relationship and influence he or she will exert on others.

Personal Benefits

The final factor in the interpersonal relationship is the attractiveness of membership in the group (i.e., the **personal benefits** of membership). The needs of the group must be weighed against the needs of each member. Each gives up something in exchange for something else. As long as individuals perceive that belonging to the group is in their best interest, the bond will remain strong. When the costs of membership outweigh the rewards, individuals reevaluate their association. The reverse is also true. When the group no longer considers a member to be advantageous, or perhaps even disruptive to its purpose, it will take steps to protect itself, including the possible expulsion of the offending individual. The benefits and rewards of membership may be monetary (pay, financial benefits), social (fellowship, acceptance), or personal (friendship, good feelings, accomplishment).

Role Expectations

Individuals bring to a group their personal abilities and talents; they also look to the group for satisfaction of their motivational needs and ambitions. These two factors, group and individual expectations, are encompassed in the **role** the individuals play in a group. Roles are acquired and assigned by forces in both the formal and informal group networks that exist in an organization.

Work group roles are determined by the job assignments, duties, and tasks that employee performs. Roles in informal groups are derived from the peer relationships between fellow members. Because of this formulation, "personal roles" have many facets that frequently result in conflicts from these competing factions. For example, a phlebotomist may be the leader of a bowling team consisting of a broad range of laboratorians yet has a subordinate position on the job, or a staff technologist may take the role of representative and spokesperson for an informal group of coworkers whose common denominator is a shared unhappiness with a policy set by the section supervisor.

A major role determinant is the *status* of the individual within either the organization or the informal group. Status within the work groujp is reflected in such items as the position held by the person, degree of independence allowed in performing his or her duties, salary level, and privileges and perks. Informal group status is determined by personal factors such as charisma, social polsiton, force of personality, and the success of a member in meeting the needs of the group.

Work Group Behavior

One variation of an old joke could be: "*What opinions or viewpoints do the employees in this laboratory have in common? ... They share a parking lot.*" The underling question is: "What causes a group to change from being just a collection of individuals, each with a separate agenda and nothing much in common except a parking lot, to a fully functioning entity unto itself?" The answer lies in the inner functioning of a work group: its **synergism**, effectiveness, and teamwork. The previous section discussed why member join groups and how people relate to one another. This section looks at the resulting group as a whole unit with its own identity.

Synergism, in which the whole becomes greater (more productive, productive) the collective sum of its individual parts, results from the bonding of the members into a viable and effective unit with a common mission and goals. To understand this force, two aspects for the synergistic process need to be examined: (1) determinants that bring about cohesiveness and operative functionality and (2) dysfunctional factors.

Work Group Functional Factors

The successful coherent work group has its genesis in the reason all groups come together: the shared mission, goals, and needs satisfaction of its members. Work groups fulfill these criteria through the following feature of the organization: nature of work and task being performed; skills and social equality of its members; reward system; competence of management; and, spatial factors such as the size of the group, physical working conditions, and types of equipment involved in the work process.

The term **emergent behavior**
describe the efforts of the group as a whole: *the behavior that "emerges" from the internal interaction of the group members*. Emergent behavior is the result, or sum total, of three forces: (1) the types and requirements of work perfumed (tasks behavior); (2) the everyday conduct of business necessary to ensure an ongoing enterprise (maintenance behavior); and, (3) the behavior of the individual members as they act in their own interests (peer and informal group-induced behavior). The emergent group behavior from the combination of there forces determines the success or failure of the work group in reaching its goals.

The following list contains factors that contribute to and enhance work group performance, synergism, and effectiveness by nurturing positive emergent behavior.

- Shared values of the member and their commitment to the goals and objectives of the work group.
- The success of the group in achieving its mission. This can be self-driven force in that success breeds success*: the more successful the group, and the more this success is recognized, the more this factor influences and encourages positive emergent behavior.*
- The status of the group within the organization as viewed by its members and peers.
- The amount and quality of participation in the decision-making process. This includes the level of creativity encouraged, as well as the degree of conformity enforced.

Work Group Dysfunctional Factors

Most of the conditions that can bring about an efficient work environment and enhanced worker commitment can also wreak havoc if not properly managed. Matched with the mismanagement of positive forces, the factors listed next can disrupt the effective functioning of a work group, with breakdowns in emergent behavior.

- Lack of self and group-esteem, or low status of the group within the organization.
- Failure in reaching goals.
- Poor physical working conditions.
- Dictatorial management styles that discourage creativity and participation.
- Members with divergent and conflicting social and personal norms.
- Personal inequalities in social and organizational status.
- Friendship and informal group clashes.
- Disagreement with or opposition to the goals of the group.
- Disagreement with how things are done.
- Difficulty in relationships with other groups and organizational competition for limited resources.

In addition to developing a strategy to build a strong, closely bonded team with a high level of commitment to work performance, the group must be placed within the context of the whole organization. To remain a viable entity, each unit and work group must be adept at interfacing with other members and teams to accomplish their own and the organization's goals.

Group Interaction

This section looks at how a group interacts with other groups. This topic, like personal relationship and internal group functioning, is many-faceted. It depends on the relationship between members of each group, because a group consists of its members, and on the nature of the group itself. An example of this dichotomy of relationship is how the laboratory interfaces with and views nursing or the purchasing departments. The departments themselves may have a positive working relationship, but two individuals involved in a telephone conversation may view each other negatively. The success of the particular transaction (lab result or purchase order) greatly depends on the people involved in the actual interchange.

As a group, such as the Hematology section, becomes a coherent entity it assumes some of the characteristics of individual persons and develops a personality of its own. One of these features is **ownership**. Ownership involves issues of identify and possession. This mentality is contained in the concepts of image and turf. For example, if Hematology, which occupies neighboring floor space with Chemistry, gets wind that Chemistry is acquiring a new instrument and will need additional space into which to expand; Hematology may typically respond by developing a strategy designed to ensure that there is no encroachment into its territory.

Although this conflict and competition may initially be seen as adversarial, it may in actuality be a positive force that brings the Hematology section into a closer kinship as a tight-knit group committed to common goals. This example demonstrates the need for both skilled leadership and an understanding of how groups interact with each other.

Factors Influencing Intergroup Relationships

In examining the preceding scenario, several questions about intergroup relationships become apparent: What issues bring groups in contact? What factors influence group relationships? What strategies are appropriate for managing these relationships?

As subsystems in the organization, groups are required to interact with other parts of the system. One of the main characteristics of a system is the interdependence of each unit on the other and the importance that the smooth operation of each subsystem has for the success of the organization as a whole. This reliance may be total and direct —for example, the laboratory's dependence on the nursing and the medical staff for test requests — or remote — for example, the staff's contact with the board of directors, which many people in the lab many not even know exists but which is still crucial to its success. The degree of dependence and active interface defines the extent of power exerted by one group over the other and the level of cooperation required from each.

Factors that may influence intergroup relationships include the following.

- The status or prestige of one group within the organizational hierarchy. This includes the professional qualification of each group's membership and their place in the bureaucracy.
- The amount of dependency or power one group has in relation to the other.
- Any conflict-of-interest issues, including the competition for budget priority, space, and credit or blame for success or failure of a project.
- The ability to communicate and deliver goods and services to each other.
- The personal relationships between the interfacing members of each group.

Union-Management Interaction: An Example of Intergroup Relationships

Many aspects of labor policies, particularly management –union interaction, demonstrate intergroup relationships. Although the legal issues surrounding union activities are reviewed in Chapter 11, the group-to-group contact provides an excellent example of how two parties with different perspectives may resolve conflicting agendas and deal efficiently with each other. Labor relations and unionization are topics that are becoming increasing important in the laboratory and health care community, and all managers are expected to be familiar with them.

Group Formation: Why Do Employees Join Unions?

Unions allegedly represent employees to management. It is also a stated purpose of management, particularly first-line supervisors, to be the link between the employees and the owners of the enterprise. Labor unions come about when management fails in this responsibility and for the same reason that all groups form: a perceived need on the part of the members; a mission or purpose; agreement about how things should or should not be done; and, a belief by the members that success in reaching these objectives is being served by the group (i.e., the union).

Research has identified the following reasons that workers find union membership attractive.

- To provide security, including employment, maintenance of pay levels, and safe working conditions.
- To ensure fairness in personnel practices.
- To be involved in the decision-making process.
- To accede to peer pressure from coworkers

People have chosen not to join unions for similar reasons; they have faith and confidence in management; they distrust the union movement or the local organizing agent; they lack the opportunity to join a union; or, are generally satisfied and complacent about current conditions.

Management-Union Relations

How management and unions relate depends on many factors; not the least of these is the background and philosophical approach each brings to the relationship. If management and union leaders see each other in a positive light, both benefit. If management hold the union movement in contempt and sees it as an invasion of management prerogatives, or if union leaders see managers as an inherently had and self-interested lot, then they have difficulty in cooperating. This feature is shared by all groups in intergroup relationships.

Readers may hold their own opinions of the merits of unionization and the perceived values of each type of organization. A summary of the common arguments for and against unionization follows.

Arguments in Favor of Unions

- Provide a mechanism to offset or balance managerial power.
- Allow employees to gain some control over their future and everyday work life.
- Ensure fair and equal treatment of all employees in the application of company policies and procedures (hiring, firing, promotion).
- Provide security in employment and improvement in wages and benefits.
- Provide social opportunities for members.

Arguments against Unions

- Cause loss of managerial control over timely implementation and adaptation of company strategy in the changing market environment.
- Lose competitive advantage to other geographic areas or foreign countries that have significantly lower wage scales.
- Interfere with and cause trouble in the labor relationship between the company and its employees.
- Create philosophical conflict over collectivism and individualism.
- Dislike of poor image and reputation of the union movement.

Management of Groups

The purpose of a supervisor is to build an energetic and cohesive team, committed to the goals of the organization. As well as the smooth internal functioning of the group, managers must also ensure that the group successfully interacts with other units and works with them in close coordination and support to accomplish the overall mission of the institution.

Group Building and Teamwork

A manager can intervene in three areas to build a strong work group: the leadership style of the supervisor, the bureaucratic structure of the work group and the organization, and the level of success achieved by the manager in building a team.

Leadership Strategies

The personal relationships between the supervisor (the formal leader) and the members of the work groups (followers) cannot be overemphasized. The techniques discussed in the leadership chapter show that leaders have two responsibilities: production (tasks) and people. A good manager gives proper respect to both. People and tasks are essential and complementary to each other, not in conflict, as illustrated in the Managerial Grid®, as well as the continuum-of-leadership model. Specifically, leaders should attempt to develop among the staff a spirit of trust and confidence in their ability to do the job assigned, which is accomplished by removing fear and fostering an atmosphere that encourages open communication and active participation by the group in the decision making process.

Structural Techniques

Just as our bodies have both abilities and limitations, the nature of the organization gives character to the types of work groups that evolve. The kinds of work performed, the skill and educational level of the work force, the technology and methodology used in the production process, and the space in which the work is performed all influence the selection of members of a work group and how well they come together as a team.

The bureaucratic structure set in place to organize these factors also plays a major role in the functions of work groups. Changes in structural format, particularly in management styles, the delegation and use of authority, and role expectations of the members, can bring about changes in how work groups perform and coalesce.

Team Building: Organizational Development Strategy

Teamwork, the goal of all work groups, arises from following the principles of good management and leadership. Sometimes referred to as *espirt de corps* or *team spirit*, teamwork gives the group a feeling of shared enthusiasm for their common mission be it winning a football game or meeting production goals. Figure 8 - 1 illustrates how crucial it is that all group members, no matter how insignificant their jobs, realize their importance to the success of the group.

YOU ARX A KXY PXRSON

Evxn though my typxwritxr is an old modxl, it works vxry wxll—excxpt for onx kxy. You would think that will thx othxr kxys functioning propxrly, onx kxy not working would hardly bx noticxd; but just onx kxy out of whack sxxms to ruin thx wholx xffort.

You may say to yoursxlf—Wxll I'm, only onx pxrson. No onx will noticx if I don't do my bxst. But it doxs makx a diffxrxncx bxcausx to bx effxctivx an organization nxxds activx participation by xvxry onx to the bxst of his or hxr ability.

So thx next timx you think you arx not important, rxmxmbxr my old typxwirtxr. You arx a kxy pxrson.

Figure 8 – 1. "You arx a kxy pxrson." [From Alder, RB: Communicating at Work, ed. 4. McGraw Hill, New York, 1992, p. 212) with permission [8th ed. (2004)].

Team building is an integral part of a management strategy call **Organization Development** (OD). The following list provides the main features of team building in the OD model.

1. Making sure that each member understands his or her duties and role in accomplishing the goals of the group.
2. Reducing and eliminating any conflict between members over issues of personal worth, jealousy, or status within the group.

3. Enhancing interpersonal relations through recognition of the contribution of each member and encouraging a sense of belonging so important in satisfying the social needs of the individual.
4. Boosting the identify of the group as a unified body by heightening the attractiveness of association through programs that advance the problem solving skills of the group as a whole, promote participation in decision making, and support personal growth.

Organization development is a long-term program that focuses on improving the attitudes and behavior of both the employees and the company, thereby enhancing the performance of the business. Human growth, personal and corporate renewal, and a synergistic approach to problem solving are the desired objectives of OD.

Intergroup Management

Although building a work group with a strong sense of identify and good team spirit is an important goal, it is just as important that the resulting group comprehends that it is a part of the larger organization and must work smoothly with other units of the system. Competition may be helpful as each group attempts to outshine each other. However, care must be taken to ensure that each department realizes it is dependent on and a part of the overall team. Success of the organization depends on preventing healthy competitiveness from becoming combative and disruptive.

This factor is illustrated in the hospital when, for example, nursing and the laboratory each attempt to blame the other for missing a timed test. Nursing may claim that the specimen was drawn late, and the laboratory may counter that it was not told the proper time for collection or that a nurse changed the time of dosage without notifying the laboratory. Avoiding this situation requires that each department be aware of the informational needs of the other section and the impact that a change in one area may have on another. Accomplishing this aim is no mean feat in an institution as large and complex as a hospital.

Although a meeting between department heads may appear to be the appropriate way to resolve this dilemma, a better solution may be to have the person responsible for collecting the specimens (phlebotomist or Phlebotomy supervisor) talk directly with the nurse to identify each other's needs and develop a solution.

The reader's initial response may be "Oh, no! Another meeting—the perfect solution!" The work "*meeting*" does, in may cases justifiably, have a negative connotation, but is only one strategy for resolving and improving intergroup relationships. Current health care management thinking focuses sharply on quality — not just in the sense of QC numbers and product standards but also from the perspective of satisfying *customer* needs and desires and eliminating medical errors. Miscommunication, fractional responsibility, and a break down in process control because components of critical care components are scatter between non-coordinated units are major contributors to patient care errors. Further examples of this emphasis on quality and error prevention include the popularity of total-quality management, quality assurance, and quality circles programs.

Intergroup management tactics include the standardization of hospital wide procedures and planning for coordinating the performance of each unit as part of the management functions design. Following is a list of additional intergroup management techniques that have proved helpful in coordinating intergroup activities:

- Integrate services that are highly dependent and must be closely coordinated. This may require braking down work by specimen and service type and crossing professional disciplines. An example is the move by the laboratory to bedside testing in efforts to provide more timely delivery of results in critical situations such as the emergency room, operating room, and intensive care units.

- Obtain mutual input and approval from a family of groups that require close coordination. An example of this method is therapeutic drug monitoring, whereby the Pharmacy, Nursing, and Laboratory meet and agree on a time schedule for giving and collecting peak and trough levels. The system becomes *impersonal* in its requirements and enforcement and allows all three departments to plan their activities accordingly.
- Designate someone to coordinate common concerns between several groups. The laboratory quality assurance coordinator and safety officer are examples of this approach.
- Develop interdisciplinary teams responsible for resolving continuing problems and issues within a department and organization. These may be temporary teams, given the responsibility of tacking specific problems or permanent committees such as Blood/Tissue and Infection Control.

Faced with conflicts between groups or individuals under their supervision, most managers attempt to have the parties resolve the differences between themselves or use one of the techniques mentioned previously. However, the manager must be ready to serve as the arbitrator of last resort when the need warrants such intervention.

The next chapter, Job Design and Job Descriptions, discusses how to apply these and other management techniques to the real-life situations of job design and work performance.

— Case Study —

Chapter Eight: Management of Work Groups

"I need your help, "Jane, the microbiology supervisor, said to Mary during a coffee break. "I don't know what to do. I just can't seem to get my staff to work together."

"What seems to be the problem?" asked Mary.

"I don't know, exactly," replied a thoughtful Jane. "I do know that part of the problem centers on Susan. She seems to block or resist everything I try to do."

"What do you mean?" asked a puzzled Mary. "Susan is one the best liked employees in the lab. She's always organizing birthday parties and making sure everyone gets flowers if they're sick or lose a family member."

"That's it exactly. ... everyone in my section always checks with her before they come to me. And worse, they all get together to support her when they don't like the way I want something done!"

"Well, what have you done about it so far?'

"For one thing, I've tried putting Susan in an area where she works by herself. But it doesn't work; her friends always seem to find a way to get to her. I've also cracked down, and I make the staff check with me before they turn out anything but normal results."

"I'm not sure you're doing the right thing, Jane," Mary answered. "Maybe you should trying winning Susan's support, rather than fighting her."

"That's easy for you to say," responded a frustrated Jane. "I do have one favor to ask your, Mary. Maybe it would also help if you try to keep your people from spending so much time with Susan. She might then focus on her job, rather than all this socializing!"

Chapter Section for Review

- Work Group Characteristics (Table 8 — 1)
- Role Expectations
- Work Group Functional Factors
- Work Group Dysfunctional Factors
- Teamwork

Questions for Discussions

1. What types of groups are in operation in this laboratory section? Who are their leaders?
2. Why is Susan able to exert such an influence in the laboratory?
3. If you were Mary, would you ask your staff to stay away from Susan?
4. What recommendations would you give to Jane to help her gain control and support of her staff?
5. What specific advice would you give Jane in dealing with Susan?

[9]

Job Design and Job Descriptions

— Chapter Nine —

Up to this point in the text the topics have been mostly theoretical and conceptual. This chapter begins the process of applying the concepts and principles presented previously. Although the reader may have been impatient to reach this stage, if the previous foundation was shortchanged, skipped, or brushed over, the groundwork and foundation essential for running a modern laboratory will have been missed.

This chapter examines the application of management and leadership skills to the designing of laboratory jobs. The *job* is actual hands on tasks we do to accomplish the duties and responsibilities for which we are paid. This process involves not only the design and development of the jobs needed in the operation of the laboratory but also matching of people to the position. The module concludes with methods for applying the analysis to strategies for determining staffing levels, scheduling personnel, and writing job descriptions.

OBJECTIVES

After completion of this chapter, the reader will be able to demonstrate accomplishment of the following objectives.

1. Explain the process of work analysis and job design.
2. Recognize the relationship between the needs of the organization, its people, and the tasks to be performed.
3. Describe the major techniques for collecting and analyzing job design information.
4. Apply the information obtained from job analysis to the staffing and scheduling of laboratory personnel.
5. Prepare and write job descriptions.

Chapter Highlights and Glossary of Key Terms

I. JOB DESIGN

Job: *A collection of task, duties, and responsibilities assigned to an individual worker.*

Job Design: *The process of organizing work into jobs.*

- A. Organizational Needs
- B. People Needs
    1. Herzberg's motivators
    2. Job behavior factors
    3. Worker selection
    4. Job enrichment

       Job Enrichment: Efforts to make work more meaningful and satisfying, especially by increasing the level of autonomy, control, and responsibility for job performance in areas that allow the worker to grow professionally.
- C. Competency Models

II. JOB ANALYSIS

Job Analysis: *The process of collecting and analyzing information about the tasks, work flow, and jobs being done in an organization so that job descriptions, work standards, and performance appraisal systems can be developed.*

A. Industrial Engineering
B. Strategies for Data Collection
C. Dictionary of Occupational Titles
D. Functional Job Analysis

III. APPLICATION OF JOB DESIGN INFORMATION

A. Staffing

Staffing: *The process of matching the number and types of people with jobs that meet the goals and structure of the organization*

B. Scheduling
C. Job Description and Performance Appraisals

IV. JOB DESCRIPTIONS

Job Descriptions: *A written statement that designates the task, duties, working conditions, and reporting relationships for a specific job.*

A. Job Description Objectives
   1. Employee objectives
   2. Organizational objectives
B. Criteria- and Competency-Based
   1. Historical requirements
   2. CLIA'88 competency rules
C. Authority Scale

   Authority Scale: *A quantitative scale that defines the specific level of independence or freedom to act in performing a job duty without immediate consultation with a supervisor.*
D. Format: Writing the Job Description
   1. Identification and job title headings
   2. Job specifications

      Job Specifications: *A summary in abridged form of the formal education, skills, and experience required to perform the duties of the job; also, included are any unusual physical requirements or working conditions.*
   3. Reporting relationships
   4. Duties
      a. Priorities of duties
      b. Format of duty descriptions
      c. Authority Scale
      d. Performance and evaluation criteria
   5. Approval signatures

Job Design

Jobs are the link between people and the organization. They encompass the expectation of both the company and the individual. **Jobs** are the mechanism through which work is done, products and services delivered, and all parties ultimately rewarded. Given this importance, close attention must be given to how jobs are constructed, who does the work, and what resources are needed to accomplish the associated tasks.

Each person within the institution — executives, supervisors, peers, incumbents, and customers — has a different perspective on exactly what a particular job entails. Design strategies must incorporate and clarify all of these views into the composition of the job.

Many factors influence the makeup of a job. The main determinants are the following.

- **Organizational factors**: these include management styles, bureaucratic structure, products or services produced, technology requirements, and the general economic health of the enterprise.
- **People issues**: these include people's skills and limitations, personal motivational needs, behavior characteristics, expectations, social mores, workforce availability, and ability to function in the conditions of the work environment.
- **Legal and union requirements**: these include legislative and labor contract rules and regulations.

This section reviews **job design** according to the needs of the organization, the needs of people, and conjunction of these needs in the context of specific job parameters.

Organizational Needs

Obviously, before any employees can be hired or assigned duties, there must be work — in other words, there must be a job available. This is not to say that there cannot be an ongoing department with people and positions that need to be redesigned and streamlined; however, for a business to hire someone, there must be an incentive to do so. Whatever the incentive, the institution has specific needs in mind when a person is added to the payroll.

To survive as an ongoing entity, the organization must be concerned with issues of *productivity* and *efficiency*. This concern is not just a greedy instinct on the part of big business to squeeze the most out of every dollar but a necessary tactic to ensure solvency. This fact has been driven home to the laboratory community in recent years, with the advent of diagnosis related groups (DRGs), increased competition for patients, and the erosion of traditional sources of revenue. The laboratory of today must be highly productive and cost-conscious, as the government, insurance carriers, and patients become increasingly intolerant of escalating health care costs and seek alternative for care.

Productivity gains are actively being sought. Promising sources in the medical laboratory include technological advances in instrument throughput, task simplification, specialization, evaluation of personnel qualifications, and user-friendly workstations. Ideas for these improvements have come from workers themselves, from industrial engineering, and by looking at workload and payroll statistics in other facilities.

Organizations need people who are technically and legally qualified to perform the tasks necessary for the production process. The goal of job design is to match the right person with the right job to achieve a work force that is productive in both volume and economics.

People Needs

The most important element in meeting the productivity and efficiency needs of an organization is a motivated and committed workforce, which is accomplished by considering people needs in job design. Because the work people perform is one of the most important factors in determining the quality of their lives on and out of the workplace, it behooves the manager to incorporate this component into the design of the job.

"How can this be done?" a manager may ask. "I have only certain work and tasks that need to be done. How can I organize each person's job so that they all are fulfilled and motivated, as the experts say I should?" The answer to this question is both complex and surprisingly simple: **job enrichment**. Job enrichment —see Herzberg's Motivators, Job Behavior Factors, Worker Selection, and Job Enrichment in the next sections — deals directly with the people issues in these questions.

Herzberg's Motivators

Herzberg's theory suggests that the following motivators should be an integral part of job design.

- Opportunity for *achievement*; that is, the feeling of making a difference and having a sense of contribution and accomplishment.
- *Recognition* for one's role in the success of the group.
- *Challenging* work that reinforces employees' confidence in their abilities.
- *Responsibility* and the feeling that one is in control of one's future.
- The chance for *advancement* and personal growth.

Not all jobs contain all of these factors, but they can offer some and provide a means to achieve the missing ones. For example, the positions of a phlebotomist or laboratory clerk may appear to be dead-end jobs with little chance of advancement. However, they provide tremendous opportunity to learn from and interact with professional staff, which can prove to be a big advantage for those who are pursuing a path of educational and personal growth [Victor H. Vroom's **Instrumentality**: *the degree of faith in the belief that current efforts may possible achieving even larger or more long-term rewards* (chapter 6: Motivation to work)]. The laboratory manager should emphasize this point as an advantage to the person assigned theses tasks.

Job Behavior Factors

Research, including the Herzberg model, has shown that there are five basic areas, or job behavior factors, in which a manager can intervene in the job design process to help satisfy human needs.

- The level of *autonomy*, independence, freedom, and responsibility that workers can exercise in performing their duties.
- The *variety* of skills, talents, and activities needed to perform the job.
- *Task identity*—the extent to which the work being done is identified with the final product; for example, the importance of the laboratory work being performed to the well-being of the patient.
- *Task significance*—the degree of significance attached to the work by both the organization and the employee.
- The immediacy and clarity of *feedback* on the effectiveness of the employee's performance.

Worker Selection

Many studies have suggested, and human nature verifies, that each individual brings to the organization his or her own set of needs, desires, and expectations. This individuality should be correlated with the wide variety of jobs available in a facility. One person may work best in an environment that encourages creativity, originality, and a rapidly changing work situation; another may seek a highly structured and stable position with precise instructions as to what and how things are to be done. Many factors guide the supervisor in this decision, including age, career stage and ambition, educational background, experience, and personality. Matching these individual needs with specific jobs is an important responsibility of management. This topic is covered furthered in Chapter 11 of the text.

Job Enrichment

The term **job enrichment** is frequently heard when the human components of job design are discussed. The term is often misused and misunderstood. All agree that job enrichment is an attractive and useful theory that brings the motivational aspect of human relations into the workplace. But *job enlargement*, not enrichment, is the usual result in practice. Although variety is the spice of life and a proposed cure for boredom, it is not an answer to professional dissatisfaction or burnout.

Job enlargement can be an effective motivational tool if it offers people the opportunity to expand their knowledge and grow professionally. However, if it is just the addition or substitution of similar tasks that do not challenge the employee or require learning new skills, it may be seen as more work that has to be done in an already-overwhelming work schedule.

Job enrichment is, in fact, increased control, responsibility, and accountability in the work situation. Specifically, it is an expanded role in the management functions of planning, directing, and controlling as they relate to the duties and content of the job. It is not something as simple as being asked an opinion of a new serology kit or reagent; rather it is being asked to investigate and recommend how the section can offer a new service or test to meet the requests of the medical staff. Such a task includes methodology selection, workplace and work low design, and personnel scheduling. Obviously, such an assignment cannot be heaped on top of current duties; the employee must be given time to assess information and resources that will enable him or her to carry out such a project.

They key points in a job enrichment program that need to be incorporated into the job design plan are as follows.

- Skill variety if several jobs are combined that require a broad range of proficiency.
- High task identify in which workers can see the impact of their efforts on the final product.
- Human interaction and respect, allowing the staff to deal directly with peers, suppliers, customers, and patients.
- Autonomy in work procedures, work flow, and quality measurements.
- Timely performance feedback.

With an understanding of the needs of both the organization and its members, the manager is now ready to proceed with an analysis of the work that must be done. From this information, the work can then be organized into discrete units, or jobs, that can be matched with people who have the necessary knowledge and skills to perform the tasks effectively.

Competency Models

Competency Models incorporates all the issues listed above, and focuses on developing a set of "competencies," which is directly linked to the goals of the organizations. Some proponents maintained that this is a separate task, different from job design and analysis; however, with its attention to the characteristics necessary to perform successfully it is an essential element of the job design process. These competencies include knowledge, personality, skills, training, performance abilities, as well as motives and personal attributes.

Job Analysis

The job design process involves analysis of the work that needs to be done and a plan to break the job down into identifiable units that can be assigned to individual workers with specific skills. This three-step process — analysis, job design, and worker assignment — culminates in a formal written document call the *job description*. However, a job description is not the ultimate goal of job design; it is a fluid, continually evolving tool that provides a means of communication between the staff and the organization about how each perceives the work that is to be done. Job descriptions are similar to organizational charts and accounting statements in that they provide a snapshot of the manager's expectations of the employee. The "*job description*" only provides a working document or representation of the person within the institution; and is not the actual breathing, evolving role that the person continually plays in the organization.

Following is a list of factors that must be considered in a **job analysis**.

- **Working conditions**: physical environment, temperature extremes, manual labor exertion (i.e., extended standing or walking, strength requirements such as heavy lifting, isolation, and extended length of work hours).
- **Technology**: methodology and instrumentation, both technical skills and physical dexterity factors.
- **Job specifications**: qualifications, skills, special knowledge, and experience.
- **Availability of labor**: types and quality (*skill sophistication*) of personnel available, both are limiting factors in job design.
- **Personal interaction**: types, frequency, and degree of coordination required with other people, both inside and outside the organization.
- **Legal aspects**: personnel and facility licensure requirements.
- **Work flow**: time of arrival of work orders and service needs, test requests, volume and predictability of STATs, routine, AM-timed, turnaround times.
- **Work itself**: actual tasks and duties that must be performed and completed to do the work.
- **Work process**: similar to methodology and work flow but deals with the steps and timing of tasks that must take place in the work process; specifically, coordination with other jobs or departments. For example, the receipt of specimens from phlebotomy and the availability of total CPK/LDH results and sample for performing isoenzymes.

Methods for job analysis can be broken into four approaches. Each has similar data collection and analytical procedures, but they differ on which aspects of jobs and work are important and how they should be measured. Industrial engineering, which is the progeny of scientific management, offers an objective and detailed time-motion study approach that emphasizes actual hands-on "*movements*." Other researchers suggest a wider selection of data sources would be more useful to fully understand the tasks being performed. Systems proposed by the U.S. Department of Labor and the U.S. Employment Service are also presented in this section.

Industrial Engineering

The branch of management that claims the role of job analysis is industrial engineering. Although it has been bitterly criticized for focusing on the mechanical aspects of work and ignoring the human element, it has demonstrated its value as a productivity tool because of the concern with analyzing work methods and establishing specific time standards. Industrial engineering breaks down each task into its smallest components to identify areas in which steps can be improved, eliminate, or streamlined. The time required to complete each step is recorded. Each phase is timed and studied to see where motion and distance can be economized or eliminated. Industrial engineering is also becoming increasingly concerned with ergonomic factors; factors which deal with the physical and psychological impact of work tasks and station design on the well-being of the employee. The basic industrial engineering process consists of the following steps.

- Break each job and task down into its smallest components, with particular emphasis on the motions involved in the work.
- Time every motions involved in each step.
- Attempt to eliminate unnecessary motions, specifically by making suggestions about the layout of workstations, machinery and equipment, and the production process to improve and conserve the number of steps and motions necessary to perform a task.

Recommendations usually consist of eliminating distances that must be travel, reducing handling time, and designing workstations in which supplies are in the order needed and within easy motion reach, so that each movement of the worker is highly efficient. Industrial engineering has made significant contributions to the design of laboratory instruments and in the workbench layout of such areas a blood bank cross-match stations.

Strategies for Data Collection

There are several other methods for obtaining information for analysis.

- Interview the workers, their supervisors, and customers.
- Hire a job analysts or supervisor trained in job design methodology to make observations.
- Have workers fill out questionnaires and checklist about their work.
- Talk with experts such as industrial engineers, employees, managers, instrument manufacturers and suppliers, or peers from other laboratories.
- Get employees to maintain logs or diaries of the steps and motions involved in their tasks.
- Use a combination of these techniques.

Dictionary of Occupational Titles

The U.S. Department of Labor offers a coding system that allows for analysis and comparison of jobs based on a nine-digit code. Many companies use this system in their job design and include the code as part of the job descriptions.

The first three digits of the code, contained in the *Dictionary of Occupational Titles (DOT),* indicate the occupational category of the job, such as professional, clerical, farming, or a machine trade. The next three digits classify a job based on the degree of functional difficulty with respect to data, people, and things. Table 9 – 1 list the classifications for coding these digits. The last three digits of the *DOT* code simply lists alphabetically the descriptive tile of jobs within the same occupational category.

Data (digit #4)	People (digit # 5)	Things (digit # 6)
0 Synthesizing	0 Mentoring	0 Setting up
1 Coordinating	1 Negotiating	1 Precision working
2 Analyzing	2 Instructing	2 Operating, controlling
3 Compiling	3 Supervising	3 Driving, operating
4 Computing	4 Diverting	4 Manipulating
5 Copying	5 Persuading	5 Tending
6 Comparing	6 Speaking, signaling	6 Feeding, off bearing
	7 Serving	7 Handling

Source: U.S. Department of Labor: *Dictionary of Occupational Titles*. Washington, DC, 1995

Table 9 – 1. Difficulty Levels of Worker Functions

As examples for laboratorians, the *DOT* lists the following job codes:

Medical Technologist (chemistry)
 – 078.261-010

Medical Laboratory Technician
 – 078.381-014

Medical Laboratory Manager
 – 078.161-010

Pathologists – 070.061-010

The first two digits (07) indicate a medical and health occupation. The number _8_ in the third column (Manage, Technologist, and Technician) signifies a position in dental and medical technology, whereas the _0_ (pathologist) is used for physicians and surgeons.

The middle three digits indicate the job's functional level of difficult with respect to date, people, and things. From these codes, this system ranks these jobs as highly complex with respect to date (digit 4) and things (digit 6) but as having a relatively low level of difficulty with respect to people (digit 5) functions.

Functional Job Analysis

Another job design and analysis approach that has recently been proposed and incorporated by health care regulatory and accreditation agencies is *competency* and *criteria-based* job descriptions. To a large extent these have their origin in an approach called *functional job analysis* (FJA), which has come about because employers have needed data to support personnel decisions.

The US Employment Service has developed an FJA system that builds on the DOT but adds four additional categories.

- Worker function, (the DOT criteria)
- Work fields, an analysis of the specific tasks and methods performed in a job
- Machines, tools, equipment, and work aids used by the worker
- Materials, products, subject matter, and/or services produced in the job
- Worker traits, including temperament, working conditions, and training necessary to do the job

In an FJA system, employees are assigned to jobs for which they have appropriate training and competence, a major factor in assuring high-quality performance, especially in providing health care services.

Application of Job Design Information

Information from job design analysis serves many purposes; for example, the date can be used for planning staffing needs, setting wage rates, recruiting and selecting personnel, designing training and continuing education programs, developing performance appraisal systems, improving working conditions, and redesigning jobs. However, the three most frequent everyday uses have to do with setting staffing levels, scheduling personnel, and writing job descriptions and performance evaluations.

Staffing

Establishing the types and numbers of workers needed is an integral part of the **organizing** management function. Staffing, in turn, is the process of matching people with jobs that meet the goals and structure of the organization. Determining the variety (supervisor, technologists, phlebotomists, clerks, and so on) and ratio of which kind of employees are needed is a major purpose of job design. It is contingent on the nature and kinds of task that must be performed. Setting the number of each type is part of the operational budget process and is dependent on the volume of work to be done. Putting together these two factors, types and numbers, is the objective of staffing.

From the research and analysis conducted during the design study, requirements necessary for performance of each position can be specified. These criteria are spelled our in the job description, and specific formal requirements relating to skills and physical requirements may be abstracted into a statement referred to as job specifications. Job specifications are usually listed as a separate section on the job description and include two key components.

1. The skills, training (both formal and experience), and regulatory (licensing, unions, professional societies) qualifications necessary to do the job.
2. The physical demands of the work such as dexterity, heavy lifting, extended standing or bending, and tolerance for temperature extremes.

Specific information about establishing staffing levels and the budgeting process are provided in chapters 13 and 19 of this book.

Scheduling

Scheduling, although closely allied with staffing, is a distinct management activity requiring its own special techniques. Staffing has to do with determining the types and total number of employees needed at specific times in the production process. Scheduling builds on staffing information and focuses on matching people on a day-to-day basis with the fluctuating workload of the laboratory. It determines where and when employees work and usually results in a schedule posted on a periodic basis — daily, weekly, or monthly. The supervisor must balance the needs for the department with those of the employees who need time off for vacations, holidays, and illness. Examples of several scheduling strategies for the laboratory are presented in Module 18.

Job Description and Performance Appraisals

The formal written documents of job design are the job description and the forms used in conducting the performance appraisal system. The preparation of these two documents is highly interdependent as well as contingent on the results of the job design and analysis study. Job descriptions are discussed in the next section. Performance appraisal is coved in chapter 10.

Job Descriptions

The most basic of the job design documents, the job description, establishes the foundations for many other employment-related activities including the development and implementation of the performance appraisal system. A **job description** is a written statement that designates the tasks, duties, working conditions, and reporting relationships for a specific job. It also establishes the authority for the worker to do the job and sets the boundaries and limitation of responsibilities. This section covers the objectives of job description, criteria- and competency-based standards to be used in their preparation, authority scale assignment, and the formats recommended for actually writing job descriptions.

Job Description Objectives

First and foremost, job descriptions are a communications tool for assuring that the employee, supervisor, and organization understand the duties for the position. The two parties to this relationship—worker and management—bring needs and expectations to the relationship. Therefore, job descriptions serve as a means to clarify any ambiguities or misunderstandings.

Employee Objectives

From the standpoint of the employee, job description must meet the following objectives.

- Identify the duties, tasks, and responsibilities of the job.
- Provide orientation to the organization, supervisory and peer networks, and workplace assignments.
- Give guidelines and direction to the performance expectation of the organization.
- Set the limits and boundaries of responsibility.
- Assign the authority to act in performing duties.

Organizational Objectives

The goals of the organization are similar to those of the employee, but they have a different perspective, including the following aims.

- Decrease or minimize confusion, ambiguities, and misunderstanding between employees and supervisors about job duties and expectation.
- Recruit and select qualified personnel.
- Design orientation, training, and developmental programs.
- Assign staffing levels and work schedules.
- Determine performance standards and appraisal criteria and systems.
- Meet legal, professional, and labor contract obligations.
- Establish the right point at which to intervene with corrective action when performance falls below job requirements.
- Set uniform company policy around job descriptions to ensure an equitable wage and salary system and fair treatment of all employees.

Criteria- and Competency-Based Job Descriptions

Another area fraught with controversy over terminology is what to include in the job description and how to word it. Terms that have come in and out of repute include "criteria-based," "performance-oriented," and "task-specific." Now a concept which is being imposed in the laboratory by the regulations of the Clinical Laboratories Improvement Act of 1988 (CLIA'88) is "competency assessment," which must be incorporated in the job description and performance appraisal system.

All of these programs provide positive suggestions for writing job descriptions, specifically by forcing managers to think about the priorities, functions, and goals for which job description and performance appraisal systems are designed. There is a general agreement on three points regarding writing job descriptions:

1. They should be both inclusive and exclusive; that is, they should contain only those duties and tasks that the worker is responsible for and has the power to control. Describe *this* job, not someone else's.
2. They should be concise. Leave details for orientating and competency checklists, procedure manuals, or other supportive documents.
3. They should contain only items that can be measured. List duties unambiguously, using concrete language to describe competency.

Historical Requirements

Job descriptions can be viewed as a *summary* of the findings obtained from the job analysis. This point, which is absolutely crucial in the appraisal stage, uses the criteria identified in the analysis process as necessary to the successful performance of the job. Many authors and organizations, including the Department of Labor, US Civil Service Commission, Board of Registry of the American Society of Clinical Pathologist (ASCP), and the American Society for Medical Technology (ASMT), have suggested criteria guidelines that can be used in the development of laboratory job descriptions and performance evaluations. A synthesis of these proposals would contain the following job description and evaluation criteria.

- **Knowledge parameters:** the training and education ional requirements necessary to produce a product or services, specifically as related to issues of *quality*.
- **Technical abilities:** the hands-on experience and physical skills and talents needed to actually perform the tasks and duties under the environmental conditions that exist on the job, as they relate to *quantity*.
- **Judgment factors:** the degree of autonomy in making decisions and the potential impact of the decisions on the organization or its clients. These factors include planning and use of time, level of initiative and creativity, and emotional characteristics such as maturity, independence, and self-discipline.

- **Relationships:** communication routes (i.e., interaction with peers, customer, and vendors), supervision and management status, and teaching and training obligations.
- **Attendance and reliability:** expectations regarding the technical and physical demands inherent in the workload.

CLIA'99 Competency Rules

*Employee competency assessmen*t (ECA), as now required of the medical director and technical consultant by CLIA'88 regulation, should not be a new duty of laboratory management. It is a function, like QC → QA, which was already being performed, even in on an informal basis. Although this term is still in transition, many of the techniques for compliance are already in place and in most cases need only minor changes and modifications (i.e., orientation checklists and performance reviews).

A competency assessment and assurance program should consist of these three stages.

1. **Employee selection**: this involves the application (job description), candidate information solicitation (interview), and validation of qualifications and experience.
2. **Orientation:** the current orientation checklist for laboratories looks strikingly similar to the observation lists developed to meet ECA rules and serves as examples of an ECA tools already available.
3. **Continuing education and in-service training:** this program, an area in which the laboratory should already be strong, can be modified to ensure the continuous competency of the staff. An excellent example of an application of an ECA model is a training session which incorporates a wet workshop concept (i.e., the ECA observation requirement) as part of the educational evaluation. This approach allows both the instructor and the student to assess their performance and identify areas that need improvement in a non-threatening environment.

Authority Scale

An essential clarification necessary for any task listed on a job description is the level of authority and degree of autonomy the person has in carrying out the duty. This may, at first glance, seem redundant: "Why should something be on the job description if the person is not allowed to do it?" This question goes to the heart of writing a job description. Unfortunately, however, if not addressed directly, this issue may lead to future confusion and misunderstanding between the employee and supervisor.

Table 9 – 2 abstracts a few of the duties for a 3:00 to 11:00 pm shift supervisor and provides a key to the authority-level scale. One of the duties listed is responsibility for calling in additional help (overtime) if necessary. Without further clarification, supervisors may assume they have unlimited authority to call in help; however, the laboratory manager may wish to be notified before this action is taken because of budgeting constraints and to identify reoccurring problems early. By agreeing in advance on the level of authority the shift supervisor has to act before checking with the manager, controversy may be avoided. The assignment of an authority level (AL) key scale to the duty serves this purpose. The AL assigned in our example is a level 2. This means that the supervisor may call in help when needed, including overtime, without further permission, but he or she should leave a note of explanation so that this information is readily available to the manager upon arrival at work.

Another example of this system is the duty to discipline staff, which is assigned an AL of 3. At this level of authority, supervisors are expected to check with their administrator before taking action; however, they have the power to intervene if the manager is not available for prior consultation and the urgency of the situation requires immediate attention (e.g., the supervisor may send an employee home, if their presence is disruptive to the laboratory).

Task	Authority Level
1. Perform testing services according to procedure manual	1
2. Change testing protocol and policies in special cases	3
3. Reject unacceptable specimens	1
4. Perform instrument maintenance	1
5. Request service assistance from outside vendors	2
6. Call in addition (overtime) staffing	2
7. Order routine supplies	1
8. Approve special supplies or authorize rush shipment charges	3
9. Discipline staff	3

Authority level key: **1** = No prior checking or special notification required; **2** = Notify manager ASAP during normal working schedule; **3** = Must attempt to consult manager before acting, authorized to take corrective action if manager is not readily available for consultation; **4** = Not authorized to act, must refer problem to manager for resolution.

Table 9 – 2. Job Description Abstract: 3:00 – 11:00 Supervisor

Returning to the question asked at the opening of this section, there should be very few, if any AL 3 to 4 on a job description. Otherwise, someone else's job is being described. The AL 3's and 4's levels that are present should serve only to establish the boundaries and limits of employee responsibility and clarify when problems should be turned over to a supervisor for resolution. The AL 3 assigned to staff discipline, for example, signifies to a shift supervisor that disciplining staff is not their responsibility but that they are empowered to act if necessary.

Format: Writing the Job Description

There is no single acceptable method for deciding what should be contained in a job description or it order of appearance (i.e., format). The personnel and payroll departments each have their own set of preferences, and the laboratory has its priorities. Given the importance of this document as the foundation for many other activities including recruitment, wage and salary administration, staffing and scheduling, and the performance appraisal system; it should be as complete as possible, so as to serve as a quick date reference sheet while maintaining its summary nature.

> Examples found on the web [*September 2, 2006*] for a laboratory supervisor range from a very short format containing only a brief descriptive job statement with a list of minimum qualifications (license, years of experiences, etc.) at the Clinical Laboratories of Hawaii; to a more extensive design with an detail list of duties and required Qualifications (education, experience, degree level, and skills/abilities) provided by the Duke University Health System [see Internet Provided Job Descriptions in Bibliography]

Most of the items continued in the job description along with the format order, are specific to the facility (e.g., see Figures 9 -1 and 9 – 2 at the end of the chapter). The following suggested list contains basic information that should be included on the job description.

- Identification and job title headings
- Job specifications
- Reporting relationships
- Duties
- Preparer
- Date of preparation and activation
- Approval signatures

Identification and Job title Headings

The heading should include the name of the facility, the location (department, section) at which the work is performed, and a short descriptive title of the position. There may also be job classification data, including personnel and payroll codes such as salary or wage grade, job status (exempt or nonexempt), and the *DOT/FJA* code, if used by the organization.

Job Specifications

A list of **job specifications** is sometime considered a separate document, but the job description should at least contain elementary prerequisite requirements. Job specifications include the formal educational and experience qualifications (legal, union, professional requirements) necessary for employment; the technical, people, and physical skills necessary to perform the duties; and, any atypical working conditions. Working conditions are the environment (outside or inside), unusual physical or sensory demands such as temperature extremes or wearing/handling major protective equipment, and schedule hours.

Reporting Relationships

In this area, the person or position to whom the employee reports is specified (supervisor), along with the supervisory responsibilities of the job (supervisees).

Duties

This section, the heart of the document, lists the duties, tasks, responsibilities, and functions that define the job. Once again. this section should serve as a summary and outline of the parameters of the position and should not attempt to itemize and fully describe every task. Details should be covered elsewhere in procedure manuals and orientation forms.

Priorities of Duties

If a sense of priority is not built into the format, one will be assumed from the order in which duties are listed. For this reason, duties should be ranked according to their importance to the mission of the organization, the amount of time that they will require, and the degree of scrutiny they will receive for the supervisor.

Format of Duty Descriptions

Because most organizations impose a uniform formant on how job descriptions are prepared, the personnel department is usually responsible for ensuring compliance, and their priority take precedence in what is included on the form. The personnel department is interested in information that allows jobs to be classified into equitable wage and salary grades and that assists in recruitment of qualified staff. For these reasons the duty section may be organized around the *DOT*, the US Chamber of Commerce job analysis criteria, or anther criteria-based method such as the performance appraisal system. This section is facility-specific and may be arranged along a variety of lines but often contains the following factors.

- Work and task performance-related duties.
- Machinery, equipment, instrument, or specialized tools and work aids involved in the work.
- Materials and/or complicated paperwork processing and handling.
- People responsibilities, particularly meeting the public or close coordination with coworkers in performing their duties.

Authority Scale

As stated previously, each item on the duty list should be assigned an authority scale code to clarify the latitude the individual has in carrying out assignments.

Performance and Evaluation Criteria

The wording of a job duty is important because it serves as the basis for the performance appraisal system. Responsibilities must be written in a clear manner that provides an understanding of the person's duties. It is not enough, for example, to say that a technologist performs testing in the Hematology section; it must also say that the work must comply with and be measured against the standards of the department. For example:

Incomplete

Technologist performs tests and procedures on specimens received in the Hematology section.

Complete

Technologist performs tests and procedures on specimens received in the Hematology section, according to standards and protocols continued in the procedure manual.

Approval Signatures

The person who writes or revises the job description should be identified, along with the date the description was prepared or modified and the effective date. Necessary signatures for final approval should be appended. These may include the supervisor, laboratory manager, medical director, and the administrator responsible for the laboratory. The personnel manager may also sign the form to verify that it meets the established format of the facility.

The suggested format for writing the job description ends the chapter: *Job Design and Job Descriptions*. The next chapter deals the most controversial topic facing every manager: *Appraisal of Job Performance*.

Following are Figure **9 – 1** and **9 – 2** presented as two examples of Job Descriptions.

****

Figure 9 — 1. Job description for a Hematology Technologist

MEDICAL CENTER HOSPITAL
Anytown, Florida
Department: Laboratory

JOB TITLE/PAYROLL CODE: Hematology Technologist, LAB-023-N, Nonexempt

POSITION SUMMARY: Performs laboratory tests on clinical specimens in the Hematology Section of the laboratory.

JOB SPECIFICATIONS:

Professional Qualifications: Bachelor of Science plus graduation from an accredited school of medical technology, or training/experience acceptable to the laboratory director.

Licensure Qualifications: Licensed at the technologist level in hematology by the Florida Department of Health, Division of Medical Quality Assurance

Experience: 0 (May be eligible for employment upon graduation)

Working Conditions

- Continuous exposure to specimens and material considered to be highly infectious and hazardous
- Moderate lifting/bending, walking/time on feet
- Operation of electrical equipment/instruments containing heating and freezing components, moving parts, and high-speed centrifugation
- Use and wearing of protective garments and equipment, which may frequently be bulky, hot, and require special environmental/physical adaptations
- Schedule: Department/section staffed on a continuous basis, 24 hours a day, including all holidays and weekends. Work schedule may be modified to meet these requirements.

REPORTING RELATIONSHIPS

Immediate Supervisor: Hematology supervisor

Supervisory Responsibility: No employees are supervised in this position; However, the technologist may be asked to fill in for the Hematology supervisor during absence or provide guidance to support personnel such as phlebotomist or clerical staff

Customer/Suppler: Close consultation and coordination required with fellow laboratorians, nursing personnel, patients, and physicians.

POSITION DUTIES:

1. Performs tests and procedures on specimens received in the Hematology Section according to the protocols contained in the procedure manual or as instructed by the Hematology supervisor. AL = 1

2. Operates and maintains equipment and instruments within the section according to manufacturer and laboratory established procedures. This specifically includes: AL = 2
   - Processing/running of laboratory specimens
   - Calibration
   - Quality control
   - Preventive Maintenance
   - Basic troubleshooting procedures

3. Follows general hospital and laboratory policies concerning dress codes, professional conduct, attendance/punctually, documentation, performance criteria, and other directives as issued. AL = 1

4. Actively participates in the instruction and clinical supervision of students, in the orientation of new employees, and in the department's continuing education/in service programs. AL = 1

5. Compiles with all safety/infection control polices and procedures of the laboratory and hospital. AL = 1

APPROVAL:

Hematology Supervisor ______________________________	Date: _________
Laboratory Manager ______________________________	Date: _________
Medical Director ______________________________	Date: _________
Administrator ______________________________	Date: _________
Personnel Director ______________________________	Date: _________

EFFECTIVE DATE: Initial Approval _________________
Review/Modify _________________

Copy received by employee: ________________________________ Date: _________

Authority Level Key (AL)	1 = No prior checking or special notification required. 2 = Notify supervisor ASAP during normal schedule of any problem 3 = Must attempt to consult supervisor before acting. Authorized to take corrective action if manager is not readily available. 4 = Not authorized to act. Matter must be referred to supervisor

---

****

Figure 9 — 2. Job description for a 3:00 pm to 11:00 pm shift supervisor

---

HEALTH CARE MEDICAL CENTER
Anytown, Florida
Department: Laboratory

JOB TITLE/PAYROLL CODE: Laboratory Shift Supervisor, LAB-021-E, Exempt

POSITION SUMMARY: Responsible for laboratory operations and supervision of technical and support staff during the hours of 3:00 Pm to 11:00 pm.

JOB SPECIFICATIONS:

Professional Qualifications: Bachelor of Science plus graduation from an accredited school of medical technology, or training/experience acceptable to the laboratory director. Formal training in management and supervision is also highly desirable

Licensure Qualifications: Licensed at the Supervisor level in hematology, serology, immunohematology, chemistry, and microbiology by the Florida Department of Health, Division of Medical Quality Assurance

Experience: Three (3) years of professional experience. One (1) year in a supervisory position preferred.

Working Conditions

- Continuous exposure to specimens and material considered to be highly i infectious and hazardous
- Moderate lifting/bending, walking/time on feet
- Operation of electrical equipment/instruments containing heating and freezing components, moving parts, and high-speed centrifugation

- Use and wearing of protective garments and equipment, which may frequently be bulky, hot, and require special environmental/physical adaptations
- Schedule: 2:30 pm to 11:00 pm M-F; may require weekend duty, depending on availability of personnel.

REPORTING RELATIONSHIPS

Immediate Supervisor: Administrative Director

Supervisory Responsibility: All personnel scheduled to work during hours of responsibility; supervisor may be asked to fill in for the administrative director during absence.

Customer/Suppler: Close consultation and coordination required with fellow laboratorians, nursing personnel, patients, and physicians. Specific collaboration with nursing managers, pathologists, section supervisors, and other laboratory managers.

POSITION DUTIES:

1. Supervises methods/personnel in the performance of test and procedures on specimens received in the laboratory according to the protocols contained in the procedure manuals. AL = 1

2. Performs test and procedures on specimens received in the laboratory according to the protocols contained in the procedure manuals. AL = 1

3. Supervises the work of support personnel in the performance of their duties (phlebotomists, clerical staff, and computer operators) according to the protocols in the procedure manuals. AL = 1

4. Supervises the operation and maintenance of laboratory equipment and instruments according to manufacturer and laboratory established procedures. This specifically includes: AL = 2
    - Processing/running of laboratory specimens
    - Calibration
    - Quality control
    - Preventive Maintenance
    - Basic troubleshooting procedures

5. Prepares work schedule/assignments for shit personnel. AL = 1

6. Oversees adherence by laboratory staff to general hospital and laboratory policies concerning dress codes, professional conduct, attendance/punctuality, documentation, performance criteria, and other directives as issued. AL = 1

7. Actively participates in the instruction and clinical supervision of students, in the orientation of new employees, and in the department's continuing education/in service programs. AL = 1

8. Ensures compliance with all safety/infection control policies and procedures of the laboratory and hospital. AL = 1

9. Prepares operational budget for shift in coordination with administrative director. AL = 1

10. Advises and collaborates with other laboratory managers, specialists, and section supervisors on the preparation of policy and procedure manuals, selection of equipment/instrumentation, and work space organization of the laboratory. AL = 1

11. Develops standards and conducts performance appraisal reviews for shift personnel within the administrative process of the laboratory. AL = 2

12. Resolves operational/personnel problems that arise during hours of responsibility within the guidelines, policies, and procedures established by the department:
    - Modifies testing protocol/policies in special cases. AL = 3

- Changes work assignments or schedules due to fluctuating workload or unusual circumstances. AL = 1
- Reject, advises recollection, or makes exception to laboratory policy on unacceptable specimens upon request by attending physician. AL = 2
- Request/authorizes payment for service/repair assistance from outside vendors. AL = 2
- Calls in additional (overtime) staffing. AL = 2
- Authorizes special supplies or rush shipment charges. AL = 3
- Corrective action and disciplines staff
    - Counsel sessions for specific incidents. AL = 2
    - Suspension (employee told to report to the laboratory manager) or temporary relief of duties. AL = 3
    - Dismissal/firing. AL = 4

APPROVAL:

Administrative Director ______________________________ Date: _________
Medical Director ______________________________ Date: _________
Administrator ______________________________ Date: _________
Personnel Director ______________________________ Date: _________

EFFECTIVE DATE: Initial Approval _________________
Review/Modify _________________

Copy received by employee: _________________________________ Date: _________

Authority Level Key (AL)	1 = No prior checking or special notification required. 2 = Notify supervisor ASAP during normal schedule of any problem 3 = Must attempt to consult supervisor before acting. Authorized to take corrective action if manager is not readily available. 4 = Not authorized to act. Matter must be referred to supervisor

— Case Study —

Chapter Nine: Job Design and Job Descriptions

"Here is what I needed to see you about.'" said the laboratory manager, handing a bunch of papers to each of the laboratory supervisors. "Personnel said these job descriptions were very old and needed to be updated before the JCAHO inspection next month. Get them back to me in 2 weeks, so we can go over them before they're turned in."

Chapter Section for Review

- Job Analysis factors
- Format: Writing the Job Description
- Duties
- Performance and Evaluation Criteria

Questions for Discussions

1. Look at the Job Descriptions in Figures 9 – 1 and 9 -2. What do you like about them? Dislike? What can be improved?
2. Choose a section (e.g.. hematology, chemistry) in which you work, and list the main duties performed there. Do not worry about format, just use key words or short phrases at this point.
3. Select two of the duties you listed in question two, and write criteria-based position duty statements for each, using Figures 9 – 1 and 9 – 2 as examples.
4. Share the duty statements with colleagues and see if they are written in a clear and understandable manner (incomplete vs. complete) that can be used to develop a measurable performance evaluation.

[10]

Appraisal of Job Performance

— Chapter Ten —

> The time Mr. (Jeffrey) Davidoff *(marketing, Whirlpool)* now spends on reviews, he says, was formerly spent doing more of the marketing work himself. Now, he focuses on coaching and developing his staffers to improve their own performance. "This is how the work gets done," he says. "If you believe in your people, the time with them is literally the best way to spend your time.
>
> Erin White

Performance appraisal systems have been much maligned by critics, often with justification. Historical methods used to evaluate performance have been denounced for their destructive impact on the morale of individuals and the organization as a whole. Famous pundits of total-quality management (TQM) programs and other management gurus, such as W. Edwards Deming and J. M. Juran, have attacked performance appraisals as being especially venal and predicted their early demise. Although these critics have waxed eloquent in their condemnation, they have offered no replacement or suggestions for alternatives to this critical management tool.

In similar fashion, there was a move against the word "control," as in "quality control." The word "*assurance*" was substituted by many laboratories and agencies. Quality assurance is certainly much more the QC; however, the traditional tools of QC —statistical analysis techniques—a re seen as crucial in the evaluation of quality. The same is true with performance evaluations. Adherents and disciples of TQM and other management programs continually attempt to come up with other tactics for letting people know what is expected of their performance and methods for measuring accomplishment of job goals. They avoid at all costs the words "appraisal" and "evaluation" and substitute such terms as "feedback conferences" and "participation sessions."

Whatever terms or words you prefer; this chapter reviews the application of job design information to the preparation and performance of four important management tasks.

1. Letting employees know what they are supposed to do (i.e., their job descriptions, as reviewed in Module 4).
2. Obtaining agreement on what is expected (performance standards).
3. Providing and receiving feedback on how they are doing (performance appraisals).
4. Discussing how things are going (evaluation interviews or conference)

These topics are actually part of a single group of tasks, in which the preparation of a single document is so dependent on the completion of the others that changes in one must be reflected in all of the forms. For example, a duty should not be listed on the job description without stating how successful completion of the duty will be measured. If this is not determined in the early stages of job design, the remainder of the process is impaired.

OBJECTIVES

After completion of this chapter, the reader will be able to demonstrate accomplishment of the following objectives.

1. Describe the key design elements of a performance appraisal system.
2. Develop and write job performance standards.
3. Design a performance appraisal measurement instrument.
4. Use the appraisal measurement instrument in evaluating and judging worker job performance.
5. Plan and conduct a productive evaluation review.

Chapter Highlights and Glossary of Key Terms

I. PERFORMANCE APPRAISALS

Performance Appraisal: *The formal communication system used by an organization to assess and provide feedback to employees about job performance expectations.*

II. PERFORMANCE STANDARDS

Performance Standard: *An item (statistic, statement, model) against which the performance or behavior of an employee can be compared to obtain a relative measurement.*

Performance Criterion: *A standard, test, guideline, or rule upon which a judgment can be based.*

A. Source of Performance Standards
B. Writing Performance Standards

III. PERFORMANCE APPRAISAL MEASUREMENT INSTRUMENT

Performance Appraisal Measurement Instrument: *The formal system (forms, paperwork, checklist) used by an organization to document the results of the performance review and feedback conference.*

A. Appraisal Focus
   1. Scale rating methods

      Scale-Rating Methods: *Predetermined standards or criteria against which performance or behavior is matched, including descriptive statement, rating scores, and defined terminology checklist, usually in a preprinted graphic format.*

      a. Forced-choice method
      b. Critical incident method

         Critical Incident: *Behavior in some aspect of the job that results in unusual success or failure*

      c. Behaviorally anchored rating scales (BARS)
      d. Mixed-standard scales
      e. Laboratory scale-raking performance appraisal model
   2. Peer comparison

      Peer Comparison: *Procedures that compare the behavior or performance levels of an employee with his or her coworkers.*

      a. Ranking method
      b. Forced distribution
      c. Point allocation method
      d. Paired comparison.
B. Format: Performance Appraisal

IV. JUDGING PERFORMANCE

Performance Judgment: *The actual decision or rating assigned to an individual about job performance and the recording of the result.*

A. Judgment Problems
B. Qualifications to Judge
C. Appraisal Selection

V. EVALUATION INTERVIEWS
A. Conference Suggestions
B. Types of Evaluation Interviews
C. Questioning and Discussion Strategy

Performance Appraisals

The **performance appraisal** process represents the formal communication system used by an organization to assess and provide feedback to employees about job performance expectations. To be effective, a performance appraisal system of any kind must have five components.

1. A person expected to perform a job with a designated job description.
2. Standards and criteria that clearly state what is expected and how it is measured.
3. A measurement instrument to compare actual performance with the desired behavior.
4. A judge or assessor trained and competent in using the measurement instrument to do the appraisal.
5. A feedback mechanism (conference, information report, interview) to share the results of the review, identify corrective action. And arrive at an agreement on a plan for the future.

Wayne Cascio (pp. 334-336) summaries these factors as: relevance (link between standards and job); sensitivity (able to distinguish between performance levels); reliability (consistency of judgment); acceptability (supported by those who use them); and, practicality (ease of use). Job description was covered in Chapter 9. The next four aspects of performance appraisal are discussed in the following sections.

Performance Standards

Laboratorians are quite familiar with the concept of standards. Standards provide a measurement against which a similar object can be compared. In chemistry, standards are used to calibrate procedures so that values on patient samples can be obtained. In another instance, the control results are compared against the accept-reject criteria before a batch run on a laboratory instrument is accepted. One level of controls may fail the ±2 standard deviation (SD) standard, but a decision or judgment to accept the run may be appropriate if it meets the established QC criteria for both levels, such as the 1_{3S}, 2_{2S}, or R_{4S} guidelines in the Westgard rules.

In a similar process, management uses standards as targets, or performance criteria, against which to gauge performance. A **criterion**, by definition, is a standard, test, guideline, or rule upon which a decision or judgment about job performance can be based.

Source of Performance Standards

Standards for a particular job are derived from the information obtained through job analysis and the duties listed on the job description. This knowledge is then combined with the management plan of the institution to develop performance standards for each level of employment.

For example, the laboratory may have a turnaround standard of 40 minutes for a STAT glucose from the time the request is received by the department to the reporting of results. This time period needs to be divided, and supportive standards assigned to jobs that are involved in the process. For example, the phlebotomist may be expected to collect and deliver the specimen to the chemistry technologist within 20 minutes of notification; and the technologist may then be expected to deliver the results to the nurse within 20 minutes of the time the specimen arrived in Chemistry. By assigning a goal, such as "90 percent of the time," to the performance standards, criteria can be developed by which the success of the department, the section supervisor, and each member of the staff can be assessed. This data can then be used to identify any problems and take corrective action by further refining the performance review process.

Performance standards are major component of the management control function and of many management programs such as management by objectives and total-quality management. A crucial element of these programs — and a point continually emphasized in this text — is the importance of participation by all members of the organization in the development and design of objectives and performance standards.

The perpetual and cyclical nature of the management process tied to the development of job standards is demonstrated in the following schematic model:

Management plan:
→ Job analysis and design
→ Job description and management plan
→ Job standards and measurement instrument
→ Actual job performance
→ Feedback
→ Corrective action:
management plan,
job analysis and redesign,
revised job descriptions,
and so on ...
→ Job standards

Writing Performance Standards

Performance standards and criteria must clearly define acceptable performance, detail work that falls below expectations, and recognize exceptional achievement. These standards are sometimes also referred to as *dimensions* of performance. To meet theses specification, performance standards should satisfy the following four goals.

1. Be *relevant* to the actual job and task being done.
2. Allow for *fair comparison* between different positions; one person or group should not be held to higher or more difficult standards than other peers. For example, the staff of a STAT lab cannot be held to the same productivity (number of test per hour) standards as a section that processes only batch tests. Neither can an area that must produce a huge volume of tests be accountable for the turnarounds time expected of a STAT laboratory which may have an instrument dedicated and available to the receipt of single samples. Each site should have criteria that measure the specific job expectation and allow for comparative measurements that recognize the performance achievements of each sec-

tion. The importance of productivity in one area, for example, may be compared with turnaround time in defining success for another unit.

3. Ensure *consistent* application of organizational programs for which the performance appraisal system is used. They can include salary and wage administration, promotions, and other employment recognition plans.
4. Be *objective*, which is not only a goal of fairness but also a requirement for compliance with the laws and regulations of such agencies as the Equal Employment Opportunity Commission. Objectivity depends on documentation of performance and the avoidance of vague and subjective observations and standards. Both the supervisor and the employee must be able to agree upon when a standard has been achieved. For this reason, terms such as "attitude" are usually left off evaluation sheets and replaced with descriptive statements like "assists coworkers when own work is caught up" and "responds to request for overtime and call-in assistance." These two factors can be documented by recording events and are not based on the arbitrary opinion of the supervisor.

A performance standard or criterion is satisfactory if it links the statement to an area of responsibility (relevance), state how tasks should be performed (comparison, consistency), and includes a measurable (objective) mechanism by which to assess performance.

Here are some examples of acceptable performance standards.

- Preventive maintenance protocol, following laboratory and instrument manufacturers' policies, are completed as scheduled on the TESTMAX chemistry analyzer; 100 percent of the time.
- Fasting blood glucoses are collected and in the Chemistry section by 6:30 AM; 90 percent of the time.
- Fasting blood glucoses are reported to the nursing unit by 7:00 AM; 90 percent of the time.

Performance Appraisal Measurement Instrument

> Consultants say an unusually large number of employers have tinkered with review systems in recent years. **National Cooperative Ban**k in Washington,
> D. C., conducts more frequent reviews. Forest products firm **Weyerhaeuser** Co. and gas and electricity company **KeySpan** Corp. changed rating scales or descriptions to help fight grade inflation. Texas Children's Hospital gave employees more responsibility to draft their own goals and track progress. Some employers use technology to streamline reviews, while others, such as Whirlpool, push for more face-to-face discussions.
>
> Erin White

No matter how precisely written a criterion, it is useless if it cannot be measured. Laboratory assay standards, for example, may be specified down to the nanogram, microsecond, or millimeter, but the effort is to no avail if no ruler, clock, or scale is available for measurement. Beer's law may wax eloquent in theory, and our glucose standards may be accurately prepared, but they are of no use without a photometer or color chart against which to compare the assay.

There are two basic means for appraising individual or group performance. One is to compare results against some type of *scale*, using a quantitative rating (1, 2, 3, or 4 for example), qualitative descriptive terms (superior, needs improvement, below expectations) or a narrative format (statement). The other option is to compare individual or groups with their *peers*, either ranked (best to worst) or grouped (top, middle, lower third). Each method has pluses and minuses.

At this point two terms — "average" and "top-third phenomenon" — need to be explained. Among friends "average" (*doesn't think they are special*) can be a compliment, implying that a person is approachable, easy to get along with, needs no special consideration and enjoys everyday relationships (e.g., "You will like her. She's just an average person"). This term, however, when applied in the context of students or workplace is not considered complementary, the bell-shaped distribution curve notwithstanding. "Average" can be perceived as the ultimate insult when used to describe performance, even if used to assure employees that their work is up to standard and in line with coworkers.

The top-third phenomenon refers to our tendency to rank ourselves *and* our peers, with rare exception, in the top-third of our group. Although no formal research has verified this point, it is frequently used as an anecdotal illustration in motivational workshops. Because by definition not everyone can be in the top third and people dislike being ranked in the middle or lower levels; writers of performance appraisal system, have a creative challenge, particularly in describing the competent worker who is the backbone of the laboratory yet does not excel in a particular category.

Appraisal Focus

There are four approaches, or orientations, in measuring performance.

- *Result-oriented* approaches focus on achievement, as in MBO programs quality assessment and improvement (QA & I), and continuous performance improvement (CPI).
- *Behavior-oriented* methods, which include tools that rate the worker against descriptions of predetermined behavior levels.
- *Skills-oriented* methods, which attempt to measure the traits and skills of the worker (*focus on the performer*).
- *Peer comparison*

The fist three approaches generally use some form of scale or line graph as rating instruments. Preprinted scales and checklists are popular because of the uniform descriptions and application and relative ease of completion by the appraiser. Following are examples of several conventional methods that use scale-rating procedures.

Scale-Rating Methods

Included in this category are methods that have descriptive statements, rating scores, and defined terminology checklists that the appraiser matches against the performance of the person being evaluated. These are usually in a preprinted graphic format that allows the appraiser to mark the appropriate option. However, some methods do allow for narrative description or may even require justification comments. Discussed below are four examples for **scale-rating** methods: forced-choice method, critical incident methods, behaviorally anchored rating scales (BARS), and mixed-standard scales. Also provided is an example of a scale-rating method which applies to medical laboratory professionals.

<u>Forced–Choice Method</u>

This method requires the rater to select from among a group of predetermined descriptions the statements that best and least match the employee being evaluated. The resulting ratings are then scored by a third party. The main advantage of this system is that the form is standardized and the rater does not know the weight assigned to each statement. This helps to remove bias. A major disadvantage is the statements are not usually job-specific, and there is not place for feedback to the person being judged. Also, the value of each rating usually becomes common knowledge through the normal conversations of the workplace.

<u>Critical Incident Method</u>

Table 10-1. BEHAVIORALLY ANCHORED RATING SCALE (BARS) FOR A MEDICAL TECHNOLOGIST: – PERFORMANCE CATEGORY, – INSTRUMENT MAINTENANCE		
Rating	Performance	Description
7	Excellent	Instrument always clean and preventive maintenance protocol completed, including no downtime due to operator error, complete record documentation of calibration, QC, maintenance, and troubleshooting log. Successful troubleshooting and solving of problems within expected abilities of instrument operator, as defined by manufacturer, with minimal consultation with supervisor or vendor (troubleshooting skills).
6	Very Good	Level 7 performance, but with rare lapses in troubleshooting skills.
5	Good	Level 6 performance, but with rare lapses in documentation or tidiness.
4	Acceptable	Level 5 performance, with occasional guidance from supervisor about troubleshooting skills, documentation or tidiness.
3	Below standards	Level 4 performance, with increasing need for supervisor intervention in troubleshooting skills, documentation or tidiness.
2	Poor	Level 3 performance, but in frequent need of supervisor or vendor assistance in troubleshooting skills, documentation, or tidiness.
1	Extremely poor and unacceptable	Level 2 performance, with constant supervision required to maintain instrument, unacceptable documentation or tidiness.

This method seeks to minimize the trary nature of performance reviews by requiring supervisors or appraisers to cite specific examples (i.e., critical incidents) of behavior, both positive and negative, in support of their conclusions. A **critical incident** occurs when behavior in some aspect of the job results in unusual success or failure. Documentation and illustrations that clarify good or bad performance are the strength of this system. The "black book" implications of keeping records on all employees and the time required to record the entries are the major drawbacks.

Behaviorally Anchored Rating Scales (BARS)

This technique incorporates the critical incident method into a system that identifies key job dimensions or tasks and develops a behavior description with a graphic scale to measure elements of the job that are crucial to its success. In this procedure, BARS are developed by committees that include workers as well as supervisors to ensure that both terminology and performance expectations are acceptable to each group. In a BARS presentation, a behavior category critical to the success of the job is described and ranked along a scale ranging from **7** (*excellent or outstanding performance*) to **1** (*extremely poor or unacceptable*). Table 10 – 1 illustrates a BARS for measuring preventative maintenance (PM) activities required for a staff medical technologist.

Mixed–Standard Scales

This method modifies the BARS procedure by assigning only three levels of performance options to each critical job dimension or task. In this simpler model the employee either exceeds, meets, or fails the behavior expectation, which is plotted on a 3-point scale. The most common rating are either a 3–2–1 or 2–1–0 scale signifying level of behavior achieved (Table 10 – 2). The factors are then usually weighted according to their relative importance, and the total for all critical tasks tallied to provide a performance score.

The apparent advantage of this system is that the rater must choose between only three behavior choices; however, it does not improve on other methods that are designed for the convenience and perspective of the appraiser and does not allow for active feedback and participation by the employee in the review process.

The methods used in management by objectives programs are similar to mixed standards in that the employee either achieves or fails to meet the specified objective. For this reason, MBO is frequently detailed in the discussion of performance appraisal methods, even though MBO involves much more that the final review of results.

Laboratory Scale–Rating Performance Appraisal Model

Scale	Performance Description	Measurement Criteria
2	Exceeds expectations	Upon request: assists 75% of time or three times in a 6-month period
1	Meets Expectations	Upon request: assists 50% of time or twice in a 6-month period
0	Fails expectations	Upon request: assists less than 25% of time or fewer than three assists in 1 year

Table 10 - 2 MIXED-STANDARD SCALE FOR THE JOB DIMENSION OF AVAILABILITY

Below, is an example of scale-rating code being assigned to the performance standards listed previously? In all situations, health care generally and the laboratory specifically, the definition and meaning of the terms associated with each option on the scale is crucial. Many formats may use a grading system which ranking ranging for "*Exceeds expectations*," to a low of "*Unacceptable*." The rating codes in this example use a modified mixed-standard scales approach that attempts to address the issues of average and the top-third phenomenon discussed previously. Using this model only two performance levels are normally assigned and printed on the form. There are two additional options which are available for discretionary use by the rater, when a situation may warrant special consideration.

The following text box provides a list which defines each level of performance rating.

Competency Assessment and Performance Rating Codes Key

Essential The core and heart of the department. Meets and usually exceeds performance standards. A high-caliber worker who consistently makes a major contribution to the success of the laboratory. Has satisfactorily demonstrated competency in performing duty(s).

Deficient Has problems meeting the standard or frequently fails to achieve performance expectation. Following the improvement plan developed between the employee and supervisor is anticipated to bring behavior up to expectations.

Discretionary Rating Codes

Exemplary The top employee for this criterion, who could be held us as the model for others to emulate.

Warning Employee has received written warnings of unacceptable behavior and is presently in a corrective action program. If performance is not improved immediately, further corrective action, including possible dismissal, may be forthcoming.

These two choices along with the discretionary codes parallel the performance standards presented in an example of St. Vincent's Hospital (Fried and Johnson, p. 107) with lists three performance rating definitions. They only require comments for "Role Model" and "Unacceptable" ratings, and "unacceptable" require the review of the evaluator's supervisor

Role Model: The associate's performance and/or behavior can be held up as an example for others to follow.
Commendable: The associate's job performance and/or behavior meets the high standards set by this organization.
Unacceptable: This associate's job performance and/or behavior consistently falls to meet the standards required by this organization.

The final format chosen by an organization may have an extensive design that lists in descriptive detail every item to be measured or a succinct format that provides only the measurement criteria, with a separate document that provides a definitional key to the nomenclature being used. After the measurement instrument has been developed, a trained assessor must know how to properly use it. The selection and training of assessors in the performance appraisal system techniques and forms is the topic of the next section.

Peer Comparison

Evaluations using procedures that compare employees with coworkers are more often used to identify candidates for promotion, staff reduction, and merit pay or recognition programs than for providing feedback to employees on their job performance. Because of the importance of these business decisions, it is imperative that the manager be aware of ranking techniques. Below is a listing of the four main comparative methods.

Examples of acceptable performance standards and competency assessment and performance rating

- Preventive maintenance protocol, following laboratory and instrument manufacturers' policies, are completed as scheduled on the TESTMAX chemistry analyzer; 100 percent of the time.
  Essential _____ Deficient _____ ______

- Fasting blood glucoses are collected and in the Chemistry section by 6:30 AM; 90 percent of the time.
  Essential _____ Deficient _____ ______

- Fasting blood glucoses are reported to the nursing unit by 7:00 AM; 90 percent of the time.
  Essential _____ Deficient _____ ______

Ranking Method

In this most direct method, the supervisor or rater is asked to rank staff from best to worst. This method is considered highly subjective, and frequently the opinions of several appraisers are solicited in attempts to overcome this problem. The procedure also fails to shed any light on the relative worth of a particular worker because the difference between the performance level of employees ranked above or below may be insignificant or represent great disparity in ability.

Forced Distribution

This method attempts to overcome the top-third phenomenon by forcing the rater to recognize that not everyone can be ranked at the top and requiring some employees to be rated low. Employees are sorted in different categories (top, middle, bottom; top 10%, next highest 20%, middle 40%, next 20%, lowest 10%) for either overall performance or specific job parameters such as quality and quantity. This technique has been particularly unpopular with both supervisors and employees because some staff members may be unjustly ranked higher or lower than they deserve. It also has the differential problems mentioned in the direct-ranking method.

One of the most notorious, and public, examples of the impact of a Forced Choice Ranking system on both managers and staff is provided in a program which was used at **Enron**. Kurt Eichenwald [*Conspiracy of Fools*; Broadway Books; New York; 2005] describes one opinion of a senior executive:

"Vince Kaminski was furious. Once again he was being forced to put his analysts through the wringer of the Performance Review Committee, the PRC, and the outcomes were inane. These were top minds in their field, but now Kaminski was almost required to designate a portion of them as average or below." **...** "They call it forced ranking." *(p. 462)*

How did efforts to avoid favoritism work at Enron?

"Every senior executive participated in the PRC; several days of ranking and debate decided everyone's bonuses and promotions. *(Mr.)* Skilling had pushed it on the theory that wide input meant an executive couldn't be held back by a single boss. But it didn't always work that way. Most members of the PRC didn't know employees in other divisions." *(Eichenwald, p. 132-133)*

A brief description of the system at **Enron** emphasizes the "forced" nature of the method:

"Rankings were one through five—ones being worthy of fat bonuses and big promotions, five needing to get their act together or move on." ... "Only a set percentage could be at each level, usually meaning that some had to be moved down. (*Eichenwald, p. 212*)

Point Allocation Method

This system attempts to overcome the relative-worth problems of the two previous procedures by assigning points to each employee according to the perceived value of his or her contribution to the organization. The appraiser is given 100 points that must be allocated among the staff, with the best member receiving the highest score. The resulting ranking is supposed to reveal the "relative worth" of each worker in relationship to his or her peers.

Paired Comparison

This complex method requires the assessor to go through a process of comparing each individual against *every other* individual, based either on overall performance or some other criterion of accomplishment. The results are developed into a ranking matrix, based on the number of times each individual was found to be superior to his or her peers. The top employee is the one who is "preferred" the most often.

Format: Performance Appraisal

The format for performance appraisals is as varied as that for job descriptions. Both, however, have certain section in common. These include the following items.

- Identification information such as the name of the person being evaluated, title of the position, job grade, category, salary, date review is due, and possible information about longevity (i.e., date of hire/years of service) of employment.

- A list of objectives from the previous review period.
- A section with the appraisal measurement instrument.
- A place for setting goals and objectives for the next review cycle and for comments by the assessor.
- An area for comments by the person being appraised.
- A closing section related to promotion, salary incarcerates, date of next review and signatures of the employee, evaluator, and administration.

These common elements are a further illustration of the ways in which the performance appraisal system builds on the foundation laid through the collaborative process of job analysis, design and description, as well as the management approach of the organization and its leaders.

Judging Performance

The stage at which most of the criticism of performance reviews is focused is on **performance judgment**. This criticism centers around three issues: (1) problems in judging, particularly the subjective nature of the review; (2) the qualifications of the evaluator to judge; and, (3) the person who is in the proper position to do the judging.

Judgment Problems

Both the strengths and weaknesses of any performance review system stem from the fact that people are being evaluated and people are doing the judging. Both parties may agree with the range of possible performance levels which are represented on the scale but the employee may react defensively when a fellow human being actually marks their score. This human relationship factor is magnified in the review process and results in distortions in measurement and judgment decision that are called *rater biases*. They may work for or against the person being assessed.

- To avoid charges of favoritism, the appraiser may simply mark all individuals and scores toward the center of the scale, avoiding either extremely high or low ratings. This results in *errors of central tendency*.
- *Errors of leniency*, in which everyone is given high marks, may be committed by evaluators seeking to avoid confrontations. The reverse is also true; one rater in the organization may be stricter than other appraisers.
- A *halo effect* occurs in the performance level of one factor is so strong or weak that it affects how other items are graded. For example, a technologist whose behavior is frequently disruptive may still be scored satisfactory in this area, if he or she is very good at troubleshooting or always willing to work an unpopular shift.
- *Recency phenomenon* is the tendency to make rating judgments based on recent events or unusual isolated incidents that had a profound impact on performance at the expense of a balanced overviews of the entire review period. These events may either be strongly positive or negative. This bias is admittedly difficult to overcome because of the salience of these events in the memory of the assessor. It is also a frequent complaint of person being evaluated.

Qualifications to Judge

"Passing judgment" is something we have been socialized to avoid because of the implications of our own shortcomings; however, it is a task that each manager must come to grips with. In spite of this taboo, judging is a common and respected component of many parts of our lives — for example, the justice system, academia, sporting events, art and music shows, and business decisions. The judges in all of these activities are expected to be prepared by formal training and appropriate experience — hence <u>qualified</u> for the role of <u>judge</u>. The same should be true in performance appraisals.

Four qualification are necessary to be an effective appraiser.

1. Intimate *knowledge* of the intricacies and realities of the job or work being done.
2. *Proximity*—physical and informational—to the person being judged.
3. *Skill* and *training* in three areas: use of the measurement instrument, observation of performance, and communications and feedback mechanisms.
4. *Time* to dedicate to the process.

Unfortunately, in the majority of instances, raters are exclusively chosen on the basis of the first two criteria (job knowledge and proximity); the second two (assessor training and time) are either neglected or ignored outright.

Appraiser Selection

Appraiser selection raises the question of who should do the appraising. Appraiser options include the following.

- The *immediate supervisor* appears best situated to conduct the review because of direct access to knowledge of the job and the worker.
- *Higher-level managers*, such as the department manager or division executive, may do the evaluation to ensure consistency, relying on the recommendations of the supervisor.
- The *employee* may be assigned to do a self-evaluation based on performance and accounting data. This method is in entitled a **self-appraisal.**
- *Coworkers* may be asked to assess their peers on the assumption that they are in the best position to know the details of the job. However, these attempts have been fraught with charges of being "popularity contests."
- The opinions of *subordinates* may be solicited to gauge the performance of supervisors, usually through such techniques as questionnaires and surveys to avoid the "popularity contest" criticism.
- The most sought but elusive input is that from *customers* and *suppliers* (the TQM model) who, understandably, are reluctant to provide direct comments out of fear of offending. This method is referred to as a **350-degree appraisal**, and attempts to make a more comprehensive assessment of performance by obtaining feedback from all persons which the employees comes into contact or may have a relationship representing the business.
- In an attempt to achieve a more objective evaluation and deal with the issues of training and time, *independent experts* from assessment centers outside and inside the organization have been asked to conduct performance appraisals. However, this approach has suffered greatly because of their lack of firsthand knowledge of the work and unfamiliarity with the people being evaluated. For this and other distance issues, independent experts are usually only used in situations were the employee may be under consideration for promotion or transfer.

Each of these options, or a combination of methods, may be suitable for use in certain performance appraisal situations, such as selecting candidates for promotion and merit programs. However, the best reviewer in one-on-one relationships still appears to be the supervisor, who meets the following criteria.

- Has the qualification and training in observation and evaluation skills previously identified (knowledge, proximity, skill and training, and time).
- Operates with a well-designed performance appraisal system.
- Is an integral part of a management philosophy that focuses on participation and continual feedback.

Once the performance measurement instrument is prepared and the appropriate appraiser is selected and trained, an evaluation can be conducted. The process can move to the next and most important stage: communicating the results to the employee and getting feedback.

Evaluation Interviews

> The moment most feared by the Hematology supervisor and technologist has arrived. It may have been delayed and postponed repeatedly by both parties in efforts to avoid the inevitable, hut here it is. Each is determined to get it over quickly, with as little pain as possible. The employee wants a raise, and the supervisor wants to get the personnel department off his or her back.

What's wrong with this description? Does it sound familiar? Why should this scenario be the most frequently cited example of the performance appraisal meeting? Haven't these people been working together for the past year; communicating, solving problems together, developing solutions, each knowledgeable about how he or she has performed? Why should there be any suspense now? Isn't the conference viewed as the culmination of a year's work, at time of recognition and rewards, a time to set in motion the plans for the future? **These questions go to the heart of performance reviews and lead to the *first* and *primary* rule of the feedback session: *no surprises*!**

If there are surprises, the problems go far beyond the evaluation interview. The manager has failed in achieving the goals of the four basic management functions (planning, organizing, directing, and controlling). In this situation, particularly given the negative feelings or responses that may justifiably result, the best strategy for the conference is to attempt to open communication channels and dialogue between the individuals and establish a working relationship on which to build. A person could not help but to feel betrayed, if they are ambushed by an unexpectedly negative evaluation.

Conference Suggestions

Even in the best of circumstances, there is still major apprehension about the formal documentation of a person's performance record. The following suggestions are designed to make the conference as productive and rewarding as possible.

- Emphasis should be on behavior and performance *improvement*, not a tally of weaknesses, transgressions, personal characteristics, or discipline.
- *Time* should be allocated to an unhurried and complete review and explanation of the measurement instrument.
- Sufficient *advance notice* should be given to allow for preparation, including supplying the employee with the information upon which the review will be based. ***No surprises*!**
- The appraiser should convey to the employee a feeling of importance and that his or her concerns and presence are a top priority for the appraiser. The place and setting of the meeting should be familiar and comfortable to the employee. The appointment should consider the scheduling needs of the employee. There should be no interruptions from the telephone or visitors.
- Remove furniture, noise, and distance barriers, and be sure that body language and nonverbal clues and signals match verbal expressions.
- Remember that *feedback* mean input from both sides. The appraiser should be asking questions about how to improve performance and should be looking for suggestions about improving working conditions, eliminating bothersome policies, and correcting supervisor idiosyncrasies.
- Be *specific* and *consistent*, citing examples when discussing poor performance or giving criticisms in areas that needs improvement. Avoid expressing vague, arbitrary, and unfounded opinions. ***No surprises*!**

- *Listening* is far more important than speaking. Be especially alert to the need for listening if you as the appraiser seem to be doing all the talking.
- Remember that this is only one part of the *total communication loop*, a course correction and verification map check, not the feedback and communications journey itself.
- Open and end on the *positive* aspects of the employee's performance and contribution to the success of the organization.

Types of Evaluation Interviews

Following these guidelines, the appraiser should be able to conduct an interview that is fairly relaxed, non-threatening, businesslike, and beneficial to both parties.

Norman R. F. Maier, a well-known authority in this area, has identified three types of appraisal interviews. The particular format selected by the appraiser should match the temperament of the employees.

- **Tell-and Sell method**: The strategy in this session is to inform the worker of the results of the performance appraisal and then persuade the person to change. This method is considered useful only in dealing with young or inexperienced employees.
- **Tell-and-listen method**: The key here is to share the results of the review with the employee and then actively solicit his or her opinion and feelings. The meeting is designed to be a give-and-take session, with each participant graining from the encounter.
- **Problem-solving method**: The focus of this meeting is on the mutual identification and solving of problems, with particular emphasis on stimulating the growth and development of the employee.

One method which incorporates both a self-evaluation approach and aids conversation exchanges during the interview session is call the **Negotiated Performance Appraisal**. In this system the employee is asked to bring their thoughts on three aspects of performance*: (1) areas where the employee performs well; (2) areas where the worker has shown recent improvement; and (3) areas where the worker feels weak, or thinks his supervisor would like to see improvement." [Encina]* As pointed out above, the employee should be given sufficient notice of the appointment to properly prepare. One variation is to actually provide the employee with a blank copy of the evaluation form to complete, and then a comparison can be discussed between the viewpoints of both parties.

After deciding on the style and type of evaluation interview that is best for the conference, the manager should use skill in selecting and designing questions and follow-up strategies to stimulate the desired depth of discussion and feedback.

Questioning and Discussion Strategy

Techniques designed to bring the employee into the conversation focus on how questions should be worded. Because a primary goal of the review is to have employees assume responsibility for the establishment and achievement of performance goals, their active participation in the conference is essential. The following suggestions apply to most situations in which one person is being questioned by another to gain information and feedback on a topic, including job and customer interviews. The interviewer should choose a strategy that fits the specific objectives.

- *Open-ended* questions which require expanded responses, as opposed to queries that require only a yes or no answer: "What is your opinion?" ... "How do you view the situation?' ... "If you were to organize the program, how would you go about it?" Bad examples of questions: "Is this OK with you?" ... "Shall we go with this program?" This approach shows interest in their opinions and confirms that you value their ideas.

- *Reflective* questions that demonstrate that you have been listening to their comments. This method repeats an important part of a statement and asks for further elaboration: "That's an interesting suggestion, but what makes you think that approach will work?" . .. "It sounds like a good idea, but won't it put more work on the evening techs? What will they say about shifting more work to them?"
- *Directive* questions that solicit addition information or seek to clarify a point. In this method the interviewer waits until the speaker has finished, then follows up, to advance the conversation: "What steps would you take to implement your program?" ... "How do you think the 11:00 to 7:00 shift will react to the change?"

At the conclusion of the evaluation conference, each party should have a clear idea of how each views the accomplishments over the past review cycle, and what is expected in the next period. The paperwork is completed and a copy provided to the employee. The performance appraisal process is only a part of the overall management strategy, but it plays a crucial role in ensuring that the expectations of the organization are effectively communicated to the workers and that vital feedback is obtained about the perceptions of the employees.

____

Talking daily, communicating continually, each other understanding what is expected, are all essentials of any *Appraisal of Performance*. ***No surprises*!**

Next chapter: *Human Resources Management: The Personnel Process.*

— Case Study —

Chapter Ten: Appraisal of Job Performance

"Why do you look so down, Bob?" asked Terry. "You haven't spoken the whole time we've been here, and you're barely touched any of your food."

"I'm not looking forward to this afternoon. I have to do John's evaluation. It won't be good news for him, and I know he won't like it. It took two months for him to get over last year's review, with just a little criticism and he got one of the best raises in the lab."

"What's the problem?" Terry inquired. "You've told me often enough about how John likes to wander around to other sections and nursing stations when he finishes his work and how he doesn't like to help other people, especially now that he is divorced. I've even asked you to speak to him about staying out of my area."

"That's just it. John is excellent about getting his work done, he's a great troubleshooter on the instruments, and he's always willing to work overtime when needed. The couple of times when I have confronted him about his wandering problem, he has become very upset about how slow the other staff is and how they need to get the work done instead of poking around. He holds a grudge for months, and retaliates by ignoring problems he usually will jump right in and fix. I don't want to cause any more trouble; but Jill [the lab manager] told me that I must document this problem on the evaluation this year and give him a smaller raise because of the disruption it causes in other areas of the lab and hospital."

Chapter Section for Review

- Writing Performance Standards
- Halo Effect
- Evaluation Interviews (no surprises)
- Conference Suggestions
- Questioning and Discussion Strategy

Questions for Discussions

1. What do you think is Bob's real problem? What rule about evaluation interviews has he broken?
2. Could this confrontation have been avoided or handled better at another time?

[11]

Human Resource Management: The Personnel Process

— Chapter Eleven —

The human resources or personnel department is the organizational entity charged with guiding the institution in its relationships with its employees. The activities necessary to accomplish this mission include designing and overseeing wage, salary, and payroll functions; recruiting and hiring staff; planning and budgeting for personnel; administering benefit programs; handling grievance and discipline problems; assuring compliance with laws and company policies; and, maintaining employee records.

As illustrated in Figure 11 – 1, the personnel process represents the individual's relationship with the organization from recruitment to final separation. This chapter details this association.

Needs Assessment
|←— Job specifications
|←— Budget authorization
↓
Recruitment
|←— Application pool: file/advertisements
|←— Employment tests
|←— Reference/records verification
|←— Legal/regulatory requirements
↓
Selection
|←— Qualifications review
|←— Job offer: salary/benefits
↓
Employment
|←— Pre-employment screening
|←— Payroll registration
↓
Orientation
|←— Company/department policies
|←— Job descriptions/duties↓
|←— Workplace/staff
↓
Human Resources Management
|←— Salary and wage administration
|←— Staffing/scheduling
|←— Performance monitoring/evaluation
|←— Labor relations
|←— Professional growth and development
↓
Separation
|←— Exit interview
|←— Payroll severance
↓
Employment Termination
|←— References
|←— File maintenance
↓
Needs Assessment

Figure 11 – 1. The Personnel Process

OBJECTIVES

After completion of this chapter, the reader will be able to demonstrate accomplishment of the following objectives.

1. Prepare a recruitment campaign that meets the personnel needs of the laboratory and complies with regulatory requirements.
2. Conduct an effective employment interview.

3. Make an informed decision regarding selection and placement of a job candidate.
4. Develop and implement a laboratory orientation program.
5. Participate in the design and monitoring of the organization's wage and salary administration plan.
6. Explain the role of human resource management in the successful operation of a laboratory and the functions of the management process.

Chapter Highlights and Glossary of Key Terms

I. PERSONNEL NEEDS ASSESSMENT

II. RECRUITMENT, SELECTION, AND EMPLOYMENT

A. Legal and Regulatory Requirements

Disparate Treatment: *Discrimination that occurs when a member (individual) of a protected class receives unequal treatment.*

Disparate Impact: *Discrimination that occurs when an employer's actions affect a protected class differently from other groups.*

B. Recruitment

1. Labor Market

Labor Market: *The total number or pool of potential employees qualified to perform a job.*

2. Inside sources
3. Outside recruitment

C. Reference Checks

D. Employment Tests

Employment Tests: *Standardized measurements of the attributes and/or skills of potential job candidates—typing speed, ability to deal with stressful situations, dexterity, and similar evaluations.*

Pre-Employment Tests: *Tests, such as medical and drug screens, that are par of the registration process of new employees who have already been selected and offered a position.*

E. Preliminary Screen of Applications

F. Employment Interview

1. Interview strategy
2. The interview process
   a. Preparation
   b. Establishing rapport
   c. Questioning and information exchange
   d. Listening
   e. Closing and follow-up
   f. Evaluation

G. Selection: Matching Jobs With People

H. Job Offer and Hiring Decision

III. ORIENTATION

Orientation: *The formal introduction of new employees to the organization and their duties.*

IV. HUMAN RESOURCE MANAGEMENT

Human Resource Management: *The process of managing and integrating human resources with the goals and objectives of the organization.*

A. Wage and Salary Administration

1. Components of a wage and salary plan

Cafeteria Benefits Plan: *A program that offers a group of benefits from which the employee can pick and choose, according to his or her own wishes and needs, rather* *then the traditional approach of providing the same benefits package to all employees regardless of their personal situations.*

2. Regulations governing employee compensation

B. Wage Determination Methods

1. External comparison

Wage Surveys: *A survey that seeks to learn what competing organizations are paying their workers.*

2. Internal analysis
3. Incentive programs
4. Other wage-determining factors

C. Staffing, Scheduling, and Performance Monitoring

D. Labor Relations

Labor Relations: *In the formal sense, the company's dealings with organized labor unions.*

E. Professional Growth and Development

1. Training needs assessment
2. Education Sources

V. CORRECTIVE ACTION AND EMPLOYEE DISCIPLINE

VI. SEPARATION AND EMPLOYMENT TERMINATION

Exit Interview: *Interview conducted during the final week of employment as a method of identifying why personnel are leaving the organization.*

Personnel Needs Assessment

At the root of any employment decision is a *need*. The need for a worker could have come about because of another employee's departure, an increase in workload, or a change in the work process that requires the recruitment of a person with special skills or training. Whatever the reason, the manager must be prepared to specify the type of person required, justify the need, and obtain authorization to fill the position.

The groundwork for needs assessment and justification should have been completed during the job analysis process and in the preparation of the job description. From this information managers can supply their supervisors and the personnel department with a job specification sheet.

A job specification sheet is usually abstracted from the job description and contains only the qualifications (i.e., knowledge, skills, professional or legal certifications, physical attributes, and working conditions) necessary to design a recruitment plan. If this position has already been authorized during the budgeting process, obtaining approval may be only a formality. If the manager is seeking to increase staffing levels because of changes in either workload or technology, a more detailed justification procedure is required.

Recruitment, Selection, and Employment

This topic, often referred to as the hiring process, is a major function of the human resources department. Its responsibilities are two fold: (1) to ensure that the organization complies with federal, state, and local requirements and regulations and meets the social and ethical issues involved in hiring personnel; and, (2) to fulfill workforce needs by recruiting qualified candidates.

Legal and Regulatory Requirements

Myriad laws, executive orders, rules, and regulations govern the relationship between an organization and its employees. These mandates touch every aspect of the management process: initial hiring of staff; workplace design and safety; schedules, breaks, and lunch; working conditions; labor union contracts; on-the-job behavior; promotions; discipline; compensation; benefits; and, separation. In all of these areas, government regulations define what an employer can, must, and cannot do. These regulations are directly reflected in and strongly influence the design of the application form, the recruitment strategy, and the conduct of the employment interview.

Table 11 – 1 provides a summary of the major labor laws and regulations. Until the 1960s the emphasis was on the rights and limitations of the labor union movement. The emphasis has since changed to the protection of civil rights and the correction of past deficiencies through affirmative action programs, particularly in the areas of race, sex, religion, age, handicap, military status, and national origin. The federal agency responsible for enforcing these rules is the Equal Employment Opportunity Commission (EEOC), formed in 1965.

The EEOC, as well as court rulings, forbids questions at any time, especially during the application or interview process, that may reveal, either directly or indirectly, information about areas in which discrimination Is prohibited. Questions about the following topics have been ruled inappropriate by the EEOC and the courts, unless the employer has specific evidence and documentation that the information is essential and crucial to the actual performance of the job. Even in those situations, the employee must be careful about the wording, so as not to force job candidates to reveal information about themselves that may be considered discriminatory.

- Height and weight
- Marital status, number of children, and childcare arrangements
- English language proficiency
- Arrest record
- Military service
- Citizenship (However, *all* applicants must supply evidence that they are eligible to work in the United States)
- Credit history
- Availability to work on specific religious holidays or weekdays
- Property ownership (home, auto)
- Date of birth or age
- Organizational membership

The EEOC has identified two types of discrimination that must be avoided: (1) **disparate treatment**, which occurs when a protected class of individuals (i.e., discriminates against a specific person) receives unequal treatment; and, (2) **disparate treatment**, which occurs when an employer's actions affect a protected class differently from other groups. The EEOC requires employers to have aggressive plans in place to assure that discrimination does not take place and that past transgressions are immediately rectified.

Recruitment

Recruiting is the process of locating and attracting qualified job applicants. It is a searching stage, designed to build a pool of candidates from which to select the person best suited to fill the position.

1911	Workers Compensation
1935	Social Security Act Title IX of the act covers unemployment compensation
1935	National Labor Relations Act or Wagner Act Established the National Labor Relations Board (NLRB) Recognized the right of employees to organize Health care excluded until 1975 (Public Law 93-360) Established collective bargaining rights
1938	Fair Labor Standards Act (FLSA) Minimum wage Workweek (>40 hours OT) Child Labor laws
1947	The Taft-Hartley Act or Labor Management Relations Act Title I Amended the Wagner Act Title II Established federal mediation council to prevent work stoppages Title III Provides enforcement authority Title IV Establishes labor-management commission Title V Gives workers right to refuse to work under dangerous conditions
1959	The Landrum-Griffin Act or Labor-Management Reporting and Disclosure Act Regulates labor unions
1963	Equal Pay Act Outlaws discrimination in pay based on the sex of the worker Applies to employers engaged in interstate commerce
1964	Title VII of the Civil Rights Acts of 1964, amended in 1972, 1978, and 1991 Outlaws discrimination in employment based on race, color, religion, sex, pregnancy or nation origin Sets up the Equal Employment Opportunity Commission (EEOC) to monitor and enforce the act Applies to employers with 15 or more employees
1964	Executive Order 11141 Prohibits hiring discrimination by government contractors on the basis of age
1965	Executive Order 11246 (1965) and amended by Executive Order 11375 (1966) Prohibits hiring discrimination by government, contractors on the basis of age
1967	Age Discrimination in Employment Act Outlaws discrimination against those between the ages of 40 and 65 (now 70) Applies to employers with 20 or more employees
1969	Executive Order 11478 Prohibits discrimination by governmental agencies, including the Postal Service, on the basis of age, race, color, religion, sex, handicap, or national origin
1972	Equal Employment Opportunity Ace Amended Title VII (1964) to strengthen EEOC's enforcement powers Extended Title VII to cover government employees, higher education employees, and others
1973	Vocational Rehabilitation Act Requires affirmative action in hiring of handicapped persons by government contractors
1974	Vietnam-Era Veterans Readjustment Assistance Act requires affirmative action in hiring of Vietnam-era veterans by government contractors
1978	Pregnancy Discrimination Act of 1978 Broadens the definition of sex discrimination to include pregnancy, childbirth, or related medical conditions
1986	Immigration Reform and Control Act of 1986 (IRCA) prohibits companies from hiring ineligible aliens and prohibits discrimination against noncitizens.
1990	Americans with Disabilities Act
1991	Civil Rights Act
1993	Family and Medical Leave Act
1994	Uniform Services Employment and Reemployment Right Act

Table 11 – 1. Summary of Labor Laws and Regulations

Labor Market

Obviously, this recruitment objective is highly dependent on the conditions of the **labor market**. In dealing with an acute shortage of personnel, such as for medical technologists (i.e., a *tight* labor market), the recruitment strategy has to be highly creative and aggressive and the selection options are limited. If, however, the pool of applicants is large, (i.e., open labor market), the focus is on selecting the right person for the job from the existing applications on file.

There are two sources of recruits: those who are already known to the manager or human resources department, either through personal knowledge or because their applications are already on file; and, candidates solicited through an internal or external recruitment campaign. Recruitment strategies will center on techniques that are targeted toward candidates inside (interest in promotion or transfer) or outside the organization.

Inside Sources

Although some employees are simply looking for a change in duties (a *lateral* move, or transfer), most inside recruitment efforts focus on identifying persons who want to improve their positions (i.e., promotion). Candidates may acquire new skills and jobs through in-house, on-the-job training programs (such as phlebotomist, computer operators, or other laboratory assistants) or by obtaining a promotion either by obtaining advanced credentials within the laboratory, or out-side training schools (a *vertical* move). The database of employees seeking lateral and vertical moves should be available from the performance appraisal systems and the employee development program, in which the attributes and aspiration of an employee have been identified and become part of the individual's and the organization's long-term plans. In addition, inside candidates may be found through:

- Personnel records such as application files and transfer requests
- Job posting and bidding, whereby current employees are notified of in-house opportunities
- Recall from layoff
- Promote-from-within policies

Most institutions prefer to promote from within because it rewards dedicated and deserving employees and demonstrates an organizational commitment to staff development. It can also boost morale. There are other advantages to promoting from within:

- Continuity in administration and services is insured, particularly if the company likes the way things were done by the previous manager.
- Current employees may have already shown their loyalty and long-term commitment to the firm.
- The company takes advantage of its investment in the individual.
- Minimal orientation and training time and expenses are needed because the employee is already familiar with operations and culture.

Outside Recruitment

There are reasons and advantages to looking outside the organization as well—some more legitimate than others.

- Acquisitions of new skills, knowledge, and expertise.
- Need for improvement in performance; that is, management is unhappy with the way things are going.
- No suitable in-house candidate.

- Low moral, group dissension or rivalry.
- A worthy candidate who deserves a chance may be somewhere else in a large corporation.
- First-time managers have a high failure rate (80 percent of new supervisors fail in their first management situation because of lack of training and commitment by the organization).

The need to recruit outside the organization is usually an expensive and time-consuming operation. This factor is magnified by the availability or shortage of suitable candidates. Some of the more common approaches to conducting an outside recruitment campaign are listed below.

Advertising: The strategy usually focuses on professional journals or trade magazines such as *MLO*, *Laboratory Medicine*, and *Advance*; newspapers; and career fairs that offer international, national, or wide regional coverage. Most personnel managers avoid help-wanted ads in local newspapers as futile; believing that anyone who was looking for a job would already have applied. However, such ads are a visible sign to the current staff, who may be struggling from the overload created by the personnel shortage and who see those local ads as positive evidence that at least management is trying to find help.

Sign-up or referral bonuses: This method is gaining in popularity because it offers an attractive inducement to speed recruitment efforts. *Networking* the professional job grapevine for recommendations and referrals among colleagues, has become the job-finding system of the 2000s, and this strategy taps this potential source. Bonuses can be offered to both new (sign-up) and current (referral) employees to encourage them to spread the word through their professional networks and among their peers.

Employment agencies: Government employment agencies may be a good source for staff that can be trained on the job. Private placement agencies and executive search firms specialize in recruiting professions. They are usually very expensive, with fees that range up to 30 percent of a year's salary.

Educational institutions: Institutions that have medical laboratory training programs offer excellent recruitment opportunities. In addition to informing current students about your facility, the faculty and college job service may provide leads to alumni looking for work.

Unsolicited applications or chance walk-ins: The personnel department is always receptive to application for open positions. However, this method can be slow and highly inefficient way of building a candidate pool to fill a current need. It is best used to maintain a file of applications interested in future openings.

Professional organizations: These groups usually have several recruitment opportunities, including journal advertisement, employment referral programs, and meetings (local, state, and national), in which recruitment activities can be conducted. Labor unions may also be a source of potential employees.

As the application pool begins to grow and the recruitment drive draws to a close, the selection process begins. At this point the collection of applications must be sorted and a preliminary screen conducted. The stage eliminates any person who does not obviously meet the job specifications and identifies those who will be referred to the responsible manager for further consideration. The next step may include a check of references, testing, and an invitation for an interview, depending on the type of employee being selected.

Reference Checks

Background reference investigations have become increasingly controversial and are often viewed as a waste of time by many personnel experts. The reasons for this include:

- The understandable reluctance of past employers to provide a negative recommendation or comment because of threats of hard feelings and litigation
- The tendency of applicants usually to list only names of people who will speak positively about them
- Rules and laws that protect the confidentiality of personal background information such as employment records and credit history.

For these reasons, most employers verify only dates of employment in writing and do not issue a written recommendation. Letters of reference are usually considered only a formality with no particular value other than possible support for the accuracy of the statements and information provided by the application.

Many managers and companies are just as reluctant to give a verbal assessment of a former worker unless confidentiality can be positively assured or the inquiring party is personally known to them. In spite of these considerations, reference checks remain an important verification of the training and experience claimed by an applicant.

As a significant number of high profile cases of misrepresentation have made the news, checking and verifying credentials has taken on even a more important urgency. This has included outright falsification of degrees and experience by business executives, football coaches, and even people masquerading as physicians. A Scripps Treasure Coast Newspaper *(Fort Pierce, Florida)* in their Thursday, March 2, 2006 edition *(page D2)* report that:

"almost half the job seekers in a new study lied on their resumes [It found 'significant inaccuracies' in 42.7 percent of them]."

All colleges and licensing agencies will verify degrees, licenses, and date awarded; and, most employers will confirm employment dates even if they will not provide information on performance.

Criminal background checks have also come to the forefront. There is considerable controversy over both doing, and not doing these types of investigations. The issues usually surround problems of accuracy and confidentiality of information. Specific details (name, court document numbers, nature of charges, etc.) must be available if inquires are made to governmental agencies; and commercial search sources have had extensive problems in reliability. Obviously, the more relevant or sensitive the situation in which the person will be employed (e.g., data security, handling of money, sexual vulnerability), the more important the background check.

Employment Tests

Employment tests are common for jobs that require specific manual skills such as typing, computer processing, or machine tool work. These are also occasionally used in assessing candidates for top management positions to measure their analytical and decision-making skills and their emotional temperament. They are rarely used for testing the knowledge level for professional positions, because competence has already been demonstrated through academic achievement, certification, and licensure protocols. The EEOC and state agencies have strict guidelines about the tests that can be administered, requiring these tests to be directly related to the duties that are performed in the job.

Employment tests are designed to be standardized measures of the attributes and skills of potential employees. They are different from *pre-employment tests* such as medical and drug screens, which are part of the registration process of new employees who have already been offered a position.

In addition to the requirement that test content be pertinent to job duties, testing methodology must have established validity. For these reasons, most employers use standardized tests produced and administered by professional testing services. Tests offered by commercial testing services cover the following areas.

- General (academic, scholastic) mental abilities
- Mathematical and verbal skills
- Dexterity
- Polygraph or lie detection
- Drug abuse
- Clerical skills, such as typing and computer processing
- Mechanical aptitude
- Personality evaluation of emotional adjustment confidence, and perseverance
- Attitudes, perceptions, and decision-making skills purported to measure supervisory and managerial potential
- Personal-interest inventories

Preliminary Screening of Applications

Once the necessary reference checks and employment tests have been completed and the recruitment objective of building a pool of qualified candidates has been accomplished, the selection process can continue. Usually an initial screening selects those who appear on paper to be best suited for the position and who will be invited for an interview. The number of persons interviewed depends on the strength of the applications, the attractiveness of the position available, and the receptiveness of those issued an invitation. The next section reviews the methods for conducting an effective interview.

Employment Interview

An employment interview is a formal conversation, designed to achieve the following general goals:

- Meeting and beginning a relationship
- Exchanging information
- Verifying credentials
- Comparing with other candidates
- Evaluating suitability
- Predicting performance and probability of success

Preferably, the interview is conducted in person but may frequently involve telephone contact when a candidate lives a long distance for the facility. Another interview method is for a third party (personnel staff, search firm) to do the personal interview at conventions or during recruiting trips; the information is then followed up with a call from the manager. Either method makes use of the following strategies.

Interview Strategy

Three basis types of employment interviews can be used, according to the kinds of information desired and the type of position being filled.

1. *Structured* or *patterned* interviews, which have a predetermined format and list of questions, usually with a standardized checklist or interview form. The advantage of this approach is that it allows easier comparison between candidates. This form is common for third-party interviews; however, it often hinders the free flow of conversation and information.

2. *Unstructured* interviews with a broad agenda, in which each party is free to discuss any issue in depth and follow up on responses. This strategy allows spontaneity and candor; however, it requires considerable skill by the interviewer to ensure that the desired information is obtained.
3. *Stress* interviews, which take many forms and are designed for specific purposes. They are most often used in formal testing procedures to identify traits and characteristics needed for jobs in which the individual will be exposed to highly dangerous or intimidating situations, such as with police officers and military personnel. Another method classified as a stress interview is problem-solving sessions, which focus on a job-related problem that the applicant is expected to solve.

These three interview techniques can be used either by a single interviewer or in a *team* approach. Many job counselors recommend that applicants avoid, if at all possible, being subjected to group interviews; they cite the stress of the situation, lack of control, inability to focus one's response to one individual, and the possibility of encountering numerous hidden agendas. As an illustration of the validity of this description and problems which may be associated with group interviews, panel interviews are frequently listed as a stress-interview technique.

The Interview Process

Employment interviews have six components that correlate with interview goals: preparation, establishing rapport, questioning and information exchange, listening, closing and follow-up, and evaluation.

Preparation

Preparation includes reviewing information about the job (job description) and the data submitted by the candidate (application, resume, references, and communication contacts). By becoming familiar with this material, the interviewer can identify specific items and information gaps that need to be addressed and avoid duplicate and redundant questions.

Establishing Rapport

Any person being interviewed for a new job is naturally nervous, and it is incumbent on the interviewer to make the candidate as relaxed and comfortable as possible. This deference demonstrates the importance you place on the person's application. Remember, the candidate is also in the process of forming an opinion on the attractiveness of working in you laboratory.

Questioning and Information Exchange

Because the primary goal of the meeting is to allow both parties to obtain as much information as they can to make a decision about employment, the order and wording of the questions become a priority. Always keep in mind the list of topics that may be considered discriminatory.

As detailed in Appraisal of Performance module, there are three types of questions: open, reflective, and directive. Readers may want to review these questions as part of understanding the interviewing process.

Listening

Listening is the crucial communication element. It cannot be stressed often enough. It assures understanding, clarifies intent, and demonstrates interest.

Closing and Follow-up

At this point a brief review to clarify pertinent information is in order, and the interviewer may formally provide candidates with the opportunity to ask any questions they may have. The next step in the selection process should be explained, along with a specific time frame for notification and follow-up. Both participants may be interested in the impressions of the other; if possible, either the manager or the applicant may state reasons for not pursuing the application process further. It would save considerable time and anxiety for both parties if employment consideration has been ruled out. Remember, this is a business meeting, so ending the session with a strong sense of congeniality and a clear understanding of what to expect is important to both sides.

Evaluation

As soon as possible after the close of the meeting an evaluation and assessment of the results should be conducted. Many companies have a checklist or fill-in section on the application form for the interviewer to complete. This list may ask for information and impressions of the candidate, along with a recommendation about employment.

Selection: Matching Jobs with People

The selection process matches the right person with the right job. The criteria for selection have been determined through development of the job description and specifications, and these criteria should be matched to the pool of qualified candidates that has been collected during the initial screening and interview stages.

Comparing the needs of the laboratory with the available applicants can be a frustrating responsibility. The decision has a direct impact on both the success of the department and the future employee. There are two basic selection methods to aid in this deliberation.

1. The process of *elimination* or *comparison* in which applicants are weeded out and the most desirable person is identified, based on the predictive weight given to their qualifications and interview ratings.
2. A *prioritizing* or *ranking* procedure, in which the candidates are placed in order according to their desirability, as determined by the manager making the hiring decision.

In conducting this final selection review, personnel experts have warned against certain errors.

- The *halo effect*, in which a particular aspect of a candidate's qualifications overshadows—either favorably or unfavorably—other factors.
- Making decision based on *inferences* derived from the biases and perceived stereotypes of the evaluator.
- The *recency effect*, in which applicants interviewed during the end of the selection process are given inappropriate stronger consideration because they are fresh in the memory of the manager.

Job Offer and Hiring Decision

Once the selection process has been completed, the decision about the nature of the job offer (salary, benefits) can be made. If the candidate accepts the offer, the hiring process can be concluded. If not, and an agreement cannot be negotiated, the process may begin again or an offer may be made to the next choice. This step includes determining the salary level for the job, setting a starting date, completing any pre-employment tests, and signing up for benefits and payroll registration.

Orientation

Orientation is the introduction of new employees to the organization and their duties. It is the beginning of the process of professional development and training. At this point in the relationship, the rights, privileges, responsibilities, and expectation of both parties should be clarified. The success of this initiation period forms the foundation for the future.

The three aspects to the orientation program are a general organizational review of the policies and procedures that apply to all employees, department policies and rules governing behavior, and specific job duties. The items and topics that are usually covered in each area are listed in Table 11 – 2. Orientation is also the second stage, after employee selection, of competency assessment and assurance.

A key objective of the orientation program is to familiarize and socialize the new employee into the institution by assimilating the worker into the group and reaching a consensus on shared mores, beliefs; and, values crucial to the success of an organization.

Most facilities use a combination of the following four general methods for conducting the orientation program.

1. Formal meetings and training sessions, which usually focus on broad institution-wide programs such as risk management, infection control, and fire and safety procedures.
2. Supervisor-directed sessions, in which the employee is personally led through the process.
3. A checklist approach, which gives primary responsibility to new employees for completing the program by ensuring they understand all the items listed on the sheet.
4. A buddy or sponsor system, in which new workers are paired with colleagues who assist them in adjusting to the new environment, show them the ropes, and smooth their socialization into the group.

The first few days on a job are stressful for new employee, and everyone in the institution has an obligation to make this transition as smooth as possible. It is especially important for the supervisor to ensure that the employee has the support and attention he or she needs during this time. There are a few trouble spots the supervisor should be alert to, along with some guidelines about how to ease the transition path.

- *Cooking in someone else's kitchen.* Remember that even the best chef (i.e., technologist) must know where things are stored and needs directions about new equipment and technologies. This area also covers pet peeves and protected turfs.
- *Being overwhelmed with information.* The orientation should be well organized so that time is allowed for absorbing, learning, and adjusting to the new environment.
- *Assigning menial tasks.* It may be tempting to put the new employee in an area that involves simple, repetitive task, especially those that the other techs dislike. This tendency may be encouraged by a philosophy of "let them pay their dues;" however, it can also give the person a negative impression about how the laboratory operates and the staff is treated.
- *Missing information gaps.* Gaps can be particularly devastating if the new worker is left to "assume" important facts or figure things out for himself or herself.

ORGANIZATIONAL OVERVIEW
- Company history and mission
- Products and services
- Organizational structure—introduction of company executives, names-to-faces identification, and organizational charts, and department interrelations
- Tour of facilities
- Salary and wage program
- Benefit plans
- Employee recognition programs
- Payday
- Quality improvement philosophy and program
- General fire and safety plans: infection control, risk management, fire and evacuation plans, and OSHA requirements
- Employee handbook: code of conduct, probationary period, discipline and appeals procedures, grievance procedure, and Equal Opportunity Commission policies

DEPARTMENT ORIENTATION
- Welcoming (feel-at-home/part-of-team) functions
- Tour of department
- Organization of laboratory: management/supervisory personnel and network, organizational charts
- Introduction to staff and coworkers
- Safety rules and enforcement penalties: specifically fire, evacuation, and infection control procedures; safety data sheets; and, applicable OSHA requirements.
- Quality improvement program
- Dress code
- Scheduling policies
- Purchasing and supply requisitioning
- Training and continuing education opportunities
- Time card, or punch in/punch out records
- Locker, breaks, and restroom facilities

JOB DUTIES ORIENTATION
- Job descriptions
- Performance standards
- Orientation agenda and schedule
- Reporting network: supervisory, problems, and assistance
- Performance appraisal system: quality and quantity expectations, appraisal format (forms, time frame, and measurement criteria)
- Tour and introduction to workplace: people, instruments, equipment, workstation, supply requisitioning and storage, and location of procedure and instrument manuals
- Work assignments
- Relationships to coworkers and other jobs
- Scheduling policy (work, vacation, holidays, call-in)
- Breaks and lunch periods
- Leaving the premises
- Task orientation and competency assessment worksheets

Table 11 – 2. Orientation Topics

The transition from recruit to productive worker, combined with the pressure of the probationary decision, can be a tedious but rewarding journey. The outcome of this passage establishes the pace and tone of the future alliance that develops among the employee, manager, and organization.

Human Resources Management

Orientation is only the start of the relationship between the individual and the organization. The supervisor and personnel department have the responsibility to ensure the well-being of this association and the productivity and coherence of the workforce. This activity is referred to as human resource management and consists of the following four components: wage and salary administration; staffing and scheduling; performance monitoring; and, labor relations.

Wage and Salary Administration

Compensation management is the most visible aspect of the personnel process. Both the institution and the employee are reminded of this fact every payday. In addition to the direct material rewards of the paycheck, this activity represents the physical evidence and reinforcement for the employees of their individual worth to a company. Establishment of the wage and salary plan has a tremendous impact on the economic and motivational well-being of both the organization and its employees.

The goals and objectives of the wage and salary admonition program include:

- Recruiting a highly skilled and qualified staff
- Maintaining a stable workforce
- Maximizing productivity thorough incentive plans that reward desired behavior
- Controlling labor costs
- Complying with legal regulations
- Meeting social and cultural expectations and goals

The nature of the objectives helps to explain why the compensation plan is usually closely aligned and monitored through the performance appraisal system. "*Perhaps the most important objective of any pay system is fairness, or equity.*" The author continues to point out that equity can be assessed on three dimensions, or "relative" comparisons: internal equity; external equity; and individual (compared to others doing the same job) equity (Wayne Cascio, p. 419).

This section contains a review of the components (salary, benefits, prerogatives) of the program, regulations governing employee compensation, and methods for setting pay rates.

Components of a Wage and Salary Plan

The total compensation package consists of three elements: the actual paycheck; the benefit package; and, the perquisites associated with the position. The *paycheck* represents reward or amount of money the employee can take home for their efforts. A more formal definition of the wage and salary paycheck incorporates the concepts of total reimbursement (gross amount) and discretionary income. The *total reimbursement* is directly the hourly wage multiplied by the number of hours paid [worked and benefit (vacation, holidays, etc.)]. *Discretionary income* ("*take home pay*") is the net amount left after mandatory payments (taxes, etc.). Discretionary income also includes deductions over which the employee has control or makes personal choices; i.e., such items as optional insurance and retirement contribution.

Benefits are an important part of the total compensation package and are supplements to the cash payment of salary and wages. Some are mandated by law (Social Security, unemployment insurance, and workers' compensation taxes), and other are costs incurred by the employer as a means of providing increased employee security and making the company a more attractive place to work. Federal and local governments also encourage benefits programs through tax incentives.

Historically, employers provided a uniform benefits package to all employees, regardless of their individual needs or lifestyle. It is now common for businesses to offer a group of benefits from which employees can choose. Under this **cafeteria benefits plan** the employer provides a designated amount of money or credit that can be allocated among a selection of benefits options, depending on the family and personal needs of the employee. These may include selection of more family coverage for medical benefits or even allow employees to opt out of medical insurance completely if they obtain this benefit through their spouse's plan. They may then select other benefits, or in some cases even receive reimbursement credit for funds they do not use. Major governmental changes have also encouraged businesses to set up accounts were employees can make tax free contributions to help cover out-of-pocket expenses for childcare, education, and medical costs.

Organizations frequently provide the following benefits:

- Medical, disability, and life insurance
- Retirement plans, including contributions from both employer and employee
- Paid time off for sickness, vacations, holidays, and continuing education
- Tuition reimbursement
- Social Security, unemployment, and worker's compensation insurance

Rounding out the total compensation package are certain perquisites ("perks"), which can range from the blatant display of trappings to subtle advantages. The list may include job title, private secretaries, use of a company car, offices with a view and attractive furniture, travel on the company's private jet, a personalized parking place, or even country club membership.

Regulations Governing Employee Compensation

The first legislative attempt by government to intervene in the economic well-being of its citizens was the federal Workers Compensation Act of 1911, which required employers to contribute an additional percentage of wages to a fund that paid employees if they were injured on the job. Responsibility for administering this program has since been passed on to state governments.

Much legislation intended to protect and improve worker welfare was passed in the 1930s. The Social Security Act was passed in 1935; Title IX of this act provides for unemployment compensation. The National Labor Relations Act, which gives workers the right to organize into labor unions, was also passed in 1935. The Fair Labor Standards Act (FLSA), commonly referred to as the wage-and-hour act, was enacted in 1938 and has been amended many times since. The main provisions of FLSA are:

- **Minimum wage rate**. Currently set at $5.15 an hour (1997), many states and some cities required a higher rate. [It is of some interest to note that the first rate established in October, 1938 was $0.25] http://www.dol.gov/esa/minwage/chart.htm [connected July 9, 2007]
- **Child labor provisions**. Workers under the age of 18 can be employed only in nonhazardous work. Hazardous work includes mining, logging, woodworking, and meat packing. Workers under age 16 must obtain a permit from the Department of Labor unless they are working for a parent or guardian. Parts of the this law govern the number of hours a week minors can spend on a job, as well as how late they can work on a school night.
- **Overtime payment**. There are two methods for determining if an employee must be paid overtime. The 40-hour rule states that an employee must be paid time and a half for any hours worked over 40 hours during a week [the definition of a week may be modified from the traditional calendar timeframe (Sunday – Saturday) with specific permission of the Labor Department and proper notification to the employee, to another seven day period (e.g., Saturday/Friday to Sunday/Saturday)]. The 8/80 rule, frequently used in health care facilities, allows employees to work up to 80 hours in a 2-week period with no limit on the number of days worked in a row without being paid overtime; however, they must be paid overtime for any time that exceed 8 hours on any given day. Other provisions allow some employees to be exempt (hence the terms *exempt* and *nonexempt* employee) from being paid overtime. The exceptions relate to the professional status of the job (e.g. physicians, attorneys), the level of salary paid, and the amount of time spent doing supervisory or staff-level work.

In the 1960 (See Table 11 – 1) major legislation attempting to prohibit and correct discrimination in hiring, pay rates, and promotional opportunities included an amendment in 1963 to FLSA, the Equal Pay Act, which required wage rates to be set on an equal-pay-for-equal-work principle and not on the sex or head-of-house status on the individual. Other laws further banned wage and salary discrimination based on age, pregnancy, race, color, disability, religion, or national origin. Many states also have rules that are frequently more stringent than those imposed by the federal government.

Wage Determination Methods

Based on the objectives desired for the wage and salary administration program described previously, wage determination methods can be grouped into three broad categories.

1. *external comparison*, which focuses on recruiting and keeping personnel;
2. *internal analysis*, which seeks to establish equity between jobs, recognize the relative worth of the position to the success of the organization, and maintain a stable workforce; and,
3. *incentive programs*, which are designed to motivate performance and reward desired behavior.

These three categories are in a hierarchical relationship in that each builds upon the work of the other. For example, the prevailing rate being paid by all companies wishing to attract a worker must be met before internal factors can be addressed. In turn, issues of equity and worth must be resolved before incentive programs can become effective.

External Comparison

The foundation for all wage programs is the alignment of institutional rates with those of neighboring facilities. This is accomplished by conducting wage surveys to learn the amount that competing organizations are paying their workers. Information for external comparison of wages can be collected from the following sources.

- Written or telephone questionnaires may be sent to organizations in the same geography service (commuting) area which are employing similar staff.
- Department managers may conduct their own informal survey by talking with their professional peers.
- Professional organizations, journals, and trade magazine make periodic reports of salary levels for their constituents.
- Data can be collected from employment and exit interviews about salaries offered at other laboratories (e.g., "*how much did the other job offer to pay*").

A wage survey may appear to be a relatively simple and straightforward way to gather this information; however, it is fraught with problems. There are issues of validity, which become greatly magnified when companies are competing for scarce personnel and are therefore reluctant to reveal their pay scales or recruitment incentives.

Problems with survey accuracy also arise from terminology and comparability of job titles, timeliness of the information (i.e., by the time all the forms are returned and compiled, the market could have changed significantly), and discrepancies between official and actual wages (e.g., at what rate in the formal pay scale are new employees being hired, or how much credit is being given for "experience"). For example, personnel clerks may become confused over terms such as technician, technologist, tech, specialist, clinical laboratory scientist, or senior tech — most of which have different definitions in different laboratories, or the title may not exist at all in one institution and the clerk just fills in the questionnaire the rate they think may fit.

Another issue may develop when a survey conducted by the laboratory manager does not agree with the findings of the personnel department. Administration and laboratorians may become suspicious about the motivation behind each section's data. Unfortunately, for these reason, the bottom-line verification that a laboratory's wage schedule is out of line is that retention problems become acute because workers are leaving to accept better-paying jobs elsewhere.

Internal Analysis

Determining the wage schedule based on internal analysis finds its foundation and tools from the techniques of job analysis and design, as well as the resulting job descriptions and performance appraisal system. The bottom line, as well as the overall framework of the wage schedule, has already been established from the external comparison. The remaining issues to be resolved are:

1. The salary range for each position, particularly the differential between new recruits and senior workers.
2. Alignment of the pay scale according to the relative worth of each job to ensure equity in the wage program.
3. The time frame for review of wage schedules and the interval between raises.

Of these issues, determining the relative worth of a job to the institution, in relationship to the work done by other members, is the most controversial. It is especially difficult, given the interdependent nature of work and the need for proficiency among all employees.

Job evaluation is one tool used to determine the relative worth of jobs. Jobs evaluation builds on the information obtained during job analysis (job descriptions, performance appraisals). The four most common methods for conducting a job evaluation are as follows:

- **Job ranking**. In the simplest and most direct method of comparison, each job is ranked subjectively according to the weight given to the work by the person doing the judging. There are usually no formal guidelines as to the value of specific skills, efforts, or working conditions using this approach. The number of employees supervised and the educational levels of the incumbents are the two criteria usually given the highest priority under the system.
- **Job grading or job classification**. This method classifies jobs according to a predetermined scale. This scale ranges from work considered simple and repetitive to work believed to be highly complex. This system is more complex but is still imprecise because it depends on the subjective grouping based on general classification descriptions.
- **Point system**. This method is the most popular because it attempts to consider all the components of a job in comparing one job to another. The typical model allocates points to four broad groups of factors: skill, effort, responsibility, and working conditions. These factors are then broken down further into detailed subfactors for comparison. For example, "skills" can have points assigned to subfactors such as education, experience, creativity, and training.
- **Factor comparison**. This method focuses on determining the relative worth of a job by comparing it to other jobs in the organization on a scale that assigns a dollar amount to each factor. The monetary value of each factor is then totaled to give the wage rate for a specific job. This system is similar to the point method, but it differs in that each job is compared to specifications developed from analyzing a group of "common jobs" performed throughout the organization. Determinants frequently evaluated in the factor comparison method and assigned a monetary value include responsibility, skill, working conditions, and mental and physical efforts. Following is an example of how this system might appear for laboratory positions.

Critical Factor	*Phlebotomist*	*Clerk*	*Technologists*
Skill	$3.00	$3.00	$10.50
Working conditions	2.00	1.00	3.00
Mental efforts	2.50	2.00	6.00
Physical effort	2.00	1.00	1.50
Total wage/hr	$9.50	$7.00	$21.00

Incentive Programs

The purpose of incentive programs is to reward and encourage behavior considered desirable from the perspective of the employer. The overriding goal of most incentive plans is to maximize productivity based on the volume of work done or sales generated. To a much lesser extent, merit programs may promote quality enhancement and public relations activities such as community service and staff morale. Following are several examples of incentive programs.

- **Piecework**. Pay is tied directly to the amount of work performed or units produced, a highly controversial system, you may recall, which was at onetime used in the laboratory to encourage cytotechnologists to read more slides.
- **Commissions**. A pay-plus system whereby the employee receives a basic salary plus additional pay determined by volume, or commissions may constitute the entire paycheck. Laboratory supply salespeople and reference laboratory representatives commonly are paid this way.
- **Bonuses**. Although usually reserved for executive level managers, all employees may be allowed to participate in stock purchase plans, profit-sharing programs, and rewards for cost-reduction suggestions. Bonus plans range from direct cash payments, travel, to stock options.
- **Merit rises**. The amount of salary increase is based on the results of the performance appraisal.
- **Maturity curves**. This method puts employees in pay scales with different top-rate ranges or salary caps, based on performance and experience. This approach is often used in industry for technical and professional workers who, because of the nature of their job (research and support activities), do not usually qualify for other incentive programs, particularly promotion through the administrative routes. This technique is used for assigning pay scales to the parallel career ladder programs now gaining popularity in the health care field (see Table 11 – 3 for an example of a laboratory career ladder model).
- **Perks and Perquisites**. Simple and inexpensive recognition programs give awards such as designated parking places and small cash gratuities to, for example, the employee of the month. At the executive level, however, these perks can become expensive and be viewed as signs of power and prestige. Company cars, location and furnishings of private offices, and dues to country clubs are examples of executive privileges rewarded according to the position or performance.

Other Wage-Determining Factors

The most notable of alternative methods for determining wage rates is the collective bargaining process, the negotiation process conducted between a company and a union. In addition, special circumstances may make a person especially attractive to an origination, and a salary agreement may be reached through personal negotiations between the parties. Personal negotiations are more common at the managerial level, at which the factors determining the worth of a position are more subtle and subjective. The *employment contract* is an example of an agreement between the employer and the new hire, listing the length of employment, terms (salary, benefits, perquisites, etc.) and usually specifying the reasons under which the contract may be terminated, Non

—competition or solicitation of customers, and the protection of confidential information may be another reason for an employment contract agreement.

In times of high inflation, cost-of-living adjustments (COLAs) to the basic pay schedules may become necessary to maintain a stable workforce and keep the staff from seeking employment elsewhere in efforts to protect their basic standard of living and purchasing power.

Pay scale and authority rank	Bureaucratic route	Technical route
Pay grade A	Administrative director	Technical director
Pay grade B		Technical scientist
Pay grade C	Assistant administrative director	Associate—technical scientist
Pay grade D		Assistant technical scientist
Pay grade E	Section Supervisor	
Pay grade F		Senior Medical Technologists/CLS
Pay grade G	Assistant Supervisor	
Pay grade H		Medical technologist/CLS

Note: As a matter of simplification and to allow for institutional needs and difference, the specific qualifications have not been delineated. A suggestion for achieving the technical scientist category may be graduate education, professional competence, and contributions to the profession in forms that bring both technical expertise to the laboratory and prestige to the reputation of the institution. Positions in the bureaucratic route would have administrative authority over those in a similar grade or below. Simultaneous rank may be achieved in both paths. For example, a technical scientist may also occupy the position of a section supervisor or be the administrative director.
SOURCE: Varnadoe, LA; Upward Mobility, MT Today 2:16, 1992

Table 11 – 3. Model Career Ladder for the Medical Laboratory

Staffing, Scheduling, and Performance Monitoring

These two components, staffing/scheduling and performance monitoring, of the personnel process represent he everyday relations and interaction between the organization and its members. They are a major part of the *directing* function of management, the most visible activity in the life of both employees and managers.

Labor Relations

The term **labor relations**, in the formal sense, refer to the company's dealings with labor unions. However, it should not be limited to this agenda. Labor relations really encompasses the way an organization views and treats its employees — particularly the way it handles grievances and applies its policies in a fair, equitable and consistent manner. Included in Table 6 – 1 is a list of the laws and regulations that cover the rights of employees to organize and bargain collectively with an employer.

Several terms are used to discuss and describe the topic of labor relations: "*Open shop*" means that employees do not need to be members of a union to work there. "*Closed shop*" is used to signify that union membership is required to be employed. Right-to-work laws in some state prohibit unions from setting up closed shops in their contracts.

Professional Growth and Development

An essential ingredient of any business plan is a talented and well-trained staff, prepared and ready to meet the challenges facing the organization. Attempting to hire qualified help only at the moment when the situation dictates, rather then keeping them on staff or developing current employees may seem like a good strategy that allows an institution the flexibility to obtain specific expertise when needed. However, it entails the risk of missing business opportunities and failing to have critical skills in place in time to avert a crisis. It may also alienate current employees who see it as proof of a lack of genuine interest in their personal growth.

Lifelong learning is imbued in the laboratory mentality and culture, as demonstrated through its emphasis on high-quality patient care, educational and training institutions, and the tenants of inspections, accreditation and personnel certification agencies. Most acutely, however, it is driven by the rapidly changing nature and the advances made in the technology and knowledge base of the profession. To ensure that the laboratory has a staff capable of delivering the service expected on it, managers must pay particular attention to the continuing education of their employees, which is achieved through a well-designed and executed plan that natures the professional growth and development of both the laboratory and its workforce. The most desirable and important characteristic of this program is that it is a *continual* and *ongoing* commitment by the laboratory and its staff to employees' personal and professional development. Such a program must identify and meet the specific training needs of the department and its employees.

The importance of education and training to the core success of the laboratory is discussed further in the next chapter dedicated to this purpose.

Training Needs and Assessment

An active continuing education program, based on the objective assessment of needs, is a requirement of all agencies that regulate medical laboratories. It has gained additional urgency under the competency assessment rules implemented under CLIA'88. Ideas for additional training and documentation can be derived from the following activities.

- Suggestions and requests from staff members
- Results of internal and external proficiency testing programs
- Orientation and competency assessment reviews
- Performance appraisal systems
- Inspection, accreditation and licensure surveys
- Quality management monitoring activities

Educational Sources

Continuing education resources for laboratorians are abundant. Bellow is just a few of the opportunities available.

- **In-service training**, including competency assurance programs and educational sessions presented by staff members and experts hosted by the laboratory. Journal clubs as well as material produced by instrument manufacturers, educational institutions, profes-

sional societies, and laboratory suppliers are examples of in-service training opportunities.
- **Intensive training** by instrument specialists, either on site or in the manufacturer's facilities.
- **Conferences and seminars** hosted by local laboratories and colleges or, at the state and national level, by professional societies. The key element in sending a person to an educational session away from the laboratory is that the information obtained be shared with coworkers upon return.
- **Formal college courses** that update not only the changes in the laboratory field but advances in the underlying academic fundamentals of biology and chemistry or other relevant sciences. They can be obtained either by on-campus attendance or through alternative instructional access (correspondence, internet, concentrated sessions, or self-study material).

Corrective Action and Employee Discipline

One of the most difficult and distasteful decisions faced by a manager is how to deal with an employee who continues to have problems complying with the policy and procedures of the laboratory or who fails, despite all efforts, to meet minimum performance expectations. There are no easy answers in this situation, and the action taken depends on the history of the employee and the nature of the problem. The key to an effective corrective action and disciple program, however, is equability and fairness — a thorough investigation of the cause of the problem (whether technical, work environment, schedule disruptions, or personal), combined with a helpful spirit of offering whatever assistance and guidance may be appropriate to the situation.

Table 11 – 4 details a corrective action and discipline step program that many laboratory managers have found useful and is a common procedure for institutions. Seeking the advice of senior managers, human resource experts, and colleagues who have had similar experiences is also a wise strategy. Obviously, the seriousness of the problem in many cases dictates the options available to the manager, but all action should be designed with the wellbeing of both the laboratory and the employee in mind.

If the situation is chronic such as tardiness, absentees, tidiness, or low productivity; documentation and follow-up of the incidents will be crucial. Records should be matched with genuine efforts of managers to provide assistant to the employee. Documentation is an essential ingredient in any plan, particularly for situations which are chronic. If the manager only addresses the problem out of the frustration caused by the latest incident, and has not maintained a history, he or she may not be able to get the employee to see the seriousness of a pattern, or pining down the employee to a specific "reoccurring" problem.

An example of management willingness to help a person deal with the situation would be offering the employee an alternative work schedule if possible, and reviewing the work place circumstances to make sure that latent errors (i.e., management caused problems such as poor or failures in planning, organization, or staff training) have been addressed. Counseling tools such as a "*Last Chance Contract*," may help clarify the seriousness of the problem for the employee.

Acute problems, such as falsifying records or testing, or illegal activities must be dealt with immediately and usually results in dismissal (Step 6). Again if this action is necessary, the manager is responsible to precisely document the incident and obtain approval from any designated administrator (e.g., notify human resources).

Table 11 – 4. CORRECTIVE ACTION AND DISCIPLINE STEP PROGRAM

Unacceptable behavior Incident occurrence		Action
1.	Awareness	Informally, make sure employee is aware of problem and check to see if any assistance is needed
2.	Troubleshooting	Informally, at the supervisory level, talk with employee about the problem, attempting to identify the causes and offer assistance in correcting the situation.
3.	Verbal warning	A formal counseling session, by either the immediate supervisor or laboratory manager about the serious nature of the problem; offer assistance, guidance, and a plan of action for correcting the situation. Notes and records of the conference are maintained by the manager, but employee is not asked at this point to sign any documents.
4.	Written warning	A formal counseling session, where the employee is given written notice that specified behavior cannot continue, with warnings of further action if behavior is not corrected. Assistance, guidance, and plan of action are continuously reviewed.
5.	Suspension	Employee is suspended for 2 days without pay, with warnings of possible dismissal if problem is not corrected. Assistance, guidance, and plan of action are continuously reviewed. This step may also include a last chance contract.
6.	Dismissal	Employee is dismissed.

Note: Nature and timing of corrective action are dependent on the seriousness of the problem. This model is intended for chronic situations in which violations of laboratory policies continue despite normal supervisory intervention.

Separation and Employment Termination

The final aspect of the personnel process and employment cycle is the conclusion of the formal relationship between the employee and the organization. It may be either voluntary, as when an employee retires or accepts a position at another laboratory; or, involuntary, such as a disciplinary dismissal or layoff resulting from a hospital wide reduction of personnel.

This stage includes the routine paperwork associated with removing the person from the payroll and maintaining the records for any possible future use. For example, potential employers frequently request reference check. Many companies have a policy of verifying only dates of employment; and, possible, salary levels because of treats of litigation arising over an evaluation given about work performance.

Exit interviews may be conducted during the final week of employment as a method of identifying why personnel are leaving an organization. The information gained from these interviews may be used in assessing the overall efficiency of the organization's human resource management system to include such issues as sense of job security, quality of management and supervision, satisfaction with the performance appraisal system, working conditions, fairness of company policies, general attractiveness as a place to work, and the perceived equity and competitiveness of the wage, salary, and benefits plans. Because a single individual may have had a bad experience with or hold a grudge against a particular supervisor or department, these findings are usually batched to identify trends and problems with a department or policy rather than dealt with as isolated incidents.

This completes the chapter on *Human Resource Management: The Personnel Process.* The next chapter will cover the needs assessment and training techniques of *Education and Training of the Laboratory Professional.*

— Case Study —

Chapter Eleven: Human Resource Management: The Personnel Process

"I have to have someone I can depend on for the 11-7 shift," remarked the laboratory manager to the personnel director as she signed the forms to terminate the tech just dismissed because of attendance problems. "I know everyone has family, health, and life problems where they must miss work sometimes, but we must be able to depend on them to be at work. The is why we have a job for them in the first place."

"I understand," replied the personnel director. "Make sure you cover this point when you hire a replacement. I know dismissing the tech was hard on you, with her sick child causing her to miss so much work, but you must have someone who can show up for work regularly. I'll go through the files and start looking for a replacement."

"Thank you," nodded the laboratory manager as she departed.

(One week later)

"Hello," said the laboratory manager, answering the phone call from the personnel director

.

"I think I've found the perfect tech for you," announced the personnel director. "She just came into our office and has recently moved into the area. She has excellent qualifications and experience. She even worked the night shift at her previous hospital, and she prefers it. She is also available immediately."

"Great, send her over!"

(In the laboratory manager's office during the interview)

"Why did you leave your last job? It looks like everything was going great for you there," asked the laboratory manager?

"It was. ... I loved the laboratory. However, we heard that my husband was going to be transferring here, and I decided I would take a few months off and enjoy being with my baby until we were settled. Here's a picture of him. Isn't he beautiful?"

"He certainly is," said the laboratory manager, admiring the picture the tech handed her.

Chapter Section for Review

- Legal and Regulation Requirements
- EEOC inappropriate interview topics
- Disparate Treatment
- Interview Strategy
- Correct Action and Employee Discipline

Questions for Discussions

1. Was it against employment laws to have dismissed the first tech because of attendance problems caused by child care? Was the employee protected form dismissal because her problems were caused by her children?
2. How can the laboratory manager find out about the attendance record of the person applying for a job without violating employment laws? What questions or interview strategies might be appropriate to explore this topic?
3. Now that the job candidate has volunteered her family situation, can the laboratory manager ask further questions about child care arrangements?
4. Can the laboratory legally consider this information in the hiring decision?

[12]

Education and Training of the Laboratory Professional

— Chapter Twelve —

The National Accrediting Agency for Clinical Laboratory Sciences (NAACLS), supported by examination content guidelines of the Board of Registry (ASCP) and the National Credentialing Agency (ASCLS), expect that professional laboratorians should be skilled in the training and education of their peers and patients. Specifically these agencies have standards for instructional areas and curriculum criteria that must include the following subjects.

- Educational principles, techniques, terminology, and methodology
- Technical training and clinical instruction.
- Continuing education and staff development.
- Monitor compliance to regulatory requirements for education and technical competence documentation.
- Evaluation of the effectiveness of training and educational programs.
- Teaching and training responsibilities of management.
- Job orientation.
- Assessment of training needs.
- Self-improvement and professional development.

These topics will be reviewed in this course in three sections: 1) the teaching and training responsibilities of laboratory management; 2) developing a program of continuing education and staff development; and, 3) principles of educational and instructional methodology in the preparation and presentation of teaching programs. Special attention will be focused on the process and techniques of topic/subject selection, teaching goals and objectives, instructional strategies and presentation methods, learning activities, training material, and evaluation tools used in didactic and clinical teaching.

OBJECTIVES

After completion of this chapter, the reader will be able to demonstrate accomplishment of the following objectives.

1. Explain the teaching and training responsibilities of laboratory management.
2. Assess the educational and training needs of the laboratory.
3. Monitor compliance to regulatory requirements for education and technical competence documentation.
4. Develop a program of continuing education and staff development.
5. Identify needs and topics for continuing education and staff development.
6. Evaluate and improve effectiveness of training and educational programs.
7. Incorporate principles of educational and instructional methodology in the design and development of teaching programs.
8. Describe the learning process in relationship to the adult/professional student.
9. Write instructional objectives.

10. Select an instructional strategy for a CE program.
11. Develop course content parameters.
12. Use the tools of presentation.
13. Present a professional CE program.
14. Prepare a subject mastery demonstration method.
15. Design a program evaluation instrument.

Chapter Highlights and Glossary of Key Terms

I TEACHING AND TRAINING RESPONSIBILITIES OF LABORATORY MANAGEMENT

II. CONTINUING EDUCATION AND STAFF DEVELOPMENT
- A. Assessing Educational and Training Needs of the Laboratory
- B. Identifying Needs and Topics for Continuing Education and Staff Development
- C. Evaluating and Improving the Effectiveness of Training and Educational Programs
- D. Continuing Education and Staff Development Resources

III. PRINCIPLES OF EDUCATIONAL AND INSTRUCTIONAL METHODOLOGY IN THE PREPARATION AND PRESENTATION OF TEACHING PROGRAMS. (Educational and Instructional Methodology)
- A. The Learning Process
- B. The Audience (Adult/Professional Student)
- C. Instructional Objectives
  1. Objective Design
  2. Format of Writing an Instructional Objective
- D. Instructional Strategies
  1. Teacher-Centered Approaches
  2. Student-Centered Approaches
- E. Course Content
- F. Classroom Support
  1. Handouts
  2. Visual Aids
- G. Presentation Skills
  1. Physical Facilities
  2. Your Appearance
  3. The Delivery
  4. Script or Outline
  5. Stage Fright
- H. Objective/Criterion-Reference Mastery Demonstration
- I. Program Evaluation Instrument

Teaching and Training Responsibilities of Laboratory Management

The laboratory manager may frequently find themselves actively involved in both meeting the training needs of their staff, and also with providing facilitates and formal participation in the clinical portion of a laboratory educational program with local colleges. Both of these responsibilities are important. Not only, does a professional have the social responsibility to *"train those who come after them;"* but these two programs are mutually supportive and assist each other in providing resources, personnel, and learning opportunities.

To emphasize the priority which education and staff development have on the daily operation of a laboratory it is important to note a key point. Teaching and training are an integral part of the tools which a manager has for implementing a plan or obtaining the desired performance *(i.e., tools of persuasion and tools of control)*. *Tools of persuasion* are a basic avenue for executing a plan and education is at the core of the management process.[1 p. 10]

Outside of the formal personnel corrective action and discipline program of an institution and the normal operational process of running the lab (*management and leadership*); the teaching and training roles of managers provide the most direct mechanism for taking action in intervening with a specific individual, the staff as a whole, or the operations of the department. It provides a positive avenue to present new information, communicate policy goals, and provide individuals with the means to understand, and the tools with which to achieve the performance expectations of the laboratory. Failure to have a sound educational and staff development program may be indicative of a breakdown in the communication system of the organization.

In addition to daily operations, the teaching and training responsibilities of laboratory management must meet specific accreditation and license requirements. These programs are part of the administrative duties of the organization and normal process of job performance. Company and job orientation, annual personnel educational requirements (*e.g., fire, safety, patient rights, risk management, incident reporting, HIPAA compliance*), new instrument and procedure implementation, performance reviews, and technical competence documentation are examples of educational programs specified in the standards of accreditation and licensure agencies and which are included as part of the human resource (*personnel*) functions of the institution. Monitoring compliance with regulatory requirements for education and technical competence documentation is a specific responsibility of laboratory management.

The laboratory also has educational responsibilities to its patients, healthcare users (*nursing staff and physicians*), and to the institution if it is part of a hospital or clinic. All of these entities are dependent on the laboratory providing information and training in the proper utilization of its services. The College of American Pathologists (CAP) lists this duty as one of its accreditation standard (Standard I: A(12)) as a responsibility of the director: *Provide educational programs for the medical and laboratory staff, and participate in educational programs of the institution.*[2] The preparation and distribution of ordering and specimen collection manuals for patients, nursing, and doctor's offices are an example of the application of this educational responsibility. While the writing of policy and procedure manuals is not the topic of this lesson, all of the concepts presented below are important in accomplishing their mission: *a clear message, a mechanism (i.e., a written procedure) to reach the intended audience, and obtaining feedback to ensure that the participants understands the instructions.*

Laboratory manuals should be frequently supplemented with training sessions for all users, particularly as part of new employee orientation and when there are changes in services.

Continuing Education and Staff Development

As pointed out in the section above, the continuing education (CE) and staff development program provides a positive avenue to present new information, communicate policy goals, and provide individuals with the means to understand, and the tools with which to achieve the performance expectations of the laboratory. In fact, it is the foundation of the communication process of the organization.

The basic concepts of continuing education and staff development are closely aligned with the professional practice of management. They are both a continuous process of interacting functions, each dependent on the other, which must work together for the organization to be successful in achieving its mission. Teaching and training is imbued in the functions of the *management process* and is the key implementation tool for each step:[1 p. 8]

- Planning
- Organizing
- Directing
- Controlling

This relationship is illustrated in the **planning** function which consists of seven steps that are closely correlated to the methods necessary to prepare and present a training program which are covered in this course.[1 p. 8]

1. Determine the goals the organization wishes to accomplish.
2. Collect information and evaluate the current situation, compared with where the enterprise wishes to be.
3. Establish a time frame or period in which to achieve the goals.
4. Set objectives that will move the company toward the desired future.
5. Forecast needs and the use of resources.
6. Determine the steps necessary to implement the plan.
7. Provide for a feedback mechanism to continually review the success of the plan and to implement necessary revisions.

Assessing Educational and Training Needs of the Laboratory

Attention to the needs, and plans for each phase of the continuing education and staff development program must be in place. There are specific content guidelines and documentation methods (*e.g., checklists*) which are designed to address the issues and goals associated with almost every stage. Some of these have components which are dictated by administration and regulatory agencies (*e.g., orientation*) but most are developed from information identified during the normal operational process of the laboratory and the employment experience of the professional. A general idea of what types of programs will be necessary may be illustrated from even a cursory review of each period of the staff's relationship with the laboratory:[1 p. 115]

→ Recruitment (qualifications)
→ Hiring decision (initial introduction to the organization)
→ Institutional orientation
→ Laboratory (department) orientation
→ Job duties orientation
→ Competency assessment
→ Laboratory operational improvement process
(policy/procedure feedback and updates)
→ Job progression
(new instruments and tests training)
→ Individual professional growth
>>>>>> *and continues*
→ Competency assessment
→ Laboratory operational improvement process
(policy/procedure feedback and updates)
→ Job progression
(new instruments and tests training)
→ Individual professional growth
>>>>>> *continues ...... until*
Separation and Employment termination

The education and training of the laboratory involves assessing the needs of the laboratory within the framework of its current goals and objectives; and, those of the staff, both as individuals and as members of the group. To accomplish this mission and fully utilize this valuable management tool, every aspect of the laboratory's operations must be incorporated into the process of identifying topics, selecting presentation channels, and ensuring that the intended message is received.

Identifying Needs and Topics for Continuing Education and Staff Development

The first step in any management process is to identify any problem and determine what is needed to correct the situation. How to develop and implement a plan usually becomes evident after this initial recognition of a problem and corrective decision is determined. Selecting the topic or subject for a training session follows this pattern. The subject is derived from the needs assessment, and the needs assessment is derived from reviewing the information flow arriving in and generated by the laboratory everyday. This includes trouble points found during reviews of quality control records, incident reports, inspections, proficiency surveys, laboratory performance (*turnaround times, missed tests, etc.*), corrective action/discipline sessions, safety programs, annual personnel appraisals, and instrument troubleshooting. Investigation of complaints and concerns, along with the suggestions received from nursing, physicians, patients, and staff will be an excellent source of ideas for course topics.

The point is: all functions and information sources should be funneled into the continuing education and staff development strategy of the laboratory. From this information stream, specific ideas and programs can be created to remedy the problems identified and turn the negative factors into a positive approach of resolution. For example, the chemistry supervisor may identify a training topic because staff continues to need assistance in performing tasks associated with instrument maintenance. The hematology department may develop a session for Techs who do not feel secure in performing body fluids differentials. A program on the proper collection of microbiology specimens may be suggested because of the frequent rejection of samples collected by nursing personnel.

This process of identifying and developing topics for inclusion in the continuing education and staff development program of the laboratory is illustrated in the model below.

Staff topic suggestions
Proficiency testing
Orientation
Competency assessment
Performance appraisals
Inspection Surveys
Quality monitoring
Risk Management
Safety program
Hiring and Recruitment
Instrument Troubleshooting
Corrective Action/Discipline
Problem Resolution plans
Incident Reports

→

Continuing Education And Staff Development Program

Evaluating and Improving the Effectiveness of Training and Educational Programs

The model outlined above also serves to evaluate and improve the effectiveness of training and educational programs. If turnaround times are reduced, Techs work more independently on instrument maintenance, and the number of nurse collected specimens which are rejected are decreased, this will be a measure that the continuing education program is accomplishing its goals. However, if there is an increase in deficiencies or no improvement is observed; perhaps the problem should be evaluated in greater detailed (*root cause analysis*) and more specific topics targeted toward narrower factors which influence the situation.

Feedback on each session or communication effort should be actively solicited to assist in evaluating and improving the effectiveness of training and educational programs. Course evaluation forms, staff inquiry, performance standard measurements, and monitoring compliance with regulatory training requirements are four examples of methods which may be used to appraise success, obtain suggestions for improvement, and identify additional topics for future presentation. Remember, the continuing education and staff development program is a continual cycle of needs assessment, course development, presentation, and evaluation.

An additional strategy to ensure the quality of continuing education programs is to obtain formal accreditation through professional and state agencies. These groups have standard for developing and presenting courses and provides the student with a record of their participation. Credit and recognition may be accomplished by obtaining either provider or course approval though such laboratory organizations as the American Society for Clinical Laboratory Science (PACE), or American Medical Technologists (AMTIE). Several states, including Florida issue licenses for approved CE providers. Universal standards and guidelines for continuing education units [CEU(s)] are also provided by The International Association for Continuing Education and Training (IACET).

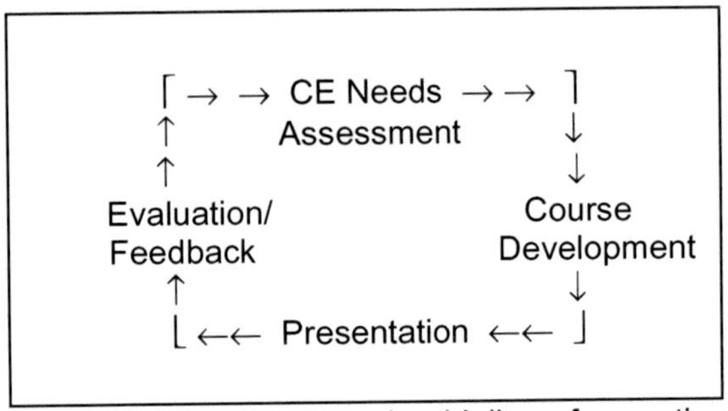

Continuing Education and Staff Development Resources

Learning opportunities are almost unlimited in the laboratory community, and is one of the attractive features of our profession. Tapping these resources and funneling them into an organized plan is a major task of management. National, regional, state, and local conferences presented by professional laboratory organizations are an obvious resources, as well as programs offered by local colleges. However, while their advantages are obvious; they tend to be broad based subjects, and may not address the specific needs of a laboratory.

Manufacturer sponsored programs, both for instruments and products may provide training for laboratory staff directly related to performance needs. An important issue with these types of programs is to make sure that the information reaches all persons in the lab. This can be accomplished by having the Tech who attends a conference or training program outside the lab present the material to the staff when they return, or making sure that classes are offered at times when all members can attend.

In-service sessions (*i.e., on-site programs sponsored by the laboratory*) are a specific strategy for meeting continuing education and staff development program needs. These are frequently presenting by pathologists, specialists, supervisors, outside experts, vendors, and staff member.

They can be customized and designed to address problems which have been identified during CE needs assessment efforts.

Including all members of the laboratory team as potential faculty enriches both the individual and takes advantage of the talents available in the organization. From personal experience and discussion with other professionals, being responsible for teaching a subject is probably the best learning technique available (*e.g., research, organization, preparing supporting material such as handouts and overheads, and lecture practice*). It requires, and affords the instructor the opportunity to learn the subject at a greater depth then they ever would as a student.

A major obstacle to having staff present lectures to laboratory students or other staff is providing for time to prepare and practice. This is a particularly concern with those who may be inexperienced in presenting training programs, and need extra time to prepare a topic for the first time. They may feel that expecting them to acquire these skills and prepare the lesson on their own time is unfair, while the laboratory may have trouble covering for them while away from the bench.

Another barrier is finding sources which provide information and training on how to develop and present an educational program (*i.e. "train the trainer"*). This is the mission of this course, and is the topic of the next section

Educational and Instructional Methodology

Principles of Educational and Instructional Methodology in the Preparation and Presentation of Teaching Programs

The variety of avenues and ease of accessibility for obtaining training and education programs have exploded recently, particularly with the introduction of the computer and the internet. It is now possible to obtain college degrees, including the Ph.D. entirely online. St. Petersburg College (Florida) has .... "*designed an online Medical Laboratory Technology program offering students the same line of study and 'hands-on' experience as the college's traditional campus program.*"[(3)] The July 2007 edition of Advance for Medical Laboratory Professionals has advertisements for three Online degree programs, both at Bachelors and graduate levels.

Classroom lectures, live seminars, video and teleconferences, movie and slide shows, interactive CD-ROM, online courses, hand-on workshops (e.g., *wet-labs*), plus the usual assortment of hard-copy printed material, including textbooks, magazines, training manuals and workbooks just begin to illustrate the broad range of methods and venues available to both the instructor and student. However, whatever the communication or delivery mechanism, these learning experiences do have one major feature in common:

they all have specific instructional goals, or a purpose, they wish to accomplish.

To achieve this instructional goal, each course or training exercise will usually have these eight components or areas which the trainer must prepare and which will form the topics of this section.

- The Learning Process
- The Audience (Adult/Professional Students)
- Instructional Objectives
- Instructional Strategies
- Course Content
- Classroom support
- Presentation Skills
- Objective/Criterion-Reference Mastery Demonstration
- Program Evaluation Instrument

The Learning Process

William G. Huitt presents, "A Transactional Model of the Teaching/Learning Process," which points out that learning variables can be classified into four groups, each playing a major role in the learning process:[4, also 5a]

> **Context**, or those factors outside of the classroom which may influence the learning process;
> **Inputs**, the background and characteristics which the instructor and student bring to the program;
> the actual **classroom process** itself concerning the instructional activities which occur; and,
> **Output**, which is the measurement of the achievement or performance level gained by the audience through participating in the course.

This model centers on the perception that the true measure of the learning process is based on the results which occur *within* the participant, and that success is not defined by focusing on the activities of the instructor, but those of the student. This concept is further emphasized in the clinical preceptor guidelines of the Columbia University School of Nursing who include among its key learning points that, "*Learning is an active and continuous process manifested by growth and changes in behavior*" and, "*Learning is facilitated when the student has an opportunity to test ideas, analyze mistakes, take risks and be creative.*"[6]

From these models we know that the learning process is dependent on the participant's active involvement, exposure to multi-avenues and repetitive events of sharing information (*i.e., teaching methods*), and the trainer's continual monitoring and adjustment to the progress of the student's mastery of the course objectives. The priority of continual feedback to the participant, as part of the learning process will also be reviewed in the *Subject Mastery Demonstration (i.e., Test)* section near the end of the course.

The Audience (Adult/Professional Students)

One of the first factors which must be considered in a program design is the nature of the target audience. In an educational situation involving adult professionals the focus of the training leader and program design is that of a facilitator in an androgogical model approach, with major emphasis on the active contribution and input of the content and instructional learning experience based on the needs and judgment of the participants.[7, 8, 9,10]

Specifically, designing a training exercise for professionals requires attention to the needs and educational expectations of the adult learner. In essence, teaching methods for adults requires a more participatory role for the student in deciding the topic, featured subject matter, learning strategy, length of the course (time commitments), level of instruction (basic, intermediate, advance) and even how success will be defined. In other words, the adult learner needs to feel they are in charge of their own educational agenda. This is basically different from the adolescent classroom where the teacher makes all these decisions for the student.

Marilyn Dixon (*manager*) of the Postgraduate Centre at Scarborough Hospital describes their learning strategy for adult professionals:

> *"In order to encourage intellectual and professional development of the trainees we take a process orientated and learner centred*$_{(sic)}$ *view of Curriculum. In this view education is most productive when:*
>
> - *Learners are encouraged to be self directed*
> - *The educator functions as a facilitator rather than a didactic instructor*
> - *The individual learner's needs and learning styles are taken into account*

- *A climate conducive to learning is established*
- *The learners past experiences are used in the learning process*
- *Learning activities seem to have some relevance to the learners circumstances*

The purpose of adult education is to help them to learn, not to teach them all they know and thus stop them from learning." [11]

The educational needs of the professional can often be achieved by providing them with a selection of courses topics, time periods, and variety of learning routes (*e.g., lecture, internet, workbook, video*) from which to choose. Within the individual course, the criteria for the adult student can be accomplished by placing emphasis on group discussions and the active solicitation of questions and directions to the instructor as to the participant's priority for the session and the topics which particularly interest them.

Instructional Objectives

RE: <u>At the completion of this exercise the participant(s) will be able to assess the educational and training needs of the laboratory</u>

Exactly what is the purpose of your course? Why are you spending the time to produce it? What do you expect to accomplish from both the perspective of the laboratory and the staff? What changes or improvements in the knowledge or performance of the participants do you expect? These are example of the questions the trainer must address in designing and presenting a program. The answers will direct how the course is prepared and presented.

Kerry Magruder points out that: *"Instructional objectives are specific, measurable, short-term, observable student behaviors."* [12] This description should clue the reader that writing learning objectives is an important task and requires a significant planning effort. It is — and the reason for this time commitment and attention to detail at the very beginning of the course development — because the resulting objectives defined the road map for the lesson. The objectives sets the boundaries of content *(i.e., what will/-not be included in the course*) and states exactly what is expected of both the trainer and the student.

There are basically three (3) **types** of instructional objectives and four (4) **parts** of a well written objective proposed in the literature of educational and instructional methodology.

> Three (3) **types** of instructional objectives
> Cognitive
> Psychomotor
> Affective
>
> Four (4) **parts** of a well written objective
> *ABCD's of instructional objectives.*
> *The **A** stands for **Audience**,*
> *the **B** represents **Behavior**,*
> *the **C** stands for **Condition** and*
> *the **D** for **Degree** of Accuracy.*

The three (3) **types**, of instructional objectives all relate to learning "*behavior*" or "*outcomes*," and are classified based on what is referred to as <u>**Bloom's**</u> <u>**Taxonomy**</u>. *"In 1956, Benjamin Bloom headed a group of educational psychologists who developed a classification of levels of intellectual behavior important in learning. This became a taxonomy including three overlapping domains; the cognitive, psychomotor, and affective. Each of the domains can be utilized through the interaction of media."* DLRN's Technology Resource Guide (13, 14)

- **Cognitive**: understanding, information recall, and problem solving. <u>*Example*</u>*: explain the methodology of glucose analysis, or selecting an antimicrobial battery.*
- **Psychomotor**: specific skills such as *perform a capillary puncture or perform daily maintenance on the chemistry analyzer.*

- **Affective**: Has to do primarily with performance attitudes or job conduct, much more abstract subjects as *teamwork or customer care.*

Objective Design (writing)

In the actual writing or construction of an objective, B. O'Bannon describes each of the four (4) **parts** which must be included: *"Heinich and his colleagues (2002) suggest that well written objectives have four parts. They call these parts the ABCD's of instructional objectives.*

*The **A** stands for **Audience**,*
*the **B** represents **Behavior**,*
*the **C** stands for **Condition** and*
*the **D** for **Degree** of Accuracy.*

Each instructional objective is written in sentence format and should contain the A, B, C and D." (15, 16; text emphasis added by author)

The key component of an objective is the outcome or accomplishment that is expected when the participant completes the project. Is the course design to increase the knowledge of a subject (*cognitive*), training on operating an instrument or performing a procedure (*psychomotor*), or an exercise intended to improve how a lab group works together (*affective*)? The type of session planned, will be directly reflected in the writing style of the objective.

Actual writing composition of an objective
Specifically, the **type** [cognitive[*understand*], psychomotor [*specific skill*], or affective [*attitude or job conduct*]) of learning experience may be identified by the selection of the action or behavior **verb** which will be at the beginning of the objective:

Verb examples:
Interpret ..., explain .... (*cognitive*);
perform..., calculate... (*psychomotor*);
organize..., design... (*affective*).

(This point is discussed further in the **B** (*behavior*) part of writing an objective below.)

In writing an objective, clarity of purpose and mutual understanding of the parameters of the subject are the goal. Following the **ABCD** model assists in accomplishing these functions.

Objective writing model
A... B ... C... D ...
Audience
Behavior or expectations
Condition of learning experience
Degree of accomplishment

Audience The audience is the target group or members of the class who will be participating in the session. Since the instructional objective is usually writing as a compound sentence, the audience is usually identified in the opening clause. In this example the audience is referred to as the *participant*:

*"At the completion of this exercise the **participant(s)** will be able to:"*

Behavior *... selecting the action word ... the verb ...*
Behavior is specifically defined by the **verb** that describes what the audience is expecting to be able to perform after completion of the program. The importance of this verb is obvious from the attention giving to it in the literature, and the consideration involved in its selection. The **verb** helps to identify the **type** of course and many verbs have been assigned specific definitional purpose. Selecting which **verb** to use is not intended to be a difficult process, and is actually made quite easy since the type of course is usually know and with the abundance of lists available with suggestions (*see bibliography and links*). The following examples will help to clarify this part of writing an instructional objective.

(*Verb Web link resources*) [connected July 11, 2007]
- http://www.adprima.com/verbs.htm
- http://www.usuhs.mil/che/write_objective.htm

Cognitive: An additional point is necessary in reviewing Bloom's Taxonomy. Cognitive courses may be also be classified into six *cognitive levels*. The basic imparting of *knowledge* is considered the lowest level in Bloom's classification. The other five are ranked according to increasing difficulty in levels of mental abilities: *comprehension*, *application*, *analysis*, *synthesis* and *evaluation*.[15]

Cognitive Level ... **Associated Verb(s)**
knowledge: *define.... locate.... list....state....identify*
comprehension: *classify... compute... explain... describe... distinguish*
application: *apply... calculate... locate... report...use*
analysis: *analyze... contrast ... distinguish...diagram... compare*
synthesis: *plan... write... design... compose... prepare*
evaluation: *appraise... evaluate... measure... select... conclude*

Psychomotor: *construct ...perform... operate ... repair ... demonstrate*
(Doing: as in performing a test or operating an instrument)
Psychomotor verbs are closely related to the *application level* in cognitive objective. A cognitive perspective focuses on teaching theoretical or introduction "*know how*;" in psychomotor courses is it the actual "*hands on*" performance which is emphasized.

Affective: *believe... value... respect... resolve... perceive*
(Feelings and emotions; *e.g.,* toward co-workers, patients, job)

Condition The conditions or situation under which the participant is expected to accomplish the objective can be spelled out, or is frequently implied by the topic of the lesson. For example, as in writing a job description criterion it can be stated that:

Upon completion of this training session the technologist will be able to perform routine maintenance on the FAST CHEM analysis ***(conditions implied)*** ... *with minimal supervision* **(*condition spelled out*)**

Upon completion of this training session the technologist will be able to calibrate the FAST CHEM analysis using the ... *instrument and laboratory procedure manuals.* ***(condition)***

Upon completion of this course the participant will be able to prepare and present a training session ***(conditions implied)*** ... using the model presented in ...*Education and Training of the Laboratory Professional.* ***(condition spelled out)***

Degree *of Accuracy* states the standard by which the accomplishment of the objective will be measured. Again, this may be implied by the nature of the exercise (e.g., *participation or attendance*) or specified as when the program is be used as part of the competency assessment training for the laboratory.

Upon completion of this training session the technologist will be able to perform routine maintenance on the FAST CHEM analysis with minimal supervision ... *90% of the time.* **(degree)**

Upon completion of this training session the technologist will be able to perform Type and Screens. {**(degree)** *100% of time, or competence is implied*}

At the completion of this exercise the participant(s) will be able to assess educational and training needs of the laboratory

*If this is presented as a live program with out a test or other mastery demonstration, then participation or attendance at the session is expected to demonstrate the **degree** of accuracy to be measured (see mastery section below).*

At the completion of this exercise the participant(s) will be able to assess educational and training needs of the laboratory and ... *submit a plan to administration.* ***(degree)***

Format of Writing an Instructional Objective

As previously stated, instructional objectives are usually written as a compound sentence with the audience identified in the opening clause. The actual subject criteria (...**BCD**) are then listed as bullets or numbered items. [16]

At the (*completion/conclusion*) of this (*session, exercise, class, module program*) the (*participant/student/trainee/technologist*) will be able to:

1. ...	• ...
2. ...	• ...
3. ...	• ...
4. ...	• ...

Below is a list of the objectives of the chapter which may be used as examples of for writing objectives.

After completion of this chapter, the reader will be able to demonstrate accomplishment of the following objectives.

1. Explain the teaching and training responsibilities of laboratory management.
2. Assess the educational and training needs of the laboratory.
3. Monitor compliance to regulatory requirements for education and technical competence documentation.
4. Develop a program of continuing education and staff development.
5. Identify needs and topics for continuing education and staff development.
6. Evaluate and improve effectiveness of training and educational programs.
7. Incorporate principles of educational and instructional methodology in the design and development of trainer programs.
8. Describe the learning process in relationship to the adult/professional student.
9. Write instructional objectives.
10. Select an instructional strategy for a CE program.
11. Develop course content parameters.
12. Use the tools of presentation.
13. Present a professional CE program.
14. Prepare a subject mastery demonstration method.
15. Design a program evaluation instrument.

In summary, and to repeat for emphases:

A = participant(s)

B = Cognitive (imparting knowledge): *assess/develop/incorporate/evaluate/monitor*

C = implied (*enabled from the course material*)

D = implied (*participation*), if a test is not planned as part of a *live* course, but may be required if in a self-study format..

(Here are additional web links for writing objectives) [connected July 11, 2007]

- https://www.uwsp.edu/education/lwilson/curric/behavior.htm
- http://edtech.tennessee.edu/~bobannon/classifications.html
- http://www.usuhs.mil/che/write_objective.htm

Instructional Strategy(s)

This section, and the rest of the course will focus primarily on live or "*speaker*" presented, classroom type programs. However, almost all of the information covered will also apply to writing or producing any educational project.

There are two approaches in which educational programs can be presented: ***teacher-centered*** or ***student-centered***.[15] Each approach has advantages and some disadvantages, and should be selected according to the topic and most conducive learning situation for the participants and objectives of the program. Often the educational event with use a combination of techniques, and many methods are complementary and may lead naturally into other approaches (*e.g., a training workshop with a lecture/demonstration breaking into a wet-lab session*). Deciding on which strategy depends on several factors including the nature of the subject mater, preparation or knowledge level of the student (*basic, intermediate, advanced*), the presentation skills and confidence of the trainer, and the physical resources available.

For example, when calibrating a new test on a chemistry analyzer a technologist may need:

- only housekeeping instructions (*here/where is the new calibrator, control, and documentation worksheet*) if they are familiar with the instrument (***student-centered***);
- direct, one-on-one, guidance if the test has a new methodology or calibrating procedure (***mix-strategy***); or,
- a classroom/group lecture and demonstration if it is a completely new technique (***teacher-centered***).

Teacher-Centered Approaches

In *teacher-centered* approaches the trainer is the featured performer and controls the class setting. Even though student participation is actively solicited and encouraged, the teacher is the primary provider of information and directly guides learning activities. These strategies place the instructor center stage and the attention of the student is directed toward them. [5b]

- **Lecture** The most common of all methods, the lecture permits the faculty to present specific information in a format were the time frame is defined and the student plays a passive role.
- **Demonstration** A familiar technique in the laboratory when introducing new procedures and methodology
- **Instructor directed discussion** A strategy used to direct participants toward specifically planed learning objects, or to reach conclusions identified by the leader.
- **Panel of experts**
- **One-on-one attention and training** This method is useful when working with new employees during orientation or training students at the bench

The major advantage of *teacher-centered* approaches is that a discreet body of material can be presented in an instructional unit. The harsh criticism is that it allows almost no live feedback from the audience as to their capture of the knowledge and limits participation to pre-determined instructional boundaries.

Student-Centered Approaches

Faculty in *student-centered approaches* plays a mentor or facilitator role with the student taking the lead in the educational program. This strategy provides a more natural androgogical, or participant directed style were the adult professional assumes control and responsibility for the learning exercise. Some example of student-centered approaches includes:

- **Student directed discussion** a topic of interest is discussed and explored by the group with the trainer providing only learning resources and passive direction.
- **Discovery (research) learning** the student is assigned a topic to investigate and frequently required to prepare a paper or presentation for the class.
- **Group projects** are similar to personal assignments, except performed within the context of group accountability and working in teams.
- **Individual directed learning** - textbooks, videos, instructional manuals, internet.
- **Role playing**; especially helpful in teaching soft (*people*) skills such as patient relationships, staff interaction, teamwork, and management styles. The leader sets up a scenario and allows the participants to play the key roles and gain experience in handling similar types of situations.
- **Simulation** for example, in the lab a demo instrument may be set up to provide the Techs with an opportunity to practice performing tests on extra samples and controls (*wet-lab format*).
- **Problem/case solving** is a good technique for provided hands on, practical experience working with real-live situations which the professional may encounter in the laboratory.

The major advantage of *student-centered* approaches is that it encourages the participants to be responsible for their own learning experience. Often, these strategies may require an even greater commitment in time and creative effort for the faculty. Without careful planning the sessions may wander off track, and not accomplish the mission of the learning exercise.

(*Advantages/ disadvantages of instructional strategies web sties)* [connected July 11, 2007]

- http://www.adprima.com/teachmeth.htm
- http://www.hcc.hawaii.edu/intranet/committees/FacDevCom/guidebk/teachtip/comteach.htm
- http://www.teaching.iub.edu/handbook_sect_toc.php?sect_id=s2

Course Content

There are several uses for the term: ***Course Content***. It may apply to a complete description of the course and activities which will occur (i.e., the ***syllabus***), which includes title, faculty, short descriptive sentence; objectives, topic outline, schedule, location, textbooks, test dates, and grading criteria. The term may also be used, as in this exercise, to refer to the part of the course description which contains an outline (***CONTENT/SUBJECT OUTLINE***) of the subject mater to be presented. This section will also provide a review of a few of the factors influencing the selection and design of the actual content boundaries of the course.

Since you could write volumes of books and obtain advanced degrees in almost any area (*cell morphology, e coli, Lewis antibodies, thyroid function testing, urine crystals*), developing the specific "*depth and breadth*" of what will be included in an instructional unit requires planning. Most all of these decisions concerning the scope of the subject(s) which will be included in the presentation have been made when ***writing the course objectives***. There are several additional parameters which will "*set the boundaries*" of the selected topic. These include:

Time frame – is it a one time narrow topic in-service session designed to be presented in one hour, or multiple classes such as a training program or college course which will have many meetings?

Subject/Topic – the nature of the topic itself will set the parameters expected to be covered. A narrow topic, such as RBC morphology review for laboratory professionals may be satisfied with a one session slide show; while identifying RBC parasites (*malaria*) may require several classes for the same audience.

Level of Instruction (*basic, intermediate, advanced*) - as mention in the subject/topic point, the knowledge level of the audience will also define the depth of the course content. Experienced technologists will require a minimal introduction to the topic, while novice laboratorians may desire a more elementary review.

Resources - attendance opportunities for busy laboratories, class room size and layout, projector and instructional material (*slide shows, videos, etc.*), preparation time (*must all material be created by the instructor, or are there prepared packaged programs-material available*) are all factors which will limit the boundaries of the course content.

Course Content Suggestion

The Three Point Principle – a very practice guide for presenting a one hour in-service or speaking at a conference is the "*three point principle*." This is a strategy recommended by many professional speakers' organizations like Toastmasters and National Speakers Association. [17, 18] Basically it suggests that this type of short program content be organized into five parts:

- Introduction
  - Point one
  - Point two
  - Point three
- Conclusion

For example, an outline of a course content for a slide-review of urine crystals morphology:

I. Introduction
II. Crystals which appear in Acid Urine
III. Crystals which appear in Alkaline Urine
IV. Crystals which appear in either Acid or Alkaline Urine
V. Review and ID differential tips

Trying to include more than two or three points (*e.g., like details on chemical methods to verify crystal ID or cellular elements*) in a one hour session may not allow time for a questioning and answering period, or permit the trainer to focus on an area of particular interest to the participants.

Classroom Support

Almost all of the audio-visual aids formerly common to classrooms have now been automated with the computer. Even blackboard/flipcharts (now *called an electronic interactive "whiteboard")* and overheads (*e.g., network document camera*) are now projected live onto an overhead screen, transmitted to individual computers, or posted on the web for current or later use.

What kind, and how much, support material to provide a class is a highly flexible option. Handouts and screen projects may vary from a simple outline of key points, to detail instructional and step-by-step procedures. It depends entirely on the objectives of the course, the needs of the audience, and the comfort level of the speaker. The use of highly detailed material appears to be the standard in presenting highly technical topics often offered in the laboratory.

If the session is a "*wet-lab*" type workshop where the trainer is acting mainly in a consultation or resource role, the support material may need to be highly detailed. However, if the session is a *teacher-centered* session most experts recommend the minimization of projection material so that that the audience will focus on the speaker rather than what is on the screen. In this case noted speaking and presentation expert, Reid Buckley, propose putting the money into the handout or package the audience will take with them rather then distracting from the presentation with abundant visual displays.

Buckley states *"Do everything possible to abolish slide shows, overhead projection, flip charts, and other visual aids"* [19, p54] He is speaking specifically about soft skill type presentations (e.g., *supervision/management/people skills*), and especially when persuasion or consensus building (*e.g., budgeting, new instrument selection, policy implementation/changes*) is the primary objective of the program leader.

In instructional and training situations, however, the strategy may need to be significantly different, and support material may serve to augment and reinforce the learning experience and may be essential in demonstrating the subject. In this case, detailed workbooks and precise projections may be needed to achieve the training objectives.

Handouts

Support material can be divided into two categories; Handouts and visual aids. *Handouts* refer to any material which the participant can use during the presentation and take with them from the class. Handout content may be duplication of the visual aids used during the presentation or include extensive support material such as copies of articles and step-by-step workbook. The key to preparing handouts is to provide material which will support the instructional strategy of the faculty, while not distracting participants from the activities being presented.

Visual Aids

Visual aids may range from material which has been previously prepared for the class by the instructor, or they may be used concurrently in the classroom to record and illustrate the instructional activity. Slides, overheads, pre-printed flipcharts, and programs like PowerPoint (® Microsoft) may be produced before the class and allows the instructor to customize each presentation. Writeable flipcharts, overheads and blackboards are available both as standard items and electronic devices to use live during the session. There are advantages and disadvantage of each method, and they should be selected to support and reinforce the learning experience of the participants. Their use is obviously also governed by the facilities available and the experience of the instructor. Additional suggestions may be found in the books listed in the bibliography and websites *links* listed here. [connected July 11, 2007]

- http://www.hcc.hawaii.edu/intranet/committees/FacDevCom/guidebk/teachtip/visuals.htm
- http://www.ljlseminars.com/flipchrt.htm
- http://www.ljlseminars.com/transp.htm

It is common for pre-packaged training programs to be made available for the laboratory. Instrument and commercial test manufacturers often provide education material which include interactive CDs, workbooks and instructional material for in-laboratory presentations. Soft skills programs with trainer guidebooks are abundantly available, as well as packaged safety and regulatory programs. The person planning the course should not hesitate to take advantage of these opportunities.

Presentation Skills

So you are ready to do it ...

- studied, planed, created, prepared great overheads and handouts, put in a lot of practice time ...
- and now here you are in front of a group of your laboratory peers, all eagerly waiting for you to start ...

Here are a few tips for this moment.

Physical Facilities

Make sure you are comfort with the room and all equipment. Arriving early permits you to check everything in advance, and give yourself the security it will work as intended.

Your Appearance

Dress and groom comfortably, but professionally.

The Delivery

Everything combines to form the success of the presentation. Eye contact, body language, facial expressions, pacing, timing, and the energy level exhibited by the trainer all blend in communicating the message. Each of these items may be rehearsed and mastered by experienced speakers, but for the novice the important thing is being prepared and at ease with your subject and equipment.

Think about the programs you have attended. Your attention was probably focused on the topic and how well you understood the information being presented; not on judging the speaker or concerned with how they may be dressed and talk. That's the key to your delivery. There are many excellent books and websites with tips and suggestions (*see bibliography and links*) and all are unanimous in this point:

> ***be yourself**, and focus on presenting your subject with decisiveness and confidence. Remember, like you, the audience is pulling for your success.*
>
> (*Web link resources*) [connected July 11, 2007]
>
> – http://www.public-speaking.org/public-speaking-articles.htm#topic
>
> – http://www.abacon.com/pubspeak/

Script or Outline

The extent to which a speaker writes or prepare prompt notes for a presentation will depend entirely on the preference and experience of the individual. From the author's personal experience, when doing a teleconference or situation were a live audience is not physically present to provide feedback or speaker interaction (i.e., a teleconference), a scripted (word-for-word) text is recommending since there are no feedback , communication, or acknowledgement signals being received concerning how you are doing. For group sessions, especially were there may be active participation, an annotated outline or PowerPoint (® Microsoft) format may provide the most support and flexibility. The details of the notes, once again should be at a level which permits the speaker to be comfortable and able to respond with the audience flow which may develop.

Stage Fright

Here are a few words about *stage fright* and the anxiety which is the natural process of any performance. Stage fright is usually caused when the artist continues to dwell on what can go *wrong*, rather then concentration on preparing the practical aspects of the performance (*the cure*) which will build their confidence. The reader is referred to the bibliography and *links* for more specific suggestions; however, some common tips include being well rested, avoiding carbohydrates, doing something you like to ease your mind (*hobby*) before the session, arriving at the site early enough to be familiar with the room and equipment, and talking with members of the audience before starting to get the reassurance and sense of working with *"people."*

(*Stage Fright Web link resources*) [connected July 11, 2007]

- http://www.public-speaking.org/public-speaking-stagefright-article.htm
- http://www.stresscure.com/jobstress/speak.html

Objective/Criterion-Reference Mastery Demonstration

A general rule in awarding CEU *"credit"* depends to a great extent on whether the program is a live presentation or a self-study type. If a session is presented with a live interactive speaker then attendance or participation may be sufficient to demonstrate mastery of the subject material depending on the design of the course. In a self-study format, such as on the internet or hardcopy (text or workbook) then something may be needed to be submitted to the sponsor to verify completion. In programs which require documentation, it is usually in the form of a "*test*." However, a written assignment (*report*), wet lab, project (*individual or group*), observation checklist, or other method may be useful in validating that the student has mastered the training objectives.

In either situation, live or self-study, feedback and assessment should be an active part of the learning process, flowing in both directions toward the trainer and the student. North Central Regional Educational Laboratory advises for effectively Incorporating Assessment Into the Learning Process — *"To allow students to construct learning in the classroom through authentic experiences, assessment must be:*

1. *Open-ended, allowing for discussion and revision of new understanding.*
2. *Tolerant of divergent thinking and promote the notion of no 'one right answer.'*
3. *Presented in alternative modes, not just paper-and-pencil responses to limiting questions.*
4. *Designed to foster analysis, comparison, generalization, prediction, and modification.*
5. *Capable of promoting collaboration and team effort in demonstration of competence.*
6. *Ongoing and cumulative, showing growth over time."* [20]

These may appear to be challenging suggestions but in live sessions a continual strategy of *question and answer* probing provides the leader and participant with real-time feedback to gauge how they are progressing. As computer designed programs become more sophisticated and interactive, continual personal appraisal assumes an increasing important role.

There are no strict rules concerning how many questions/per contact hour is appropriate. Perusal of CEU articles and courses show that a range from four (4) to 20 questions for each contact hour awarded is common (**0.1** CEU). Logical guidelines would suggest that there be at least one question for each objective necessary to demonstrate mastery. The time needed to complete the test would also be a consideration, and this time is included in the CEU awarded. For example in an one hour program (***1*** *contact hour/****0.1*** *CEU awarded*), if a test is expected to take 10 minutes to complete, then only 50 minutes would be available for the instructional portion.

— Ten (***10***) *class or instructional contact/clock hours =* ***1.0*** *CEU.* —

Question type and length also vary. It may require a quick 30 seconds to answer a multiple choice question allowing more to be included in the test. Problems with a case or calculations may take 5 or more minutes to complete, and time allotments would allow for only a few questions. The key in writing test questions or selecting evaluating methods is to concentrate on the instructional objective(s) and documentation that it/they have been mastered.

Program Evaluation Instrument

An important tool for obtaining the participant's opinion on the class is the **program evaluation instrument**. This document provides the instructor and sponsor the opportunity to evaluate and collect suggestions about improving the course design, facilities, student handouts, and faculty. This form is frequently pre-printed by the agency awarding CEU credit, or each institution (hospital or laboratory) may have their own design.

The feedback form is usually designed as a questionnaire and asks the participant to rank each category on a scale (e.g., **1** poor/worst **...** to **...** **5** excellent/best). Opinions may be asked about:

- **Physical Facilities** (Room, temperature, layout, lighting, Rest Room, seating arrangement, etc.)
- **Course Design** (Handouts, objectives achieved, too much/little information for class time)
- **Faculty** (Knowledgeable, enough time for questions, speak clearly, respective to student's input)

Both the facilities (*air conditioning not working*) and the trainer may have a bad day, so the feedback instruments are normally accumulated and tabulated to identify trends and patterns, special problems areas, and implement suggested improvements.

Summary

To emphasize the points discussed in this exercise, the following list of Fink's Five Principles of Good Course Design is provided. It was developed by L. Dee Fink who states that *"A 'good course' is one which meets the following five criteria*:"[21]

1. Challenges students to HIGHER LEVEL LEARNING. "*... include problem solving, decision making, critical thinking, and creative thinking."*

2. Uses ACTIVE FORMS OF LEARNING. *"One learns to solve problems by solving problems; one learns to think critically by thinking critically; etc."*

3. Gives FREQUENT and IMMEDIATE FEEDBACK to students on the quality of their learning.

4. Uses a STRUCTURED SEQUENCE OF DIFFERENT LEARNING ACTIVITIES. *"Any course needs a variety of forms of learning (e.g., lectures, discussions, small groups, writing, etc.), both to support different kinds of learning goals and different learning styles."*

5. Has a FAIR SYSTEM FOR ASSESSING AND GRADING STUDENTS. "*The grading system should be objective, reliable, based on learning, flexible, and communicated in writing."*

All five of these principles must be included in the course design. To review: make sure that the subject material in the course content achieves the objectives of the course; fits into the available time limitations; consists of only two or three content points per hour; matches the knowledge level of your audience; and, uses several instructional strategies to achieve its educational goals.

This chapter, *Education and Training of the Laboratory Professional,* completes **Part II** of the book on the Management of Human Resources. Next is **Part III**: Management of Financial Resources, and begins with Chapter 13, *Revenue and Cost Accounting for Medical Laboratories.*

Due to the many examples provided within the chapter, there is no separate case study.

Bibliography (Chapter 12)

[This chapter was originally presented as a course on PriorityEd.com, and has some specific chapter bibliography provided below]

(1) Varnadoe, Lionel; Medical Laboratory Management and Supervision; F.A. Davis, Philadelphia, 1996 [1st edition]

(2) College of American Pathologists, Standards for Laboratory Accreditation, *Standard I, Interpretation*, *A.* Qualifications, Responsibilities, and Role of the Director, 12. Educational Responsibilities http://www.cap.org/lap/standards.html [initial reference source contact [December 12, 2006]

(3) Medical Laboratory Technology Online (*brochure*), St. Petersburg College (Florida), www.spcollege.edu/hec/medlab, polanskyv@spcollege.edu [connected July 11, 2007]

(4) Huitt, William G.;A Transactional Model of the Teaching/Learning Process http://chiron.valdosta.edu/whuitt/materials/mdltlp.html [connected July 11, 2007]

(5) Honolulu Community College Intranet; *Common teaching methods* (note: this is an excellent site and includes suggestions and information on many instructional related subjects)
(a) http://www.hcc.hawaii.edu/intranet/committees/FacDevCom/guidebk/teachtip/active.htm
(b) http://www.hcc.hawaii.edu/intranet/committees/FacDevCom/guidebk/teachtip/comteach.htm
[connected July 11, 2007]

6) Columbia University, School of Nursing, Clinical Preceptor Guidelines; http://www.healthsciences.columbia.edu/dept/nursing/preceptors/process.htm [initial reference source contact December 12, 2006]

(7) Assumptions about the Adult Learner; Nebraska Institute for the Study of Adult Literacy http://literacy.kent.edu/~nebraska/curric/ttim1/aaal.html [connected July 11, 2007]

(8) Gibbons, Heather S., and George P. Wentworth; *Andrological and Pedagogical Training Differences for Online Instructors* http://www.westga.edu/~distance/ojdla/fall43/gibbons_wentworth43.html [connected July 11, 2007]

(9) Probyn, Laura; *Andragogy Links* http://www.msu.edu/course/aee/806/syllabus/8061999/andrag.htm [connected July 11, 2007]

(10) Kolb, David A.; Experiential Learning; Prentice-Hall, NY, 1984 (Association of Research Libraries, Washington, DC; Adult Learning Theory and Model) http://www.arl.org/training/ilcso/adultlearn.html [connected July 11, 2007]

(11) Dixon, Marilyn (manager); Adult Learning; Postgraduate Centre, Scarborough Hospital

http://www.scarbvts.demon.co.uk/adlearn.htm
[initial reference source contact December 12, 2006]

(12) Magruder, Kerry; Teaching Tips; Writing Objectives
http://www.okbu.edu/academics/natsci/ed/398/tips.htm
[initial reference source contact December 12, 2006]

(13) Distant Learning Resource Network (DLRN); *Chapter 4: Bloom's Taxonomy*
http://www.dlrn.org/library/dl/guide4.html
[connected July 11, 2007]

(14) Krumme, Gunter; Major Categories in the Taxonomy of Educational Objectives (Bloom 1956)
http://faculty.washington.edu/krumme/guides/bloom.html
[connected July 11, 2007]

(15) O'Bannon, B.; Planning for Instruction, Writing Objectives
http://edtech.tennessee.edu/~bobannon/writing_objectives.html
[connected July 11, 2007]

(16) Confex; Guidelines for Writing Learning Objectives
http://apha.confex.com/apha/learningobjectives.htm
[connected July 11, 2007]

(17) Toastmasters
http://www.freenet.edmonton.ab.ca/toast/plan.html
[initial reference source contact December 12, 2006]

(18) National Speakers Association (NSA)
http://www.nsaspeaker.org/
[connected July 11, 2007]

(19) Buckley, Reid; Strictly Speaking; MGraw-Hill, NY, 1999

(20) North Central Regional Educational Laboratory; *Incorporating Assessment Into the Learning Process*
http://www.ncrel.org/sdrs/areas/issues/content/cntareas/science/sc3asses.htm
[connected July 11, 2007]

(21) Fink, L. Dee; Fink's Five Principles of Good Course Design;
http://www.hcc.hawaii.edu/intranet/committees/FacDevCom/guidebk/teachtip/finks5.htm
[connected July 11, 2007]

— also — "Oral Presentations for Health Care Professionals," in Swayne, Linda E., W. Jack Duncan, and Peter M. Ginter; Strategic Management of Health Care Organizations; Blackwell Publishing, Malden, MA; 2006. pp. 459 – 478.

PART 2: BIBLIOGRAPHY

This book is presented as a 2nd edition, revision, update, additional text content, and sequential of: Varnadoe, Lionel A; Medical Laboratory Management and Supervision: *Operations, Review, and Study Guide*; F. A. Davis Company, Philadelphia; 1996. Following is the initial bibliography (pp. 141, 142) plus additional current citations.

Ackerman, L: A trail through the motivation jungle with apologies to those who blazed it. Clinical Laboratory Management Review 6:3, 1992

Alder, RB: Communicating at Work, 4th ed. Mc-Graw-Hill, New Your, 1992 [8th ed (2004)].

Beach, DS: Personnel: The Management of People. Macmillan Publishing, New York, 1991. *[no updates found during internet search July, 2006]

Bette, L: Developing Performance Standards for Hospital Personal. ASCP Press, Chicago 1989. *

Best, ML: Medical technologist: Changing Roles in a Changing Environment; Laboratory Medicine 24:7, 1993.

Blake, RR, and Mouton JS: The Versatile Manager. Richard D. Irwin, Homewood, Ill, 1981. *

Blake, RR, and McCanse, AA: Leadership Dilemmas-Grid® Solutions. Gulf Publishing, Houston, 1991. *

Blumstein, Rachel; Everything You Need to Know About Public Speaking; The Rosen Publishing Group, Inc., New York, 2000

Bott, Paul; Testing and Assessment in Occupational and Technical Education; Allyn and Bacon, Old Tappin, NJ, 1995

Cascio, Wayne; Managing Human Resources, 7th ed.; McGraw-Hill/Irwin; Boston, 2006.

Charan, Ram; Know-How; Crown Business; NY, 2007

Chruden, HJ, and Sherman, AW Jr: Managing Human Resources, ed 7 [8]. South-Western Publishing, Cincinnati, 1984. *

Cook, JF: Compensation for Laboratory Personnel: Action Alert: A Tool for Laboratory Manager. American Society of Clinical Pathologists, Chicago, 1993. [ASCP]

Costa, Art; Performance Assessment [*videorecording*]; Agency for Instructional Technology, Bloomington, IN: 1993.

Dawson, KM, and Dawson, SN: The Cure for Employee Malaise—Motivation. Clinical Laboratory Management Review 5:4, 1991.

DelPo, Amy and Lisa Guering; Dealing With Problem Employees, 2nd ed; NOLO, Berkeley, CA; 2003.

Desberg, Peter and George D. Marsh; Controlling Stagefright(sic);
New Harbinger Press, Oakland, 1988

Drummond, Mary-Ellen; Fearless and Flawless Public Speaking;
Pfeiffer & Company, Amsterdam, 1993

Edelson, Paul Jay and Patricia L. Malone; Enhancing Creativity in Adult and Continuing Education: *Innovative approaches, methods, and ideas*;
Jossey-Bass, San Francisco, 1999

Elizabeth, Mary; Painless Speaking; Barron's, Hauppauge, NY, 2003

Encina, Gregorio Billikopf; Performance Appraisal;
http://www.cnr.berkeley.edu/ucce50/ag-labor/7labor/06.htm
[connected July 8, 2007]

Fleisher, Charles H.; Employer's Rights, Sphinx Publishing, Naperville IL 2004

Fried, Bruce J., and James A. Johnson, eds.; Human Resources in Healthcare; AUPHA Press, Washington, D.C., 2002

Hamon, CJ, Synder, SL, Wilson, and Speecher, CD: Job Satisfaction of Clinical Laboratory Personnel under two Performance Reward Systems. Clinical Laboratory Science 4:5, 1991

Harmening, Denise; Laboratory Management: Principles and Processes;
Prentice Hall, New York, 2003

Harvard Business Review: Appraising Performance Appraisal. Harvard Business School Publishing, Boston, 1991. *

Heisler, WJ, Jones, WD, and Bingham, PO: Managing Human Resources Issues, Jossey-Bass, San Francisco, 1988. *

Hersey, P, and Blanchard, KH: Management of Organizational Behavior, ed. 5 [8]. Prentice-Hall, Englewood Cliffs, NJ, 1988.

Hilgert, RL, and Haimann, T: Supervision, Concepts, and Practices of Management. South-Western Publishing, Cincinnati, 1991. *

Kari, KR, and Feichert, JD: Occupational reinforcers for Medical Technologists in Clinical Laboratories: 1966 and 1987. Clinical Laboratory Science 2:6, 1989.

Kirkpatrick, A.L.; Complete Speaker's and Toastmaster's Desk Handbook;
Impetus Press, Orlando, 1993

Levinson, DJ: The Seasons of a Man's Life. New Your, Knopf, 1978. *

Lucas, Stephen E.; The Art of Public Speaking; McGraw-Hill, Inc.,
New York, 1992

Maier, NRF: The Appraisal Interview: Three Basic Approaches. University Associates, San Diego, 1976. *

Manzoni, Jean-François, and Jean-Louis Barsoux; The Set-Up-To-Fail Syndrome; Harvard Business School Press; Boston, 2002

Mathis, Robert L. and John H. Jackson; Human Resource Management, 11th ed; Thomson South-Western, Mason, Ohio; 2006.

Mohrman, AM, Resnick-West, SW, and Lawler, EE: Designing Performance Appraisal Systems: Jossey-Bass, San Francisco, 1989. *

1995 Florida Employment Law Manual, Survival Guide No. 7. American Chamber of Commerce, Chicago, 1995. [Florida and Federal Employment Law Manual Survival Guide, 2006. Ceridian Publishers]

Organ, DW: The Subtle Significance of Jab Satisfaction. Clinical Laboratory Management Review 4:2, 1990.

Panning, Rick and Beverly Farrell; Performance Appraisal Process — What to expect as a laboratory professional; www.ASCLS.org
http://www.ascls.org/jobs/grads/performance_appraisal.asp
[connected July 8, 2007]

Patten, J, and Thomas, H: PAY: Employee Compensation and Incentive Plans. The Free Press, New York, 1977. *

Reisman, Karen Cortell; Speaker's Notes, *Confidence can be delivered with the right touch*; Presentations, Vol. 17, No. 8, August, 2003. p.58

Sheehy G: Passages. EP Dutton, New York, 1974. *

Sibson, RE: Compensation, ed 5*. American Management Association. New York, 1990.

Spencer, CT, and Halinski, RS: Statistical Analysis of Job Level and Job Satisfaction of Clinical Laboratory Scientists. Clinical Laboratory Science, 3:3, 1990.

Stein, David, et. al.; The New Update on Adult Learning; Jossey-Bass, San Francisco, 2001

Stoner, JAF, and Freeman, RE: Management, ed 5. Prentice-Hall, Englewood Cliffs, NJ, 1992. *

Timple, AD (ed): Performance. Facts on File, New York, 1988. [This book contains an excellent collection of articles on performance appraisals, particularly the section on appraisal feedback techniques.] *

U.S. Department of Labor; Employment Standards Administration Wage and Hour Division; *History of Federal Minimum Wage Rates Under the Fair Labor Standards Act, 1938 – 1996*, August 16, 2006; http://www.dol.gov/esa/minwage/chart.htm [connected July 8, 2007]

Varnadoe, LA: What Makes the Medtech Move? Lab World 31:2, 1980.

Varnadoe, LA: Motivation and the Medical Technologists. Laboratory Medicine 21:3, 1990.

Varnadoe, LA: Upward Mobility. MT Today 2:16, 1992.

Varnadoe, LA: Keeping Medical Technologists in the Workforce: Recruitment, Retention, and Motivation under CLIA'88. ASCP Teleconference Series 4985, October 6, 1993.

Vella, Jane Kathryn; Taking Learning to Task: *Creative Strategies for Teaching Adults*; John Wiley, Somerset, NJ, 2000

Wallace, M. Ann and Deanna D. Klosinski; Clinical Laboratory Science – Education and Management; WB Saunders, Orlando, 1988

Weisbord, MR: Productive Workplaces. Jossey-Bass, San Francisco, 1991 [sequence — Weisbord, Marvin R: Productive Workplaces Revisited: Dignity, Meaning, and Community in the 21st Century, 2004]

White, Erin; MANAGING (Column): For Relevance, Firms Revamp Worker Reviews; The Wall Street Journal; Monday, July 17, 2006, pp. B1 & B5.

Internet Provided Job Descriptions [connected July 8, 2007]

Medical Laboratory Supervisor 1/2
State of Oregon, Department of Administrative Services, Human Resource Services Division
http://egov.oregon.gov/DAS/HR/class/ccrt/spec/6825.pdf
http://egov.oregon.gov/DAS/HR/class/ccrt/spec/6826.pdf

Laboratory Supervisor
Duke University Health System Job Description
http://www.hr.duke.edu/jobs/descr_duhs/select.php?ID=5055]

Medical Technologist, Supervisor
Clinician Laboratories of Hawaii
http://www.clhlabs.com/page_server/Employment/Descriptions/2006D61558032505ED406D77F5.html

ALASKA NATIVE TRIBAL HEALTH CONSORTIUM
MEDICAL TECHNOLOGIST
http://www.anthc.org/mod/jobweb/pdf/07-167.pdf

ZRT Laboratory, LLC
Medical Technologists / Laboratory Scientist I
www.zrtlab.com/File.ashx?cid=1385

Indian River Medical Center
Medical Technologist II
http://www.careerbuilder.com/JobSeeker/Jobs/JobDetails.aspx?job_did=J7X3J66JF461588QPXZ&cbRecursionCnt=1&cbsid=29382a47ed41417cbc22762106759918-237233097-KC-5

Medical Laboratory Management and Supervision

Part 3: Management of Financial Resources

[13]

Revenue and Cost Accounting for Medical Laboratories

— Chapter Thirteen —

Business accounting has three primary aspects: (1) recording revenue (charges, fees, sales, government disbursements, donations, and so on) received and owed; (2) tracking expenditures and paying bills; and (3) analyzing financial information so that management and interested parties (banks, government, stockholders) can plan and control the operations of the business. These requirements apply to the laboratory as well as to all health care providers.

This chapter introduces the fundamentals of recording, reporting, and analyzing the finances of the medical laboratory. This topic is presented in three parts: basic accounting principles; revenue accounting; and, cost accounting. The role of accounting in laboratory management and the types of information required for both internal and external purposes are discussed. The chapter provides examples of financial statements and application of financial information to laboratory problems.

OBJECTIVES

After completion of this chapter, the reader will be able to demonstrate accomplishment of the following objectives.

1. Describe the role of accounting procedures in managing a laboratory.
2. Differentiate between financial and cost accounting and the financial documents of each method.
3. Identify sources of revenue and the accounting methods for recording income.
4. Perform fee- and price-setting techniques.
5. Determine revenue and testing volume for budgeting projections.
6. Apply the procedures available to analyze, allocate, and control laboratory expenses.
7. Use percentage and ratio methods for projecting and budgeting laboratory revenue and costs.
8. Develop a feasibility study, using the techniques of break-even analysis.

Chapter Highlights and Glossary of Key Terms

I. BASIC ACCOUNTING PRINCIPLES

A. Business organizations

For-Profit Companies: *Privately held companies in which the profits are distributed to the owners.*

Not-for-Profit Companies: Tax-exempt corporations usually organized to provide a social service (religion, charity, health care, etc.).

B. Accounting specialties

Financial Accounting: *The branch of accounting that records the financial activities of the organization.*

Cost (Managerial) Accounting: *The budgeting process of a firm that provides planning and operational information to managers.*

C. Financial accounting statements

D. The accounting equation

Accounting Equation: Assets = Equities

1. Assets

   Assets: *Resources that the firm uses to conduct its business.*

2. Equities

   Equity: *Claims on the assets of the organization, such as bills and owner interest.*

E. Recording of financial activity

1. Cash basis

   Cash Accounting Basis: *Bills are paid as they are presented, and revenue is counted when it is actually received.*

2. Accrual basis

   Accrual Accounting Basis: *An accounting method that attempts to measure net income for a particular period by "matching" expenses against revenues when services are actually rendered.*

II. ACCOUNTING FOR LABORATORY REVENUE

A. Revenue sources

1. Profit and cost centers

   Tax Equity and Fiscal Responsibility Act (TEFRA): A federal program that sets caps on the amount of revenue paid for health care expenditures.

2. Diagnosis related groups

   Diagnosis Related Groups (DRGs): A federal reimbursement system in which hospitals are paid based on the nature of the case, or illness, and not on the number of individual services provided to the patient.

   Profit Center: *A department that generates billable services.*

   Cost Center: *An area that provides services that benefit the entire institution but cannot be traced to an individual chargeable item.*

3. Sources of revenue

   Captive Revenue Tests: *Patient tests in which the patient has no choice of location.*

   Discretionary Tests: *Patient tests that may be obtained in a number of different locations, according to the patient's choice.*

4. Accounting codes

B. Fee and price setting

1. Reimbursement programs

   a. Prospective payment systems

      Prospective Payment System: *A program that pays a set amount per case or patient, regardless of the amount of care received.*

   b. Current procedural terminology codes

      Current Procedural Terminology (CPT): *A schedule of medical services and procedures listed by the American Medical Association.*

   c. Master charge description file listing

      Master Charge Description File Listing (MCDFL): *A menu of procedures and prices for services offered by a laboratory.*

2. Rate-setting techniques

   a. Hourly rate

      Hourly Rate: *A rate-setting technique in which a fee is charged based on the amount of time a service is used.*

   b. Surcharge/cost-plus

      Surcharge/Cost-Plus: *A markup is added to the cost of an item to arrive at a* *charge.*

c. Weighted-value basis

Weighted-Value Basis: *A weighted value is assigned to a test and then multiplied by a cost-per-weighted- unit factor.*

d. Historical method

Historical Method: *Current prices are increased by a specified percentage, based on estimated changes in costs and inflation.*

e. Competition and rate controls

C. Revenue budgeting

1. Growth-factor projection
2. Patient-day forecasts

Patient Day: *Each day that a patient stays overnight in the hospital.*

3. Revenue budget

III. ACCOUNTING FOR LABORATORY COSTS

A. The nature of costs

B. The behavior of costs

1. Variability of volume

a. Fixed costs

Fixed Costs: *Those expenses that do not fluctuate when the volume of work changes over a short term (e.g., daily or weekly).*

b. Semi-variable costs

Semi-variable Costs: *Costs that change in steps, based on more gradual changes in workload.*

c. Variable costs

Variable Costs: *Those expenses that respond directly to any change in work load.*

d. Total costs

Total Costs: *Total of fixed, semi-variable, and variable costs.*

2. Billable procedures

a. Direct costs

Direct Costs: *Test-specific costs.*

b. Indirect costs

Indirect Costs: *Costs remaining after direct costs have been identified and assigned.*

c. Unit costs

Unit Costs: *Total of direct and indirect costs per unit produced.*

C. Cost budgeting

1. Accounting codes
2. Cost projections and budget preparation
3. Cost comparison standards

D. Break-even analysis

Break-Even Analysis: The *identification of the point in sales volume, units, or revenue at which income matches total costs.*

1. Break-even point in test volume
2. Break-even point in revenue
3. Break-even point and profit requirements
4. Gross profit or gross margin

Basic Accounting Principles

Providing financial information is the primary task of the accounting process. An effective accounting system provides managers with three types of information (Horngren, p. 3):

1. Internal reporting to managers, for use in planning and controlling current operations
2. Internal reporting to managers, for use in strategic planning, that is, making special decisions and formulating overall policies and long-range plans
3. External reporting to stockholders, government, and other outside parties

The extent of documentation and expertise necessary to accomplish these three tasks varies, depending on the characteristics of the organization. Factors such as size, purpose, and nature of the business activities performed determine the type of accounting program necessary.

This section reviews five basic accounting principles: types of business organization, accounting specialties, financial statements, the accounting equation, and the recording of financial activity.

Business Organizations

Businesses such as hospitals and independent laboratories can be organized in several different ways, depending on whether the owner is a sole proprietorship (individual owner), a partnership, or a corporation with hundreds or even thousands of shareholders.

For accounting and tax purposes, corporations may be further differentiated. If they are privately owned and the profits from the enterprise are distributed to the owners, they are called **for-profit companies** and subject to all taxes. **Not-for-profit corporations** that are sponsored by government, charitable, religious, or educational organizations to serve a social cause have special tax-exempt status.

Many critics of not-for-profit organizations have pointed out that freedom from taxation is the only significant difference between the two concerns, because both types of institutions may offer identical services and compete for the same customer or patient. This is especially prevalent in health care, in which both for-profit and not-for-profit hospitals may operate in the same community. Their accounting methods and regulation obligations follow similar patterns, with tax reporting responsibility the only noticeable difference.

Accounting Specialties

Accounting is divided into two broad categories: financial and cost. **Financial accounting** is primarily dedicated to recording the "bottom-line" financial position of the organization; it is often referred to as the *scorekeeping function*. Its focus is on the cash flow and financial position of the firm. The end result of these efforts is recorded in three basic statements, of which the balance sheet is the most common.

The primary objective of **cost accounting** is to provide the manager with information to operate the business. *Managerial accounting* is another name given this branch of accounting because of its emphasis on analyzing and providing operational information. The most prominent document generated by cost accounting is the budget. Statements used in financial accounting are discussed next, and the budgeting process is covered in Chapter 15.

Financial Accounting Statements

There are three main financial accounting statements: the statement of financial position, also referred to as the balance sheet; the statement of income and retained earnings; and the statement of flow of funds.

The statement of financial position or balance sheet is the best known document issued by a company (Figure 13 –1). Private and public organizations frequently publish these in newspapers or mail them to their members. You may have seen a copy of the balance sheet of your local bank, church, charity, or city government. You also prepared one when you balanced your checkbook, especially if you used the form on the back of the bank statement.

CENTRAL REFERENCE LABORATORY
Balance Sheet
September 30, 2xxx

Current Assets		Current Liabilities	
Cash	$ 1,225,692	Account Payable	$ 502,152
Account Receivable	21,774,460		
Less Allowances	8,164,071	Other Current Liabilities	2,170,785
Net Receivables	13,607,389		
Supplies	1,114,387	Total Current Liabilities	2,573,420
Other Current Assets	69,775		
Total Current Assets	16,017,243		
Investments/Other Assets		Long-Tern Debt	16,173,451
Property, Plant & Equipment			
Land	501,917	Deferred Income/Other Credits	
Buildings & Improvements	12,464,920		
Equipment	12,829,392	Depreciation Fund	8,759,474
Subtotal	25,796,229		
		Retained Earnings	10,653,573
Less Accumulated Depreciation	992,484		
Subtotal: Net Fixed Assets	24,803,745		
Intangible Assets	11,867		
TOTAL ASSETS	$40,832,855	TOTAL LIABILITY & RETAINED EARNINGS	$40,832,855

FIGURE 13 —1 . Statement of Financial Position (Balance Sheet)

The statement of income and retained earnings (Figure 13 – -2) and the statement of flow of funds are less familiar because they are of interest mainly to investors. These two statements are concerned with where the company gets its cash and how it makes a profit. The next two sections explain Figures 13.–1 and 13 —2.

CENTRAL REFERENCE LABORATORY Statement of Income (Loss) September 30, 2xxx		
Revenue		
Operating Revenue	$94,050,386	
Revenue Deductions	46,418,632	
NET REVENUE		$47,631,754
Expenses		
Operating Expenses	$39,573,618	
Depreciation	1,302,154	
Interest	826,949	
NET EXPENSES		42,002,721
NET INCOME		$ 5,629,03

Figure 13 — 2. Statement of Income and Retained earnings

The Accounting Equation

The balance sheet provides a snapshot of the economic status of the business at a specific time. There are two sides to the balance sheet: assets *(A)* and equities *(E)*. Recording and balancing these two sides provide the following *accounting equation*:

Assets *(A)* = Equities *(E)*
[i.e., A = E]

Assets

Assets are the resources that the firm uses to conduct its business. They are consumed-or in accounting terminology, they *expire* — in the day-to-day operation of the enterprise. Assets may be in the form of money as cash in the bank or accounts receivable (money owed the business for services rendered) or in the form of capital such as buildings or equipment. The asset side of the balance sheet is similar for both for profit and not-for-profit businesses.

Equities

Equities consist of two parts: *liabilities and remaining value*. Liabilities are the same for all enterprises and consist of bills owed or other obligations. The remaining value of the company can be described as either stockholder equity or retained earnings, depending on the type of corporate structure. In a privately owned business operated for a profit, the assets left over after all obligations are satisfied are labeled "stockholder equity" on the balance sheet. In a not-for-profit business the money or assets remaining after liabilities have been provided for is called "retained earnings." The accounting equations for these two corporations differ as follows:

For-profit
Assets = Equities
(Equities are *liabilities* + *stockholder equity* in **for-profit** companies)

Not-for-profit

Assets = Equities

(Equities are *liabilities* + *retained earnings* in **not-for-profit** entities)

Recording of Financial Activity

One additional concept is important to understanding the principles that guide accounting. This is the method used to record and report income and costs. Two standard techniques are used for this purpose: *cash* and *accrual bases.*

Cash Basis

In this plan, bills are paid as they are presented and revenue is counted when it is actually received, with no effort to assign costs and revenues to the effort and time frame in which they were generated. Most routine expenses and low-cost items used in the laboratory such as salaries, reagents, pipettes, and small instruments under $5000 such as microscopes and centrifuges are placed in the **cash accounting basis** category. Although this method is the simplest, it does not provide any information to the manager about the operations of the company or allow for projects that may extend over a long period of time.

Accrual Basis

The accrual accounting basis attempts to measure net income for a particular period by matching expenses against revenues. To accurately determine where costs and revenues are being generated and to predict expenditures and income — in other words, to budget — activities that incur expense must be charged to revenue items.

For example, when the laboratory purchases a major hematology or chemistry instrument, the initial cost is allocated (i.e., accrued) over the expected life of the instrument (say, 3 to 5 years), rather than being charged against a single year's expenses. This picture of the actual revenues and expenses that result from the acquisition of the instrument is much more realistic. If handled on a cash basis, such a purchase would result in high costs one year and unjustified profits the next. There may also be tax consequences, both advantages and disadvantages, to the accrual decision.

Accounting for Laboratory Revenue

Recording and monitoring a laboratory's income is a crucial managerial task. Understanding the nature of income, its sources, and how it can be enhanced leads to success in operations and an appropriately staffed and equipped laboratory. This section discusses profit and cost centers and recent changes in reimbursement rules that have affected the laboratory. Fees and budgeting procedures are also discussed, along with a review of methods for determining profitability of the laboratory.

Revenue Sources

In the past, departments could be segregated for budgeting purposes into either profit centers or cost centers. The laboratory was a major revenue-generating department for the hospital. The accounting strategy and management philosophy were different for each category, specifically in budgeting for revenue and capital equipment. But with the enactment of the **Tax Equity and Fiscal Responsibility Act (TEFRA)** in 1982 and **diagnosis related groups (DRGs)** in 1983, programs that covered Medicare and Medicaid patients, the health care industry had to rethink its accounting and income game plan.

Profit and Cost Centers

A **profit center** is a department that generates billable services; areas that provide services that benefit the entire institution but cannot be directly assigned an individual chargeable item are called cost centers. Radiology, Pharmacy, Physical Therapy, Nursing, and the Laboratory were considered profit centers in the past, whereas Housekeeping, Dietary, Engineering, and the Business Office were cost centers. Of course, this accounting classification was misleading because all areas generated their share of costs.

The departments that generated revenue were expected to provide sufficient income to support all the activities of the institution. The expenses of the cost centers were the major component of what is called "overhead" and were allocated to all areas of the institution.

Diagnosis Related Groups

With the advent of TEFRA and DRGs, hospitals were reimbursed for Medicaid and Medicare patients by the case or illness rather than on an open-ended fee-for-service basis. This *prospective* payment system, as it is formally called, is now being adopted by many third party payers, such as insurance companies and health maintenance organizations (HMOs).

With this government prospective payment system, the patient's DRG code classification, service intensity weights (SIWs), Trimpoints [*the low and high "trimpoints" are needed to determine if the claim is an in/outlier*] and average length of stays (ALOS) are used by the Medicaid Program to make DRG payments to hospitals. A factor, or wage index, applicable to the area where the hospital is located is also included in the calculation to arrive at a final reimbursement.

For a specific example of DRG reimbursement per region see:

Dept of health New York State

http://www.health.state.ny.us/nysdoh/hospital/drg/

[Connected August 24, 2007]

For example, the hospital might receive $2,701.90 [DRG 90] Medicare for all the services rendered to an adult patient admitted with pneumonia without complication. If the treatment costs exceed $2.700, the hospital loses money. If the cost is less than $2,700, it makes a profit.

But this payment plan applies to only some patients; others are still covered on an open-ended basis, depending on their insurance. This creates a hybrid accounting situation for the laboratory; it is perceived by the administration as both a cost center and an attractive source for additional revenue. The impact of this hybrid situation is directly related to the percentage of patients in each category. Table 13 – 1 provides examples of DRG codes and corresponding reimbursement levels.

List of DRG Relative Weight:

http://www.med.cmu.ac.th/hospital/drg/DRG.htm

[Connected August 24, 2007]

Sources of Revenue

In hospital-based laboratories, revenue has traditionally been divided into two sources to simplify the accounting process: inpatient and outpatient. These may be further subdivided, depending on the volume generated from various sources and the sophistication of the budgeting process. A more realistic view for today's laboratory manager is to view revenue as coming either from captive revenue tests or from discretionary tests.

Code	Description	Benchmark
057	Tonsillectomy &/or Adenoidectomy	$ 4,388.64
103	Heart transplant	$77,940.18
134	Hypertension	$ 2,425.97
167	Appendectomy	$ 3,664.17
232	Arthroscopy	$ 4,439.48
238	Osteomyelitis	$ 5,533.36
302	Kidney transplant	$77,940.18
307	Prostatectomy	$ 2,648.60
355	Radical hysterectomy	$ 7,909.72
371	Cesarean section	$ 2,934.37
372	Vag delivery w/complicating diagnoses	$ 2,491.57
391	Normal newborn	$ 626.07
396	Red blood cell disorders age 0—17	$ 4,744.93
397	Coagulation disorders	$ 5,033.98

Ref: MyHealthScore.com
INTELLIMED International, Corp
Hospital Inpatient Procedures
http://www.myhealthscore.com/frame.cfm?page=consumer/inpfeesearch.htm
(connected March 4, 2007)

Table 13 – 1. Diagnosis Related Groups (DRGs) Benchmarks for Hospital Inpatients Procedures

Captive revenue tests are tests in which the patients have no choice of location. This usually means procedures requested through the hospital for inpatients, outpatients, and emergency room patients.

Discretionary tests are those in which the client may select the location. Patients may be referred by physicians, outpatient departments, insurance companies, or industrial outreach programs. As is discussed in the chapter on Marketing, these are part of the revenue enhancement strategy of the laboratory.

Code	Section
100200	Miscellaneous
100210	Hematology
100220	Chemistry
100230	Microbiology
100240	Blood Bank
100250	Urinalysis
100260	Pathology
100270	Cytology

Table 13 – 2. Revenue Codes by Laboratory Section

Accounting Codes

All line items, including both revenues and expenses, in the laboratory budget are assigned accounting codes. The code is an arbitrarily assigned number, developed by the accounting department to simplify record-keeping. It usually has several parts that identify the laboratory subsection and nature of the item.

For example, inpatient revenue for the laboratory may be assigned an accounting code of 100200. The first three digits (100) may identify this as inpatient income, and the last three digits (200) may designate the laboratory. In very large institutions the code may also identify the laboratory section such as Chemistry or Microbiology. Table 13 – 2 gives examples of a coding system for a large laboratory that differentiates its revenues by section.

Fee and Price Setting

Setting fees and pricing services may appear to be a complicated matter, but in most respects running a laboratory is no different from running any other business: income must exceed expenses or the enterprise fails. In health care, many prices are either set in advance by government agencies or negotiated with insurance carriers that have pre-established guidelines for reimbursement. The laboratory manager is often requested to provide input into these deliberations and must be knowledgeable about how these charges are generated. The main types of reimbursement programs and rate-setting techniques are reviewed next.

Reimbursement Programs

Laboratories and health care organizations receive most of their revenue from direct payment by patients and insurance companies; prenegotiated payment plans, such as DRGs and other prospective payment plans; and third-party plans that pay a set amount for specific services, regardless of the charge.

Prospective Payment Systems

There are many different kinds of prospective payment systems (PPS).
Medicare's DRG system is the most notable example, but these plans also include health maintenance organizations, preferred provider organizations (PPOs), and various other plans negotiated by institutions with insurance and industry representatives. The programs have one thing in common: payment of a set amount per case or patient, regardless of the amount of care received. These plans allow their clients to choose services from a network of participating physicians and health care organizations. Patients may go to a provider outside the system, but they are usually reimbursed at a greatly reduced rate.

Both inpatient and outpatient rates are set by these plans. For example, DRG fees provide payment for inpatients; Medicare provides a list of charges allowed for outpatient or individual procedures. The level of payment is based on the care given, weighted to account for the difference in cost at different institutions.

For example, geographical location—rural or urban, northeast or southwest—may affect cost. This component of the program is widely contested, and the laboratory spends a lot of energy to ensure maximum reimbursement. In deciding whether to participate in a PPS or a managed care program, the hospital or laboratory must be aware of its total cost and revenue needs and decide if it can benefit financially from the relationship.

Current Procedural Terminology Codes

The fee schedule for PPSs, and for all third-party payers, is built around a schedule of services and procedures listed in a book published by the American Medical Association: *The Physicians' Current Procedural Terminology*, or CPT. This publication, updated annually, assigns codes for all medical procedures grouped according to common disease characteristics. To submit a bill for services rendered, the provider gives the CPT code for the test, and the agreed fee is then assigned.

These codes provide a standardized monetary value for services rendered. However, several problems have arisen in adapting these codes to the billing process because they were developed according to disease related criteria and not payment or service procedures.

Table 13 – 3 provides some examples of common laboratory tests and their corresponding CPT codes. The code numbers are formatted to identify the department and service. Pathology and the Laboratory have been assigned CPT codes in the 80000-89999 range. The numbers also identify the subsection of the laboratory that performed the test. Individual chemistry tests are found in the 82000 range, and surgical pathology procedures are given 88000 codes.

Code	Procedure
85025	CBC with differential
80053	Comprehensive Metabolic Panel
82947	Glucose
87088	Culture, Urine
81000	Urinalysis
85610	Prothrombin Time-INR
86900, - 86901, - & 86850	Type and Screen (includes ABO, RH, and antibody screen)
84703	HCG, Qualitative (serum)
86592	RPR
88164*	PAP Smear (Screen and Diagnostic)

REF: Legacyhealth.org
http://www.legacyhealth.org/body.cfm?id=130
Legacy Health System
[connected July 12, 2007]

*Medicare Reimbursement Rates for Indiana BCCP Screening and Diagnostic Services
As of March 1, 2003
http://www.in.gov/isdh/programs/bccp/pdf/cptcodes2003.pdf
[connected July 12, 2007]

Table 13 — 3 . CPT Codes for Laboratory Tests

Master Charge Description File Listing

Master Charge Description File Listing (MCDFL) is the technical name for the lists of services and their corresponding prices provided by a laboratory or hospital. This is commonly referred to as the "price list" and is the charge sheet consulted to answer a question from a patient about the cost of a laboratory procedure. Most MCDFLs have corresponding CPT codes that can readily be provided for insurance and billing purposes.

Rate-Setting Techniques

The American Hospital Association recommends three methods for establishing fees for medical services and several other techniques are commonly used.
Five methods are reviewed here: hourly rates, surcharge/cost-plus, weighted-value basis, historical, and competition.

Hourly Rates

The **hourly rate** method is used to set charges for the use of specialized areas such as surgical suites and labor and delivery rooms. Equipment such as respirators and heart monitors are also charged under this system.

To set an hourly rate, the total costs of the department and a projection of the total hours the service will be used are calculated to establish the amount of revenue necessary to cover the expenses of the department. From this figure a charge-per-hour rate can be determined. Although not normally applicable to laboratory services, associated charges may be needed in helping to set rates for PPS and managed care programs.

Surcharge/Cost-Plus

Surcharge/cost-plus is the most common procedure for establishing a charge and the method most retail businesses use. It is used for supplies or items that can be charged individually. Pharmaceuticals and other products are sold based on the cost of the article to the hospital, plus some monetary factor to cover expenses and obtain the desired profit margin. This method is referred to in industry as a "markup." The surcharge method is frequently used in the laboratory to charge for reference or send-out tests and to set in-house test fees.

For example, a reference laboratory charges a hospital laboratory $5 to perform a test. The hospital has established a policy of marking up the fee by 100 percent, or a minimum of $25 to cover phlebotomy, billing, and clerical handling expenses. The charge for this test to the patients is then $30. If the reference fee is $40, the hospital charges its patients $80.

This procedure can also be used to recommend the charge for in-house testing. The first step is to establish the cost of doing the procedure. A markup factor is then added to arrive at the appropriate price. The following example illustrates the surcharge/cost—plus application:

Direct Costs	
Supplies/reagents	$ 0.69
Labor: tech time	0.99
Labor: phleb time	0.49
Instrument depreciation	0.12
Indirect Costs	
Laboratory overhead	5.13
Hospital overhead	6.00
	$13.42

Markup factor = 400%
Charge for CBC = $53.68 (13.42 **x** 4)

Weighted-Value Basis

Weighted-value basis is of more theoretical than practical use because of its complicated and difficult formulation. It is recommended by the American Hospital Association for use by ancillary services such as laboratories and radiology departments. It is particularly suspect because it is based on the financial goals of the laboratory, not on the individual cost of delivering a specific service.

The weighted-value basis involves the following steps:

1. The financial requirements of the laboratory are established by determining the historical direct and indirect costs expended. To this number is added the profit contribution required by the hospital or laboratory management to arrive at the total desired revenue.

2. Each test performed is assigned a relative weight based on the cost of performing that test in relationship to other procedures.
3. After the test has been assigned a relative weight, the total number of weighted units produced by the laboratory is determined. This is done by multiplying the volume of tests performed by their assigned value and then totaling these values.
4. The revenue needs of the laboratory (step 1) are then divided by the total number of units produced (step 4) to arrive at a cost-per-weighted unit factor.
5. This factor, which is in dollars, can then be used to establish the necessary charge for a procedure by multiplying the assigned weighted value by the cost per weighted unit. Figure 12-3 gives an example of this weighted-value method.

Procedure	Annual Volume	Assigned Weight Value	Total Weighted Units
Prothrombin Time	7,665	1.4	10,731
Fasting Blood Glucose	4,015	1.1	4,417
Weighted units for all other tests			757,400
Total Number of Weighted-Value Units for the Lab			772,548

Revenue Needs of the Department

Expenses (Direct/Indirect) and Overhead $10,429,398

Revenue Factor per Weighted Unit: $\frac{\$10{,}429{,}398}{772{,}548} = \$13.50$

Prothrombin Test Charge = $18.90 (1.4 **x** $13.50)

Fasting Blood Glucose Charge = $14.85 (1.1 **x** $13.50)

FIGURE 13 – 3. Weighted Value Method of Rate Setting

Historical Method

In practice, many facilities simply raise their prices annually by a certain percentage based on the rate of inflation and income needs. This is the main reason that laboratories may list a charge for a CBC at $54 when the actual incremental cost to perform the test may be only 54 cents. If you start with a laboratory charge of $5 for a CBC in 1970 and raise it by only 10 percent each year for 25 years, this would result in a charge of $59.59 in 1995. Of course, there are numerous factors that limit the laboratory's ability to just raise rates at will every year, including rate controls imposed by government agencies and, most notably, competition.

Competition and Rate Controls

Many factors determine what the laboratory may actually receive or charge for a test. Most laboratories have a sliding scale based on such determinants as volume, method of payment, competition from other laboratories, and certainty or timeliness of payment. For example, a laboratory may receive six different amounts for doing a CBC on an outpatient, with an MCDFL price of $99.00.

Medicare patient:	$ 4.90
Insurance payment:	$ 7.50
Industry negotiated:	$20.00
Payment at time of service by patient, *30% discount for cash*	$69.30
Payment from billing a patient:	$99.00
No payment (bad debt):	$ 0.00

Revenue Budgeting

Several concepts and terms reviewed here are important in establishing the revenue budget for the laboratory. These include arriving at a growth-factor projection, patient-day forecasts for hospital-based laboratories, gross profit margin calculations, and the actual revenue budget itself.

Growth-Factor Projection

The laboratory manager must make forecasts of future volume for revenue budgeting purposes. The latest year-to-date records and a growth factor arrived at by extrapolating from previous growth rates can be combined to project future volume.

For example, if the volume of testing for the laboratory has grown an average of 8 percent for the past 3 years, the manager may realistically determine that this trend will continue. This figure should be adjusted for any anticipated factors that may change this growth rate, such as new services offered, hospital expansion plans, closing of beds, or new industries that may increase the population of the town.

Year-to-date test volume = 357,199
Growth-factor projection = 0.08 (8%)
Volume budget forecast = 385,755 (357,199 X 1.08)

Patient-Day Forecasts

In projecting the amount of revenue the laboratory will receive during the next budgeting period, a prediction of volume is necessary. This volume should be obtained from the master budget predictions for the laboratory (growth factor) or the institution as a whole. Budget volume levels obtained from the institution will most likely be in the form of a projection of patient days, or average census.

Each day a patient stays in the hospital overnight is defined as a **patient day**. If there are 181 patients in the hospital on a given day, the patient days for that day equal 181. With an average census of 180 patients each day during June, the patient days for the month would be 5400 (180 **x** 30). If the average daily census for the year is 178, then the patient days for the year would be 64,970 (178 **x** 365).

Frequently other service factors, such as outpatient treatments and emergency room visits, may be included in a formula to arrive at an adjusted patient days index. The calculations and factors included in this figure depend on the individual hospital's accounting decisions.

Revenue Budget

The final step in preparing a revenue budget for the laboratory is to obtain an estimate of test volume and income. The manager should have available the total number of tests performed, the gross revenue for the laboratory, and the patient days for the current budget period if the laboratory is hospital-based. This information can be used to calculate two ratios: tests per patient days for hospital-based laboratories and revenue per test. These ratios are then available to determine the volume and gross revenue of the laboratory for the coming budget year.

Figure 13 – 4 demonstrates how to use these techniques to project the revenue and test volume budget monthly or yearly. First, the actual historical data for

<u>Actual Current Data Available</u>

Year-to-Date Patient Days (January—June)	35,940
Year-to-Date Test Volume (January—June)	357,199
Year-to-Date Gross Revenue (January—June)	$4,435,488

<u>Ratio Calculations</u>

357,199 /32.940 = 10.84 Test/Patient day
$4,435,488/357,199 = $12.42 Revenue/Test

<u>Budget Forecast</u>

Patient Days Budgeted for month of August of Next Year	6,039
Total Patient Days Budgeted for entire New Year	78,104

<u>Laboratory Budget for Next Year</u>

Month of August:

Test Volume:	65,463 (6,039 **x** 10.84)
Department Revenue:	$813,050 (65,463 **x** $12.42)

Year:

Test Volume:	846,647 (78,104 **x** 10.84)
Department Revenue:	$10,515,355 (846,647 **x** $12.42)

FIGURE 13 — 4. Laboratory Gross Revenue and Volume Budget Forecast

testing and revenue are collected. This information is used to calculate ratios, which can be applied to the forecast volume as described previously. The formula for these ratios in the example is:

$$\text{Tests/patient day} = \frac{\text{test volume (357,199)}}{\text{patient days (32,940)}} = 10.84$$

$$\text{Revenue/test} = \frac{\text{gross revenue}}{\text{test volume}} = \$12.42$$

The laboratory revenue budget for the next year can then be obtained by applying the *tests/patient-days* ratio to the forecast patient days for a specific month <u>*or*</u> year to obtain **volume** projections [e.g., 6,039 $_{\text{(patient days forecasted for August)}}$ **x** 10.84 = 65,463 tests forecasted for August]. For total revenue expected, a straightforward *revenue/test* **x** volume calculation is performed [e.g., 846,647 $_{\text{(tests forecasted for the year)}}$ **x** $12.42 = $10,515,355 for the year].

Accounting for Laboratory Costs

This section reviews the accounting procedures for allocating and controlling expenditures, surveys methods used to evaluate the nature and behavior of laboratory costs, presents budgeting techniques for projecting spending levels, and discusses the role costs play in performing feasibility studies or evaluating laboratory services.

The Nature of Costs

In any enterprise, the control of expenses is an essential management function necessary to ensure solvency. The goal of cost accounting is to track where expenses are incurred and assign responsibility for their expenditure. This is also frequently referred to as "managerial accounting." Whereas financial accounting primarily supplies information to outside parties, cost accounting is focused on the operation of the business. However, even with these different objectives, the information sources and recording techniques used in financial and cost accounting are quite similar.

The Behavior of Costs

Defining and controlling costs can be approached and analyzed from two directions: by examining the influence of variations in testing volume (production) or by looking at the expenses involved in performing an individual procedure (billable procedure). Both evaluations are important to understanding the operations of the laboratory.

Variability of Volume

One method of studying the behavior of laboratory costs is to evaluate the impact of costs based on the workload of the institution. This perspective reveals that some costs do not vary, regardless of the amount of work, whereas other costs go up in direct proportion to the number of tests performed. In this model the costs of operating a laboratory are divided into three categories based on sensitivity to production volume or magnitude of variability. These categories are fixed, semi-variable, and variable.

Fixed Costs

Fixed costs are those expenses that do not fluctuate when the volume of work changes on a daily basis. They are predictable and are usually supportive in nature. Laboratory administration, instrument leases, maintenance contracts, computer services, equipment costs, and facilities upkeep are examples of fixed costs.

Semi-variable Costs

Semi-variable costs are costs that rise in steps, based on more gradual changes in workload. For example, when the laboratory hires an additional secretary or phlebotomist, labor expenses take a proportional jump; that is, salary costs go up a whole step increment, the salary of a full-time employee, rather than increasing gradually.

Semi-variable costs are sometimes called *marginal costs*, because the decision to spend the money is based on the marginal additional benefit the laboratory expects to receive from this addition.

Variable Costs

Variable costs respond directly to any changes in workload: As the volume of work increases, expenses rise in a direct and linear relationship. These costs are considered to be the most manageable and adjustable on a short-term basis.

Laboratory managers and section supervisors are usually held directly accountable for these budget items. Labor costs and supplies are the most notable examples of variable expenses.

Total Costs

Figure 13 – 5 illustrates how these costs interact to arrive at the total cost of operating a laboratory. The fixed costs provide a baseline, which is not affected by the production volume of the laboratory. From this point, total financial outlays rise in proportion to the number of procedures performed, as the laboratory buys supplies and employs personnel in response to the workload.

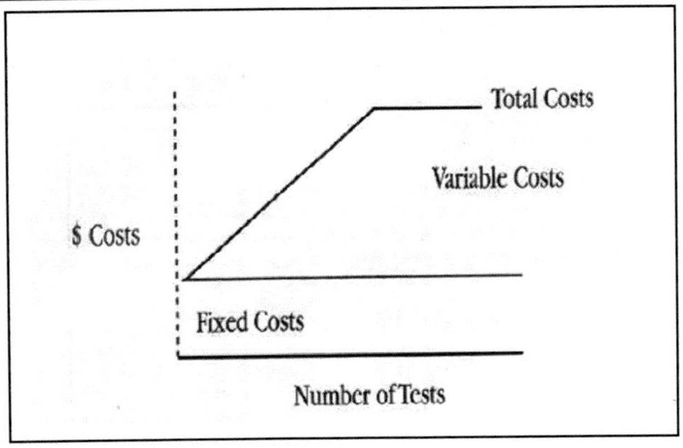

FIGURE 13 — 5. Behavior of Laboratory Costs

In applying these concepts, it is important to maintain a proper time frame. All costs, including fixed costs, are variable over the long run, as, for example, when a company goes out of business. In the same vein, variable costs are dependent on preserving a stable work force and a reliable inventory of supplies.
Even in slow times, the laboratory has to sustain a minimum level of staffing and supplies.

Billable Procedures

The other method used in evaluating financial outlays is to match the expenditures with the activity that produced the cost. A cost that can be traced to a particular procedure for which the laboratory can generate revenue is called a **direct cost**. An expense shared by many components of the institution is referred to as an **indirect cost**. These concepts are an important part of the process used in developing an operations budget.

Direct Costs

Direct costs are test-specific costs. They occur in direct proportion to the number of procedures performed or are directly attributed to the completion of the test. They are considered variable in nature and include supplies, instrumentation, reagents, and tech time.

Indirect Costs

Indirect costs are the expenditures that remain after direct costs have been identified and assigned. Hospital and laboratory administration, business office, medical records, housekeeping, physical plant maintenance, security, engineering, and utilities are examples of indirect expenditures.

Indirect costs are generally considered to be fixed or, in some cases, semi-variable, depending on the sophistication of the accounting and budgeting process. For this reason, some indirect costs are placed in a separate category, overhead. Under this system, indirect costs refer to costs that can be allocated directly to a specific area, such as the laboratory within a hospital setting. The term "overhead" then applies to institution-wide services such as administration and housekeeping, which must have their costs allocated to each area. Table 13 – 4 provides examples of methods of allocating overhead or indirect costs to individual departments.

Cost Center	Allocation Method
Utilities	Square footage occupied
Housekeeping	Number of hours needed or square footage
Central Purchasing	Dollar amount of supplies purchased
Laundry	Poundage used
Maintenance	Square footage or wok orders
Equipment deprecation	Life expectancy, usage, or straight-line rate
Human resources	Number of employees

TABLE 13 — 4 . Methods of Allocating Overhead or Indirect Costs

Also, depending on the sophistication of the budgeting process, all laboratory expenses may be considered directly or may be differentiated down to the section level. If the accounting system allows, section and department costs may be broken down into both direct and indirect costs. Tech time, consumable supplies, and other identifiable items are always assigned directly to the procedure. Supervisory time, support personnel, general quality control, educational leave, and lab computers are outlays that can be either grouped as overhead or allocated to a particular test. Because of computerization, costs are more readily categorized and managers are more aware of the source of costs.

Unit Costs

One additional term used in cost accounting is **unit costs**. By determining the total expense of performing a procedure, the laboratory can determine the economic feasibility of performing the service in-house versus sending it to a reference laboratory. Recommendations as to pricing and instrumentation can also be made. Unit costs are defined as the total of direct and indirect expenses.

For example, the unit cost of a Prothrombin time can be calculated as follows:

Direct expenses	$ 1.13
Indirect expenses	12.47
Unit cost	13.60
Reference lab charge	$10.00

By comparing these two costs, along with other factors such as turnaround time and reimbursement rates, the manager can make a more informed decision about allocation.

Cost Budgeting

This section reviews key elements in the preparation of the cost or expense part of an operational budget. The financial terms and methods associated with. this process are presented, including accounting codes, cost projection and budget preparation, and cost comparison standards from one laboratory to another.

Accounting Codes

For budgeting and recording purposes, cost items are assigned an accounting code, which is included in an accounting document called the *chart of accounts*. To an extent determined by the level of sophistication of the system, this number identifies the department or section that generates the costs and the expense itself.

For example, wages may be given the accounting code 333222. The first three numbers (333) identify this as an expense item for the laboratory, and the last three (222) assign it to salaries. Table 13 – 5 shows examples of *general ledger account control codes* with may be used for common laboratory costs.

Code	Cost Item
333222	Salaries
333333	Supplies
333444	Professional fees
333555	Educational expenses
333666	Travel
333777	Instrument maintenance contracts
333888	Instrument leases
333999	Miscellaneous

TABLE 13 —5 . Accounting Codes for Budgeted Cost Items

Indirect costs, including overhead, are prorated to the department based on an index developed to reflect the use of the service by the laboratory. Several allocation techniques are used for this purpose. Housekeeping services, for example, may be allocated based on the square footage of the department or on the percentage of housekeeping labor hours used to clean the laboratory. Personnel costs may be allocated according to the number of employees in each department. Table 13 – 4 (above) gives common indirect costs and how they may be allocated.

Cost Projections and Budget Preparation

There are three major techniques for forecasting the costs that need to be included in the budgeting process: percentage of revenue, index ratios, and actual expected (i.e., known) annual costs.

Calculating the percentage of revenue for each budget line item is a relatively straightforward method and the most widely used. Actual known costs (from contracts and so on) and the determination of a ratio for each line item per laboratory test are the remaining two options. Both the percentage and ratio methods should predict the same amount, because the revenue-volume baselines are developed from the same data (as discussed in the section on revenue budgeting).

Some projected costs such as travel, educational leave, and equipment rental and maintenance contracts should be readily available.

A sample budget projection using the percentage-of-revenue method follows:

Current year's revenue	$ 989,222	
Supplies	128,599	13% of total revenue
Reference lab	89,030	9% of total revenue
Other expenses	69,246	7% of total revenue
Projected revenue	$1,136,124	
Supplies	147,696	($1,136,124 X .13)
Reference lab	102,251	($1,136,124 X .09)
Other expenses	79,529	($1,136,124 X .07)

To this budget example would be added additional identifiable items such as service contracts, travel, and educational allowances, depending on the detailed breakdown required by the organization in the operational budget. (See Chapters 15 and 16 for further discussion of cost budgeting.)

Cost Comparison Standards

One of the most frequent concerns of laboratory managers who are evaluating and justifying their operational costs is, "How do I compare with other laboratories?" There are many methods by which laboratories can be compared. One method frequently used in the past was the College of American Pathologists' workload recording method (WLU, or workload unit). This program has now been discontinued and replaced with the more comprehensive laboratory management index program (LMIP), which offers more than 25 data areas to provide extensive information in productivity, utilization, and cost effectiveness. Other methods compare costs based on volume of tests, patient days, percentage of revenue, emergency room visits, and additional indicators of hospital size and activity.

Other indexes are frequently reported by the American Hospital Association and various other management consultant groups to compare operational factors.
The number of employees (salaries and payroll hours) per department, matched with institutions with similar characteristics (number of beds, average census, and so on) is a widely published index. The laboratory manager should be cognizant of the information available from these sources because hospital administration is familiar with these comparisons and may not understand programs unique to the laboratory.

Break-Even Analysis

Of universal concern to all managers is the economic viability of the organization in relation to financial performance and the feasibility of further projects. Cost accounting provides methods for the application of financial information to this evaluation with a group of techniques broadly referred to as **break-even analysis**. Break-even analysis identifies the point in sales volume at which revenues match total costs, and it is particularly important when calculating participation in managed care programs. If the company can expect to produce and sell products or services that exceed this point, it can expect a profit. If the revenues cannot cover the associated costs, the facility experiences a loss.

Two break-even points can be calculated for the laboratory using this system of analysis: test volume, or the number of units that must be produced and sold;
and the amount of revenue that must be generated to cover both the fixed and variable (total) costs.

Break-Even Point in Test Volume

To calculate the break-even point in test volume, use the following formula.

$$T = \frac{F}{A - V}$$

where T = number of tests that must be sold to break even
F = total fixed costs of the laboratory
A = average revenue generated per test
V = variable cost per test performed

Thus, if the laboratory has fixed costs of $40,000; a variable cost per test of $4: and, an average revenue generated per test of $21.50; the break-even point is 2,285 tests.

$$T = \frac{\$40{,}000}{\$21.5 - \$4} = \frac{\$40{,}000}{\$17.50} = 2{,}285 \text{ tests}$$

Break-Even Point in Revenue

To calculate the break-even point in revenue, use the following formula.

$$R = \frac{F}{CM}$$

where R = revenue in dollars needed to break even
F = total fixed costs of the laboratory
CM = contribution margin ratio, calculated as (A — V)/A

Thus, using the information in the example, the revenue needed to break even is $45,140.

$$CM = \frac{\$21.50 - \$4}{21.50} = 0.814$$

$$R = \frac{\$40{,}000}{0.814} = \$45{,}140$$

Break-Even Point and Profit Requirements

If the laboratory has a policy that any feasibility study must include a predetermined profit level *(P)*, then equations may be modified slightly to include this factor.

$$T = \frac{F + P}{A - V}$$

$$R = \frac{F + P}{CM}$$

Gross Profit or Gross Margin

Another ratio calculated from accounting data is the gross profit or gross margin. This ratio determines the excess of sales (charges, fees, and so on) above the direct costs involved in producing a product or service, either by individual test or for the entire laboratory.

Revenue — direct cost = gross profit

This calculation is useful in establishing pricing levels and market share. This figure can also be helpful in negotiating additional work at marginal rates. If the additional income covers the direct, or variable, costs of performing a test and makes a contribution toward covering the fixed expenses of the laboratory, it may make the project feasible. Gross profit is of limited use in determining the actual profitability of the enterprise, however, because it does not account for overhead.

For example, a nearby factory approaches the laboratory about testing its employees for $10, the same price as an out-of-town reference laboratory. The laboratory's direct cost for performing the test is $7 and total cost (fixed and direct) is $15.

Because the fixed costs of the laboratory will remain the same, the laboratory will have an additional $3 per test to help pay for this expense.

Gross profit: $10 — $7 = $3

Therefore, they should do the test.

This example completes *Revenue and Cost Accounting for Medical Laboratories*. The next chapter: *Salary and Wage Management*.

— Case Study —

Chapter Thirteen: Revenue and Cost Accounting for Medical Laboratories

"I need your help," said the laboratory manager to the chemistry supervisor. "Administration wants us to re-evaluate some of our charges based on current market conditions. She told me that we just could not keep increasing our costs by a certain percentage each year, because we were getting a lot of competition from the laboratory in the surgery center that opened across the street. We need to know just where we stand with costs and income. We thought it would be a good idea to do the basic metabolic chemistry profile (BMP) first, since that it one of the tests with the largest volume. Here's some financial information. See what you can do and get back to me soon.. We are having a meeting next week to finalize our proposal for the utility company's business, and I need them by then."

"I'll see what I can do," responded the supervisor.

"Thanks," answered the manager. "Let me know if you need any help."

Chapter Section for Review

- Rate — setting Techniques
    - Surcharge/Cost—Plus
    - Weighted—Value Basis
    - Competition and Rate control
- Break—Even Analysis
- Fixed Costs
- Gross Profit and Gross Margin

Questions for Discussion

1. Calculate the charge for the BMP using both the Surcharge/Cost—Plus and Weighted—Value Basis methods, using the figures below.
2. What is the minimum charge the laboratory can offer to compete for the utility company's business?

<u>FINANCIAL STATISTICS FOR THE BMP</u>

Supplies/reagents	=	$1.12
Laboratory overhead	=	$4.90
Revenue factor per weighted unit	=	$21.50
Instrument depreciation	=	$0.54
Labor: tech time	=	$1.79
Assigned weighted value	=	3.1
Hospital overhead	=	$7.50
Labor: phleb time	=	$0 (client will submit specimen)
Mark—up factor	=	400%

<u>SOLUTIONS</u>

<u>Surcharge/Cost—plus Method</u>

Direct Costs

Supplies/Reagents	$ 1.12
Labor: tech time	$ 1.79
Instrument depreciation	$ 0.54

Indirect Costs

Laboratory overhead	\$ 4.90
Hospital overhead	\$ 7.50
Total Costs	\$15.85
Mark-up factor	**x** 4 (400%)
Charge for BMP	\$63.40

Weighted Value Method

Revenue factor/weighted unit	= \$21.50
Assigned weighted value	= 3.1
Charge for BMP	= \$66.65 (\$21.50 **x** 3.1)

Gross Profit/Margin Analysis

Direct costs	= \$3.45
Revenue	= R (bid price for test)
Gross profit/margin	R — \$3.45r

Minimum Bid Price Option:
The laboratory must receive at least \$3.45 just to cover direct costs. Any amount above this point will contribute toward overhead and must be considered with other competitive factors. Obviously, the larger the gross profit margin, the more attractive the deal is to the laboratory.

[14]

Salary and Wage Management

— Chapter Fourteen —

Labor costs (salaries and wages) represent the largest single item in the laboratory budget. Industry surveys have shown that labor costs constitute more than 60 percent of laboratory expenditures. Therefore, salaries and wages receive significant attention in controlling and reducing laboratory expenses.

The management of this human resource is of interest not only because of its impact on the financial status of the institution but also because it is an important element in the delivery of a quality service. To ensure a well-trained, motivated, and stable workforce, the laboratory manager must look at staff needs from both motivational and productivity perspectives. This chapter looks at the nature of salary expense, productivity measurement, and the salary portion of the operational budget.

OBJECTIVES

After completion of this chapter, the reader will be able to demonstrate accomplishment of the following objectives.

1. Explain the three approaches to analyzing labor costs.
2. Identify and interpret indices to measure productivity.
3. Use productivity and financial information to make and justify staffing decisions.
4. Prepare wage and salary budget projections.

Chapter Highlights and Glossary of Key Terms

I. SALARY AND WAGE COST EVALUATION

A. Institutional labor cost evaluation

B. Technical evaluation of labor cost

Preanalytical Time: *The time involved in collecting the specimen and preparing samples and instruments.*

Analytical Time: *The time during which the test is actually performed and the results are calculated.*

Postanlytical Time: *The time in which the report is made and routine maintenance is performed.*

C. Accounting and budgeting labor costs

Total (Paid) Hours: *The total number of hours for which an employee is paid; includes actual time spent in the laboratory as well as benefits hours paid (productive plus nonproductive).*

Productive (Worked) Hours: *The actual house worked, including overtime.*

Nonproductive (Benefit) Hours: *Hours for which the employee is compensated but not available for work.*

D. Full-time equivalents
Full-time Equivalent (FTE): *An accounting calculation of the number of full-time employees represented by the payroll hours [number of hours ÷ 2080 (2080 = the number of hours a full time employee is scheduled to work in a year)].*

II. PRODUCTIVITY MEASUREMENT
A. The productivity model
Productivity Model: *Workload units divided by labor units.*
1. Selecting a productivity index
2. Selecting final productivity units
B. Billable procedures as a workload unit
Billable Procedure: *A test for which the laboratory may issue a charge.*
C. Standardized billable test
D. Weighted workload labor estimation techniques
Weighted Workload Labor Estimation: *A system that assigns a value (usually in a unit defined as 1 minute) to a specific task performed in a standardized manner, obtained by analyzing and timing each step in the production or performance process.*
1. Weighted workload procedures
2. Weighted workload value productivity calculations
E. Productivity standards

III. WAGE AND SALARY BUDGETING
A. Position control master
B. Wage Determination Methods and Budget Projections (Examples of Annualized and Monthly Projections

----

Salary and Wage Cost Evaluation

Three approaches are available to analyze labor costs: (1) institutional, which examines personnel in terms of employment relationships; (2) technical, which looks at work flow and tasks performed; and, (3) an accounting and budget perspective, which evaluates the actual labor costs of the laboratory involved in delivering a service. Each of these approaches is reviewed briefly in the following sections.

Institutional Labor Cost Evaluation

From an organizational viewpoint, the employment cycle has four major stages, each of which has specific associated costs.

1. Recruitment and acquisition costs, such as advertising and pre-employment screening.
2. Training or developmental costs, which are ongoing.
3. Productive or operational periods, when the employees are actually performing the tasks for which they were hired.
4. Cost associated with the termination and separation of employees from the institution.

For these reasons, many personnel experts claim that an employee must remain with a company for a least 1 year before hiring costs are recovered. By understanding the costs associated with the employment cycle, the manager is better able to evaluate and justify promotion from within and expenditures designed to retain, train, and encourage personal and laboratory development.

Technical Evaluation of Labor Cost

The technical approach to labor costs seeks to identify and assign labor costs to the production activities that actually generate the expenses; this enable the manager to make informed personnel utilization decisions. In the laboratory this means focusing on the analytical process from the time a test is requested to the release of the final results.

To determine the direct labor costs involved in the technical performance of a laboratory procedure several agencies and authors [e.g., CLSI, ASCLS] have recommended the following guidelines.

1. **Preanalytical Time**, which involves collecting the specimen and preparing sample and instruments; from the time the physician places the order to when the sample is ready for the instrument.
2. **Analytical time**, which includes the time in which the test is actually performed and the results are calculated.
3. **Postanalytical time**, the time in which the report is made and routine maintenance is performed.

By breaking down costs for each segment of the analytical process, the manager is able to identify where efforts are being expended and take steps to assure labor productivity and cost efficiency.

These three process steps are also important in understanding work flow and measuring productivity. This breakdown of the analytical pocess enables the manager to identify means to expedite turnaround time and decide on the most economical methodology.

Accounting and Budgeting Labor Analysis

In a financial model, salary and wage cost behavior is separated into three categories; total number of hours paid; actual hours worked; and, hours paid as benefits. This division allows many financial and managerial performance indexes to be computed and specific operational parameters to be measured. These indicators can be used to monitor staffing levels, productivity, and management performance against budget objectives.

Using the accounting and budgeting labor cost model, payroll hours are grouped into the following categories. Some very sophisticated accounting payroll systems may list each type of hours (e.g., educational, sick, vacations) in separate headings; they usually are totaled into these three categories.

1. **Total (paid) hours** equal the total number of hours for which an employee is paid, this includes actual time spent in the laboratory as well as benefit hours paid.
2. **Productive (worked) hours** equal the actual hours worked (clocked), including overtime; the time that an employee is involved in education or training is usually counted as productive hours.
3. **Nonproductive (benefits) hours** equal the hours fro which the employee is compensated by not available for work. Sick time, vacation, jury duty, and bereavement time are examples of nonproductive hours.

Total payroll hours = Productive + Nonproductive hours

During the budgeting process, projections are made by each category for use in both staffing and financial planning.

Full-Time Equivalent

An important concept in salary and wage management is the calculation of **full-time equivalents (FTEs)**, which can be used for setting and measuring budgeting and staffing goals. To calculate FTEs, divide the number of hours (total, productive, or non-productive) by 2080: the number of hours a full-time person works in 1 year (i.e., 40 hours a week **x** 52 weeks = 2080).

For example (laboratory or department) :

Total hours paid (*year*)	14,159
Productive hours	12,896
Nonproductive hours	1,263

The total number of FTEs needed to run the laboratory in this example equals:

$$\frac{14{,}159 \text{ (total hrs/yr)}}{2{,}080 \text{ (hrs of one full time person/yr)}} = 6.8 \text{ FTEs}$$

The number of productive FTEs would equal:

$$\frac{12{,}896}{2{,}080} = 6.2 \text{ FTEs}$$

Try calculating nonproductive FTEs used by the laboratory;
(1,263/2,080 = 0.61 FTEs)

FTEs may also be calculated for a month or by week. For monthly, divide the number of hours for that month by *171* or *177* depending on whether the month has 30 or 31 days (160/165 for February); or *40* if calculating per week.

Managers are held directly accountable for the number of productive FTEs in the laboratory on a daily basis. They are also responsible for controlling the total FTE staffing level, because this represents the actual expenditure used in operating the laboratory. More leeway is needed in managing total FTE goals compared with productive FTE standards because many factors, such as sick time and personal time off, are not as predictable, especially in the short run.

Productivity Measurement

The productivity index is both necessary and controversial. There are those who maintain that creativity, timeliness, and quality of professional services are beyond measurement; by contrast, others say that laboratory testing is no different than any other task. Productivity can be evaluated by examining the productivity model, billable procedures as workload unit, and weighted workload systems.

The Productivity Model

Arriving at an acceptable productivity measurement requires a definition of both a unit of work and a unit of labor. A **productivity model** is then represented by the following formula:

$$\text{Productivity measurement} = \frac{\text{workload units (WLU)}}{\text{labor units}}$$

A *labor unit* is the most straight forward: *a unit of time in minutes or hours*. For salaried employees who do not use a time clock, labor units can be measured as a 40-hour workweek standard or an eight hour day.

Determining just what to use as a workload unit (WLU) has proven more elusive. This difficulty can be illustrated by the discontinued program of the College of American Pathologists (CAP) which abandoned its WLU project after more than 20 years.

The most common measurement of productivity use one of the following baselines as the workload units:

- Hours paid per patient day or daily census
- Hours paid per outpatient and emergency room visit
- Hours paid per number of *billable* laboratory procedures
- Hours paid per weighted workload unit

Selecting a Productivity Index

It becomes obvious from looking at any of these options that none appears totally satisfactory. Not all tests require the same labor effort. Just agreeing on what constitutes a test is questionable. Is a CBC a single test or seven different tests? Do you count RBC indices as one test — or four? Should you get extra credit if you have to calculate them manually, or if the instrument includes them in the printout? A patient's visit to the emergency room can involve a minor laceration with no test ordered or a trauma that requires a heroic effort by the laboratory. For these reasons laboratory tests are commonly defined as charges or billable procedures for productivity purposes, and the other factors are considered within the managerial perspective of productivity evaluation.

An index of any sophistication usually contains some weighted factors to account for these variations. However, because of the ease and availability of accounting data, many administrators rely on simpler models, such as payroll hours per patient day. All of these methods can provide useful information, depending on their sensitivity to changes in workload.

Selecting Final Productivity Units

The final productivity measurement index can be presented in several units. Many systems that use weighted factors report their results in units of time. Under the previous CAP WLU program, for example, a unit represented 1 minute of time. A score of 60 in a time-based unit demonstrated maximum effort. Even a causal observer, would notice that any program where a participant even approached a level of 60, would appear incredulous because the tech would need to breath occasional, take breaks, answer the phone, research questions, and handling instrument malfunctions.

- The key to selecting and effectively utilizing any index to measure productivity is that it be sensitive to volume changes. It must respond and adequate reflect changes in workload. This is as workload increases the productive index must increase proportionally, and as workload drops off, it must mirror this change.

Billable Procedures a Workload Unit

A billable procedure is a test for which the laboratory may issue a charge. Using billable procedures as the numerator in the productivity equation has several advantages. Primarily, this statistic is easily obtained from financial records, and it allows an apples-with-apples comparison.

Because of the billing requirements of Medicare and insurance companies and the use of CPT codes, there are almost uniform billing standards for laboratory procedures. By law and regulation, splitting charges and panels into multiple components is prohibited. For example, a CBC or a chemistry Basic Metobolbic Panel (BMP) cannot be divided into individual tests in order to increase the number of charges and, hence, the amount of reimbursement. By counting the number of charges (i.e., the number of computer billing entries), billable procedures become an easily obtained productivity input factor.

But not all laboratorians are satisfied with this method. "*That lab reports out only automated diffs on their CBC, while we do manual diffs on ours*," some workers may say. They also rush to point out that this system does not allow any credit for quality factors, the purported advantage of the discontinued CAP WLU system and, unfortunately, one of its major downfalls

Consider the following scenario:

> You go to a store with a friend to buy identical portable tape cassette players. Your friend is charged $20, and when you bill is presented you are charged $25. Your first instinct is to cry, "*Hey! What's going on here*?" The store manager explains that your particular player was made at a different plant where they are not as automated, but they do five more quality checks than at the location where your friend's tape player was made, so you are expected to pay the surcharge.

Painful as it may be to our professional pride, government and third-party payers see laboratory tests as simple commodities in the health care marketplace (i.e., a BMP is a BMP, a urinalysis is a urinalysis, and an aspirin is an aspirin). They see no reason to pay a premium because one laboratory chose to purchase a certain type of instrument, use manual procedures, or perform more quality checks than the next laboratory.

The CPT code gives one number for a specific test, and the payers have assigned a certain reimbursement fee to this code, leaving professional decision to the individual laboratory just as we leave production decision to the manufacturer. For this reason billable procedures provide an effective market-based indicator of a laboratory's productivity.

The use of billable procedures in the productivity equation is illustrated in the following example.

Total paid hours	10,200
Productive hours	8,262
Benefit hours	1,938
Billable procedures	71,400

$$\text{Total pad productivity} = \frac{71,400}{10,200} = 7 \text{ tests/paid hour}$$

$$\text{Productive hours} = \frac{71,400}{8,263} = 8.6 \text{ tests/productive hour}$$

Standardized Billable Test Counts (SBT)

The College of American Pathologists (CAP) in their Laboratory Management Index Program (LMIP) [(1)] have addressed some of the problems of inconsistencies in how billable procedures are defined: "*Unlike other methods of test counting (relative value units [RVU] and unadjusted billable tests), the CAP standardized billable test eliminates billing, accounting, and interpretation variations across institutions*." [(2 standardized)] Referring to the standardized billable test (SBT) as "*the primary measurement of output for participating laboratories*," they defined the SBT as a test which meets these criteria:

- Ordered by a physician or caregiver
- Associated with a CPT code
- Generates a result, product, or billable phlebotomy procedure
- Performed by laboratory personnel [(2 standardized)]

The LMIP provides performance ratios in two areas: labor productivity ("*on-site test per FTE*") and overall cost effectiveness ("*manageable cost per test*"). This information is reported on the individual laboratory's data and in *comparative performance reports* which provides peer group comparison called *fingerprint cluster* (your lab with matching size and organization); geographical (*regional*); and, with labs with which have characteristics which you select (*customer defined*).

Weighted Workload Labor Estimation Techniques

A **weighted workload labor estimation** is a system that assigns a value (usually in a unit defined as 1 minute) to a specific tasks performed in a standardized manner, obtained by analyzing and timing each step in the production or performance process. For example, a glucose performed may receive a weighted workload value (WLU) of 2.0 on a manual instrument where extensive pipetting or reagent preparation is required, and a 0.5 on an automated instrument because of the time needed to perform the additional analytical steps. While this section discusses formal methods for weighted workload, laboratorians will have noticed that this is done informally every day in the lab. For example, a phlebotomist assigned to do veinpunctures on pre-op's may be expected to do four or five patients, compared to someone dispatched to the nursery to perform a heel puncture on an infant

Weighted Workload Procedures

Listed next are the four main methods used to analyze and measure workload and develop factors with which to calculate productivity within a weighted model.

- **Expert opinion**: A person knowledgeable in the field makes an estimate of time necessary to perform an activity.
- **Simulation**: A technologist performs a specific test to determine the time needed.
- **Log (diary) book**: The technologist records each step involved in the testing procedure in a log over a designated period of time. This record shows the work period (shift or time of day), instrumentation, and other important factors such as the experience of the technologist.
- **Time-motion study**: A person with special training in management engineering either directly observes the person working or develops special logs where the steps in a process can be recorded, along with the time involved. The CAP workload system used this method.

All of these methods require a trade-off between time, effort, and accuracy; the more accurate the data collection procedure, the more cumbersome and time consuming the project. This time commitment problem has resulted in other shortcuts, such as random sampling techniques and computer models, which often introduce biases that reduce their use and reliability in monitoring and defending management performance. For this reason, the value obtained from any modifications to standard methods must be carefully considered.

Weighted Workload Value Productivity Calculations

Weighted workload units (WLU) are defined as a value of one (1) unit = (1) minute. Time studies measure the time required for the initial handling of the specimen, specimen testing, recording and reporting, daily and periodic activities, maintenance and repair, and direct technical supervision. The resulting WLU is comprehensive by design. The time studies include all activities involved in the actual performance of a test and the support network necessary to operate a laboratory. This includes work performed by technical, supervisory, and clerical personnel.

The WLU assigned to a procedure is based on the specific methodology used to perform the test. Whether the analysis is performed manually, or on an instrument, and the preparation of the reagents used to to perform the test on a particular instrument are all factors used to determine the WLU for a specific procedure. Table 14 – 1 shows two examples of assigning values and determining total WLU. The WLUs are then totaled to arrive at a Workload *Value* (*WLV count*) for a department or section.

The following ratios can be used in determining productivity in weighted workload systems.

$$\text{Productivity (units per hour)} = \frac{\text{WLV court (for Lab, department, or section)}}{\text{hours (by total paid or worked)}}$$

In the following example, chemistry had a total WLV count for March of 52,213. There were 1112 total paid hours for the month, of which 1013 were hours worked:

$$\text{Paid Productivity} = \frac{52{,}213 \text{ WLV}}{1{,}112 \text{ paid hrs}} = 47.0 \text{ units/hr}$$

$$\text{Worked Productivity} = \frac{52{,}213 \text{ WLV}}{1{,}013 \text{ worked hrs}} = 51.5 \text{ units/hr}$$

To convert the WLV figure to a percentage, divide the index by 60 (the number of minutes in an hour), then multiply by 100.

$$\text{Paid productivity} = \frac{47.0 \text{ WLU/hr}}{60 \text{ min/hr}} = .783 \times 100 = 78.3\%$$

$$\text{Work productivity} = \frac{51.5 \text{ WLU/hr}}{60 \text{ min/hr}} = .858 \times 100 = 85.5\%$$

Productivity Standards

An acceptable productivity level is often very arbitrarily defined. Many variables contribute to the final score of a particular section or laboratory. These factors include the services expected on the laboratory by the hospital, extent of computerization, the benefits provide to employees, and the productivity measurement itself. For these reasons, many administrators rely on more general indicators, such as number of FTEs per patient days and billable procedures, to measure the efficiency of their managers, even though very

detailed and specific productivity data are available from programs such as the CAP Laboratory Management Index Program and the American Hospital Association. Most of these programs rank each laboratory according to a variety of financial and hospital parameters (see the standardized billable test counts section above for additional comments on the CAP LMIP).

In practice, the laboratory is held to the numbers agreed upon in the budget. If a total paid staff of 40 FTEs is allocated, the manager must be able to justify any deviation from this level. The laboratory is compared to indexes from many sources, which are monitored through the budgeting process.

Although an ideal productivity monitor may prove elusive, it is important that the indicators enable the manager to set realistic and attainable goals. Most important, the measurement must be acceptable to both the manager and the supervisor. The laboratorian should take advantage of the wide selection of productivity indexes available to assess the staffing needs and efficiency of operations.

Wage and Salary Budgeting

Salaries are budgeted and reported in the same manner as other costs, listed with a line item accounting code and expenses shown as a dollar amount. In a separate part of the budget report, cost items, labor hours, and FTEs are frequently recorded by month and year to date. Salary budgeting projections consist of two processes: (1) a document that lists every position authorized along with the name of the individual filling each job, maintained and monitored by personnel and payroll, and (2) the normal reports associated with the budgeting process using financial and accounting information.

WLU Code	Procedure	WLU Value
	CHEM 6 PROFILE on a ACI*	
**5500142.102	Automated chemistry specimen set up	3.2/specimen
5500146.102	Glucose	0.2/constitutent
5500147.102	BUN	0.2
5500148.102	Sodium	0.2
5500149.102	Potassium	0.2
5500150.102	Chloride	0.2
5500151.102	CO_2	0.2
Total WLU Value		4.4
	URINE CULTURE	
5500146.702	Accessioning specimen for bacterial culture	1.7
5500156.702	2 plates cultured	2.0
5500166.702	Processing Culture	2.0
5500176.702	Reporting bacterial culture	2.0
Total WLU Value		7.7

* "ACI" is intended as a fictitious name, used for an example of a generic automated chemistry instrument

** A code for each procedure (specimen processing, instrument operations, glucose on a specific instrument, manual diff, etc.) is usually assigned to assist in identifying a particular test processed by a specific method. It is arbitrarily assigned and any numbering system depends solely on the model used.

TABLE 14 — 1. Determining Total WLU

Position Control Master

A detailed list of the authorized position and the person assigned to each slot is maintained by the personnel department as a part of the budgeting and hiring process. This document is referred to as *the potion control master* and ensures management control of the hiring process. When the laboratory wishes to hire or replace an employee, the position control master is consulted to identify the opening and determine authorization to fill the position.

The position control master categorizes employees by department, job classification, and employment status (full-time, part-time, temporary, or as required [prn]). For example, 20 full-time technologists' positions would be listed under the laboratory with the name of each tech or with an "*open*" designation if currently vacant. This document is normally reproduced as part of the payroll process. It provides information on the number of hours worked and associated payroll data by employees and gives calmative totals in financial form and FTE figures (e.g., normal hours, overtime, benefits hours, and shift premiums).

Wage Determination Methods and Budget Projections (Example of Annualized and Monthly Projections)

The important determinant in forecasting the staffing needs for the budget year is the projected volume of work. With this information, the number of labor hours needed can be projected in ratios that calculate the tests performed per paid hours and/or worked hours.

Using the following data for the current year, it is possible to make annual and monthly projections:

Current (Actual) Year's Data

Test volume	373,332 tests
Salary expense	$399,942
No. paid hours	39,520 hrs
No. benefit hours	3,596 hrs
No. worked (productive) hours	35,924 hrs
Average hourly rate	$ 10.12

$$\text{Paid productivity} = \frac{373{,}332 \text{ tests}}{39{,}520 \text{ paid hrs}} = 9.5 \text{ tests performed/paid hr}$$

$$\text{Worded productivity} = \frac{373{,}332 \text{ tests}}{35{,}924 \text{ worked hrs}} = 10.4 \text{ tests performed/worked hr}$$

$$\text{Average hourly rate} = \frac{\$399{,}942}{39{,}520 \text{ paid hrs}} = \$10.12\text{/hr paid}$$

Next Year's Budget

(pro forma budget; i.e., budget extrapolated from historical data)

Projected* (forecasted/predicted) test volume and salary increases for the next budget cycle:

Test Volume	408,237 tests/year
	33,142 tests/month of May
5% average salary raise	

*[projected adjusted bed census **x** tests per adj. bed] *these projections are usually gleamed from the budget target set by administration and extrapolated to laboratory tests, plus any adjustment for anticipated changes in testing volume (new test, loss of patient base, etc.). (Adjusted bed census = adjusted for inpatient census, outpatient, and ER visits)*

Annualized Projections

- FTEs Budget = 20.7 FTEs (Paid)
  18.9 FTEs (Worked/Productive)
- Salary Expense Budget = $456,792

Projected Average Hourly Rate = $10.63

$10.12 (average hourly rate) **x** 1.05 = $10.63

Projected Total Paid FTEs Budget = 20.7 FTEs

$$\frac{408{,}237 \text{ projected tests}}{9.5 \text{ (tests performed/paid hr)}} = 42{,}972 \text{ paid hours needed}$$

$$\frac{42{,}972 \text{ paid hours needed}}{2{,}080 \text{ (hours work in year by 1 FTE)}} = 20.7 \text{ total paid FTEs}$$

Projected Worked (Productive) FTEs Budget

$$\frac{408{,}237 \text{ projected tests}}{10.4 \text{ (tests/work hr)}} = 39{,}254 \text{ projected worked hours}$$

$$\frac{39{,}254 \text{ projected worked hours}}{2{,}080 \text{ (hours work in year by 1 FTE)}} = 18.9 \text{ FTEs}$$

Projected Salary Expense Budget

42,972 (total paid hours) **x** $10.63 (average hourly rate)

= $456,792 salary budget

Monthly Projected Budget for Month of May

- FTEs Budget (May) = 19.7 FTEs (Paid)
  18.0 FTEs (Worked/Productive)
- Salary Expense Budget (May) = $37,088

Projected Total Paid FTEs Budget = 19.7 FTEs

$$\frac{33{,}142 \text{ projected tests (May)}}{9.5 \text{ (tests performed/paid hr)}} = 3{,}489 \text{ paid hours needed}$$

$$\frac{3{,}489 \text{ paid hours needed}}{177} = 19.7 \text{ total paid FTEs}$$

Projected Worked (Productive) FTEs Budget

$$\frac{33{,}142 \text{ projected tests (May)}}{10.4 \text{ (tests/work hr)}} = 3{,}187 \text{ projected worked hours}$$

$$\frac{3{,}187 \text{ projected worked hours}}{177 \text{ (hours work in a 31 day month by 1 FTE)}} = 18.0 \text{ FTEs}$$

Projected Salary Expense Budget

3,489 (total paid hours in May) **x** $10.63 (average hourly rate)
= $37,088 salary budget for the month of May

Wage and Salary Budgeting is the last section of *Salary and Wage Management*. The next chapter discusses *Material Management*.

— Case Study —

Chapter Fourteen: Salary and Wage Management

"It's not fair!" complained the day-shift hematology staff member to her supervisor. "We know that the numbers show that the evening shift does the same number of CBCs per person as we do, but they don't have to work-up bone marrow slides or do the special stains that we have to do. They also leave any difficult diffs for us, and don't have to any routine maintenance on the instruments, either! . I know they are real busy too, and asking for help, but it's not fair to compare them with us. We need more help!"

"I'll talk to the laboratory manager again," responded the frustrated supervisor, looking over all the work that still needed to be done. "But last time he told me that administration was only interested in billable procedures and that was how we were going to have to look at our staff. I know it's not fair to count a CBC where you have to do a manual diff the same as one where you report only the automatic one, especially one that has all kinds of abnormal cells, but that appears to be the system."

"Well, you have to do something. It looks like we are going to miss lunch again today," answered one tech, acknowledging the agreement from the other coworkers.

"Not me," announced another tech as she and a partner headed out the door. "I have to have something to eat. We are going to lunch before the cafeteria closes."

Chapter Sections for Review

- Productivity Measurement
  - The Productivity Model
  - Billable Procedures as a Workload Unit
  - Weighted Workload Procedures
  - Example of Weighted Workload Program

Questions for Discussion

1. If you were the supervisor, what would you tell the laboratory manager?
2. If the laboratory manager agreed to the supervisor conducting a review, what suggestions would you have for the supervisor in coming up with a fair study?
3. Specifically, which method would you recommend to conduct a weighted workload study in this situation? What about agreement on the results, costs, and time and labor commitment, particularly since the staff on the first and second shift will most likely have to participate?
4. Suppose after agreeing and conducting a weighted workload study, it was found that the day shift had a productivity of 52 WLU/hour (1 WLU = 1 min), and second shift had a productivity of only 48 WLU/hour. Convert these numbers to a percentage workload figure. What does the difference mean?
5. What would you do if you were the laboratory manager and you were not authorized to expand the total paid hours of the department?

SOLUTIONS

Question 4:

$52/60 \times 100 = 86.7\%$
$48/60 \times 100 = 80.0\%$

Question 5:

The difference in productivity may not be significant; however, if the class feels it is, the only options in this situation appear to be shifting of either personnel or work tasks.

[15]

Material Management

— Chapter Fifteen —

Supplies are the second largest expense incurred by the laboratory, overshadowed only by labor costs. Supply expense is a very broad category and covers most of the material purchased by the laboratory, including reagents, pipettes, chemicals, phlebotomy supplies, and even office products. This chapter presents methods for controlling, managing, and accounting for inventory.

OBJECTIVES

After completion of this chapter, the reader will be able to demonstrate accomplishment of the following objectives.

1. Distinguish supply expenses from other budget items.
2. Explain the process of material management and inventory control.
3. Describe the documents used in requisitioning supplies.
4. Select the stock replenishment method best suited to a given laboratory situation.
5. Establish appropriate inventory levels and ordering schedules, using the quantitative tools of economic ordering quantity (EOQ), economic ordering point (EOP) , and optimal reorder time (ROT).
6. Calculate the supply expense portion of the laboratory budget.

Chapter Highlights and Glossary of Key Terms

I. MATERIAL MANAGEMENT

Material Management: *The systematic process of overseeing and controlling the acquisition and utilization of supplies to ensure both availability and cost effectiveness.*

A. Goals of material management

B. Definition of supplies

Supplies: *Products that meet specific time and price criteria.*

II. SUPPLY ORDERING PROCESS

A. Purchase order

Purchase Order: *A document authorizing the purchase of a product or services from a vendor.*

B. Traveling requisition

Traveling Requisition: *A catalog of products used to order supplies stocked by material management.*

C. Standing orders

Standing Orders: *A purchase order issued for a product or service to be delivered according to a preset schedule.*

D. Product standardization committee

III. INVENTORY MANAGEMENT

A. Inventory level checks

Perpetual System: *A system that keeps account of the inventory each time a product is used or removed from inventory.*

Periodic System: *A system whereby inventory levels are checked according to an established timetable.*

Random Checks: *A method used to verify inventory levels.*

B. Stock replenishment techniques

1. Minimum-maximum
2. Just-in-time

C. Financial control of inventory

Economic Ordering Quantity (EOQ): *A formula used to determine the quantity of supplies to order at one time.*

Economic Ordering Point (EOP): *The point at which inventory should be reordered.*

Optimal Reorder Time (ROT): *The best time to place an order to take advantage of EOQ and EOP*

1. Inventory management methods
2. Inventory formulas and management tools
3. Example of inventory management methods

IV. PROJECTION OF BUDGET SUPPLY COSTS

Material Management

Material management is the systematic process of overseeing and controlling the acquisition and utilization of supplies to ensure both availability and cost effectiveness. This function consists of the purchasing or requisitioning of supplies and the oversight of products after they arrive. At the hospital level these two functions are handled by a centralized material management department organized into two sections: purchasing and stockroom. The purchasing section oversees the ordering of supplies and the processing of invoices from vendors. The stockroom maintains security and inventory levels and issues supplies throughout the facility.

These two functions are often combined in the laboratory. Ordering and inventory control may be handled by individual sections or supervisors. In other cases, an assigned individual may have responsibility for the systematic requisitioning of supplies.

Goals of Material Management

However it is organized, the purchasing plan of the laboratory should ensure that supplies meet product specifications in quality, quantity, and timeliness. The goals of material management must include steps to guarantee that the following actions happen.

- Supplies arrive in a timely manner.
- Spoilage is reduced to a minimum.
- Back orders and delays are avoided.
- Storage space is used to the best advantage.
- The most economically advantageous price is obtained.
- Financial resources are not tied up in inventory.

Within these guidelines, it is important to understand exactly what is included in material management and the process of ordering supplies.

Definition of Supplies

For budgeting purposes, products that meet specific *time* and *price* criteria are classified as **supplies.** By definition, items that fall outside these criteria are classified as capital items (see Chapter 16). The distinction between these two groups — supplies and capital expenditures — is determined as follows.

1. Items that are consumed within 1 year or have a shelf life of less than 1 year are almost always classified as supplies.
2. Items below a certain price level, as established by the comptroller, may be classified as supplies, even though their shelf life exceeds 1 year.

A product costing under $1000, for example, may be counted as a supply item, even if it can be used for several years. An automated diluter, costing $500 is actually an instrument, but for budgeting purposes it may be counted as a supply item. The cutoff amount varies widely from institution to institution and may typically range from $5,000 to as low as $100.

Supply Ordering Process

Several documents have been developed to both expedite and simplify the record-keeping process. The two most common documents are the purchase order (Figure 15 – 1), which is used to order supplies from outside vendors, and the traveling requisition (Figure 15 – 2), which provides a means to request supplies from the central stockroom. A description of these two documents, along with the use of standing orders, can serve as an overview of the ordering process.

Purchase Order

A **purchase order** (Figure 15 – 1) represents a commitment by the organization to purchase a product or service. It serves as the authorization for the vendor to ship and bill the institution. For this reason the process has to be tightly controlled.

An interim document called the *request for purchase* begins the ordering process; it is completed by the requesting unit (i.e., Hematology or Chemistry supervisor) and sent to the purchasing department, which then formally issues a purchase order. The request for purchase must be completed in exact detail; it must include the catalog number, the supplier, and a description of the product.

The purchasing department prepares and issues the purchase order for the item specified and "charges" it to the bookkeeping account of the requesting area. The supplier then ships the item requested and bills the institution.

Traveling Requisition

The **traveling requisition** (Figure 15 – 2) is a catalog of products held in stock by material management. It gets its name because the document "travels" from the stockroom to each department and back. This catalog describes the product and the unit of container (box, pack, and so on) and provides a place to request the quantity needed. These are updated on a monthly basis, and the orders are tabulated and charged to the department at the same time.

Items included on the traveling requisition are usually articles used by many departments and purchased in bulk. Examples include office supplies, cleaning materials, and patient care products such as facial tissue. They may also include nonperishable supplies such as microscope slides and vacuum collection tubes. Thousands of items are needed to run a hospital; the traveling requisition system helps to keep track of these items and to allocate charges for accounting purposes.

Central Reference Laboratories
100 Main Street
Anytown, State 100001

PURCHASE ORDER NUMBER

____

Issue Date: ______________ Account: _________________

Vendor/Supplier:
____
____
____
_____________________________ Delivery Date: _________

Catalog Number	Description	Unit	Price

Subtotal	___________
Discount/ Credits	___________
Subtotal	___________
Shipping	___________
Tax:	___________
Total	___________

Authorization Signature __________________________

____

FIGURE 15 — 1. Purchase Order

Central Reference Laboratories
100 Main Street
Anytown, State 100001

May 2008

Section: 702 Hematology Order Day: Tuesday

Contact (name) ____________________

Item #	Description	Unit	Price	(May) 6	13	20	27
6543	Slide, FR	½ gross	$ 1.25				
7238	Pencil	bx 10	$ 2.14				
8567	Tape,Trp	roll	$ 0.78				
0938	Tissue, Lt Fr	bx	$ 0.94				
8456	Pad, Legal	each	$ 1.17				
6792	Tube, 16 x100	bx 250	$15.12				
...							
...							
...							

Quantity/Order Dater

FIGURE 15 — 2. Traveling Requisition

Standing Orders

Products that have a predictable usage level or short shelf lives are frequently ordered in advance via **standing orders.** Standing orders may also be issued to reserve a single lot number of reagents or supplies. Under this procedure a purchase order is issued to the vendor with instructions to ship a specific amount of product according to an established schedule. Blood bank reagent cells and the quality control material used in chemistry are examples of products that are frequently ordered in this fashion. Standing orders are also useful for items such as phlebotomy supplies, for which a commitment can be made to buy a designated amount to be delivered according to a predetermined timetable.

Standing orders offer benefits to both the laboratory and the supplier. The laboratory is assured of the timely delivery of needed items; the lab may also be able to take advantage of bulk prices or discounts offered by the vendors and from the use of vendors' storage space. Suppliers have a commitment from the institution to buy their products; this enables them to plan their production and inventory levels on a more predictable schedule. Standing orders also play an important role in many inventory management programs, especially the "just-in-time" techniques reviewed in a later section.

Product Standardization Committee

The purpose of a *product standardization committee* is to ensure that the best product is obtained, to avoid expensive duplication of products, and to take advantage of volume discounts for generic items. The primary mission of this group, which is composed of representatives from all areas of the organization, is to review supplies that the hospital uses in large volumes, resolve differences between preferences in areas that may share a common product, and develop standards for selection and quality assurance. The purchasing section uses the recommendations of the committee to obtain bids from competing vendors for the best product and price.

Inventory Management

Inventory management is a continual process of checking stock levels, rotating stock to ensure freshness, ordering supplies in sufficient quantities to meet current needs, and minimizing the cost of carrying inventory (i.e., having too much of the organization's money tied up in items just sitting on the shelf waiting for use at some time in the future).

One of the major accounting events in a hospital is the survey to determine the value of the inventory. This inventory check, performed at least once a year, demonstrates the importance placed on controlling supply costs. The annual inventory is only one method used to manage this asset. This section reviews inventory management and stock replenishment techniques used to determine the amount of inventory that should be maintained in-house and the most economic reorder point.

Inventory level Checks

Three methods can be used to track inventory levels: perpetual, periodic, and random systems.

Perpetual systems keep account of the inventory each time a product is used. For example, when any item is taken off the shelf, the inventory checklist is adjusted by the person removing the product. When it is time to reorder, the checklist is submitted to purchasing without any need for further checks, at least theoretically. This is the procedure of choice in material management departments with a well-trained and dedicated stocking staff. However, it requires detailed attention at the time of usage, and this time commitment is not always practical at the service or bench levels, especially in the stressful work settings of the modern health care institution.

Periodic systems are more common at the bench or department level. Once a week or at another specified time the stock level is counted and appropriate supplies are ordered.

Random checks, such as the annual inventory, are used to document the value of supplies at a specific time. This "snapshot" verification procedure is a key part of financial accounting and is especially useful in confirming the accuracy of perpetual systems, which can easily become distorted if not meticulously maintained.

Stock Replenishment Techniques

Two techniques are available for determining how and when to replenish stock: minimum-maximum and just-in-time replenishment strategies. Both depend on the inventory tools described at the end of this chapter to determine the appropriate order amount and schedule.

Minimum-Maximum

One method for determining when and how much to reorder, is to establish a set point (minimum) at which inventory is to be recorded and a "reorder to" (maximum) level which is to be maintained. For example, the safety reserve (minimum stocking level) for blood bank saline may be fixed at 5 cases and the maximum stocking level at 10. When inventory is taken and 7 cases are found on the shelf, an order for 3 units would be placed to bring the count to the maximum point.

Just-in-Time

A major technique developed by manufacturers to take advantage of inventory management opportunities is a Japanese model called just-in-time ordering. This is a commitment by the suppler to guarantee delivery of an item at the exact moment of need. This limits the financial costs associated with stocking and storing inventory items. Obviously, this technique is more opportune in manufacturing, in which costs of failure are limited to monetary loss. However, its use is appropriate in health care settings in which the safety stock level can be kept at a minimum, freeing up much needed financial resources for other purposes. The standing–order programs frequently used in the laboratory for obtaining short-dated items such as reagent cells or test kits are examples of just-in-time ordering.

Financial Control of Inventory

Because supplies are the second largest cost incurred by the laboratory, much attention has been given to monitoring and controlling supply expenses. Several questions arise when managers tackle the problems of inventory management.

1. What is the most economic quantity to order, from the point of view of financial, storage, and delivery issues?
2. How can the institution take advantage of bulk purchase discounts?
3. What is the best time to place orders to both limit the amount of financial commitment and ensure adequate supplies?

To answer these questions, a specialty of management science called operations research has developed several techniques and formulas for managing inventory:

1. The **economic ordering quantity (EOQ)** , which answers the question of how much to order at one time
2. The **economic ordering point (EOP)** , also referred to as the reorder point (ROP), which provides the base or safety level for reordering inventory
3. The **optimal reorder time (ROT)** , which helps establish the best time to order to take advantage of the EOQ and EOP

In the following sections these three methods are defined and their application explained.

Inventory Management Methods

In order to determine the EOQ, EOP, and ROT, managers must understand certain underlying concepts relating to inventory.

Annual usage: Determining the level of inventory needed is based on the workload of the laboratory. Historical ordering data based on actual purchases and usage as well as predictions of future volume influences the anticipated level of supplies that must be ordered.

Average daily usage: This information can be obtained by dividing the amount of supplies ordered in a year by 365 days.

Cost of ordering: Although it may seem at first to be an insignificant point, the cost of running a centralized purchasing department is directly tied to the number of purchase orders placed and the associated work involved with keeping track of invoices as products are shipped and received. This figure is obtained by dividing the expenses of the purchasing section by the number of purchase orders issued.

Annual holding cost: This is a crucial determination. It involves decisions based on bulk orders, space utilization, and whether it is better to have the product on hand or in the supplier's warehouse. When the vendor is holding the stock, the institution's money is available for other purposes. Also called *cost of carrying* inventory, its value is determined by considering the interest lost by not having the money in the bank or the rate charged when the laboratory must borrow money to cover inventory expenses. Annual holding costs should also account for the expense of maintaining a stockroom for storing material not needed immediately.

Cost per unit: Cost per unit is a straightforward calculation once the decision has been made as to the best price available. Factors such as quantity discounts and container size (i.e., box, case, truckload) affect this decision. Dividing the purchase price by the container size provides this value.

Lead time: The amount of lead time, or advance notice, needed between placing an order and its arrival is an especially important consideration. It influences the minimum inventory that must be kept in stock, as well as the quantity that needs to be requested.

Inventory Formulas and Management Tools

Using these definitions and concepts, the following formulas are derived for EOQ, EOP, and ROT.

- $\text{EOQ} = \sqrt{\dfrac{2\ x\ (\text{annual usage}\ x\ \text{cost of ordering})}{\text{annual holding cost per unt}}}$

- $\text{EOP} = \dfrac{\text{annual usage}}{365\ \text{days}}\ \boldsymbol{x}\ \text{lead time in days}$

  <u>or</u>
  EOP = (average daily usage **x** lead time) **+** safety level

- $\text{ROT} = \dfrac{\text{EOQ}}{\text{annual usage}}\ \boldsymbol{x}\ 365\ \text{days}$

Example of Inventory Management Methods

Using the following figures we can calculate the EOQ, EOP, and ROT:

Annual usage = 11,000 20/pk blood agar plates
Cost of ordering = $25 per order
Annual holding costs = $2.50 per year
Lead time = 7 days

$$\text{EOQ} = \sqrt{\frac{2\ x\ (11{,}000\ packs\ x\ \$25/order)}{\$2.50 holding\ costs/yr}} = \sqrt{\frac{550{,}000}{\$2.50}}$$

$$= \sqrt{220{,}000} = 469\ \text{packs/order}$$

$$\text{EOP} = \frac{11{,}000\ \text{packs}}{365\ \text{days}}\ \boldsymbol{x}\ 7\ \text{days} = 211\ \text{packs}$$

$$\text{ROT} = \frac{\text{469 packs/order}}{\text{11,000 packs}} \times \text{365 days} = \text{15.5 days/order}$$

Thus, for maximum financial benefit and storage space utilization, order 469 packs of plates each time the inventory drops to 211 (about every 16 days). Several commonsense modifications should be made once this information is available. Adjustments may be made, based on such factors as a weekly ordering system and bulk sizes. However, the farther the ordering system strays from standards, the fewer the economic benefits.

Projection of Budget Supply Costs

Supply costs are projected for budgeting purposes by using the percentage-of-revenue method, with an adjustment factor for anticipated inflation (see chapters on revenue and salary budgeting). The next chapter covers preparation of the operational budget of the laboratory. The following example illustrates the calculation of supply costs as projected in the budget using the percentage-of-revenue method.

Year-to-date
- Current supply costs = $234,124
- Current laboratory revenues = $1,533,626
- Cost/revenue = 0.153

Budget projection (includes factor for expected inflation).
- Budgeted revenue = $2,127,000
- Supply cost projected = $325,431 ($2,127,000 X 0.153)

Cost-per-test information can also be useful, as illustrated in the following example, and may be more helpful in determining supply expenses for smaller units of the laboratory, such as the blood bank or Histology.

Current year cost per test = $1.56
Tests projected = 23,150
Supply cost inflation factor: 4%
Budget projection:
- 23,150 ***x*** $1.56 = $36,114
- $36,114 ***x*** 1.04 = $37,559

End of *Material Management*. Following is *The Laboratory Budget*.

— Case Study —

Chapter Fifteen: Material Management

"You wanted to see me?" The histology supervisor asked, entering the laboratory manager's office.

"As a matter of fact I do. Have a seat, while I get some papers here," replied the laboratory manager, looking through the cluttered desk. "Yes, here it is. You remember 'just-in-time' inventory management, don't you? We talked about it in our last supervisors' training in-service. "

"Well, yes, . . . but, I don't think you can take advantage of it in a situation like the laboratory. We have to make sure we have enough supplies to take care of our patients at all times, **no matter what**!"

"That's certainly true," answered the laboratory manager, handing the histology supervisor some papers. "However, I think there are some features there that may help us control our supply expenses. I believe a good place to start is your section, with microscope slides. The standing order is about to expire and I want you to evaluate our inventory levels and needs before we agree to a new contract. You use a lot of them in a year, and we may be able to save some money and have an example for the rest of the lab to use. Here is the old contract and information on our usage over the past year. Oh . . . here is another copy of the calculations for the inventory management formulas in case you misplaced your copy. Let me know if you run into a problem. I'll check with you sometime next week to see how you're doing."

Chapter Sections for Review

- Standing Orders
- Just-in-Time
- Inventory Management Methods
    - Economic Ordering Quantity (EOQ)
    - Economic Ordering Point (EOP)
    - Optimal Reorder Time (ROT)

Questions for Discussion

1. Use the information below, provided by the laboratory manager to the histology supervisor, to calculate the EOQ, EOP, and ROT for the microscope slides used in histology.

Annual usage:	540 (½ gross boxes)
Cost of ordering:	$24.00
Holding costs:	$3.10
Lead time:	3 days
Histology supply ordering day:	Tuesday
Supply delivery day:	Friday
Current safety level:	20 boxes (2 cases)
Current standing order delivery schedule:	10 boxes every Friday

2. Consider the following additional information: due to having to issue only one purchase order, the cost of ordering per shipment (or billing charge) is reduced to $15 for an annual standing order. Given this savings, would this laboratory be better off with issuing a standing order or converting the slides to a Minimum-Maximum inventory system set up using the figures from the formulas?

3. If, due to other factors, such as ordering all supplies from a single vendor, the laboratory does not want to set up a standing order for the microscope slides, what would be the most economical reorder point (i.e.. safety reserve/minimum stocking level) and reorder to inventory level? How frequently would an order be placed, if the current vendor was used? Assume that there had only been two I-week backorders in the past 3 years, and that other departments (i.e., hematology) and a nearby hospital also used these slides.

4. Would/could a "just-in-time" inventory program work in this situation?

SOLUTIONS

Question 1:

$$\text{EOQ} = \sqrt{\frac{2\ x\ (540\ boxes\ x\ \$24/order)}{\$3.10\ holding\ costs/yr}} = \sqrt{\frac{25{,}920}{\$3.10}}$$

$$= \sqrt{8{,}361} = 91.43 \text{ boxes [or 9 to 10 cases } {\scriptstyle (10 \text{ boxes to a case})}]$$

$$\text{EOP} = \frac{540 \text{ boxes}}{365 \text{ days}} \times 3_{(days)} + 20_{(safety\ level)} = 1.5 \times 3 + 20 = 24.5 \text{ boxes}$$

$$\text{ROT} = \frac{91.4 \text{ boxes}}{540 \text{ boxes}} \text{ x } 365 \text{ days} = 0.25 \times 365 = 91.25 \text{ days/order}$$

Summary:

Economic ordering quantity (EOQ) = 91.43 boxes, or 9 — 10 cases
Economic Ordering Point (EOP) = 24.5 boxes, or 2½ cases
Optimal Reorder Time (ROT) = 91.25 days, or every 3 months

Question 2:

A savings of $520 is available from this strategy ($10 X 52 weeks) if supplies are ordered once, rather than weekly. Compared this to the $100 it would cost to order according to the ROT (4 x $25), using the Minimum-Maximum inventory system.

Question 3:

From this information, safety levels could probably be lowered to 10 boxes, making the EOP or reorder point 15 boxes (4.5 + 10 boxes). With an ROT of 3 months and EOQ of 10 cases, the most economical strategy would be to check the inventory level once a week and order 9 — 10 cases when the inventory dropped to 15 boxes. *(Note: factors such as storage space where included in determining the "holding costs".)*

Question 4:

Given the long ROT, rare back orders, and possibility of procurement (borrowing) of supplies from other close sources; along with the potential of negotiating significant savings in storage and cost of items, this appears as a good candidate for exploring a *just-in-time* inventory system.

[16]

The Laboratory Budget

— Chapter Sixteen —

This chapter brings together the topics discussed in the previous chapters of Part 3 for the preparation of two documents: the operational budget and the capital budget. Revenue and cost accounting, salary and wage management, material management, and future building projects and instrument acquisition are all reflected in the preparation of these budgets. The tools and techniques for predicting future revenue, expenses, and financial requirements and the format are summarized and demonstrated in this chapter.

OBJECTIVES

After completion of this chapter, the reader will be able to demonstrate accomplishment of the following objectives.

1. Distinguish between different budgeting alternatives and select the appropriate method for the laboratory.
2. Explain the steps and schedule for preparing an operational budget.
3. Prepare an operational budget for a laboratory.
4. Describe the purpose of a certificate of need.
5. Classify expenditures as capital or supply items.
6. Define minimal and major capital budget categories.
7. Prepare a capital proposal using narrative and qualitative tools for justification and financial feasibility studies.
8. Explain the methods and options available to finance a laboratory project or purchase an instrument.

Chapter Highlights and Glossary of Key Terms

I. THE OPERATIONAL BUDGET

Budgeting: *The process of planning, forecasting, controlling, and monitoring the financial resources of the organization.*

Operational Budgeting: *The process of planning for the laboratory as an ongoing business concern; accounting for everyday needs and expenditures.*

A. Types of operational budgets

Capital Budget*: Plans for the acquisition and completion of specific equipment and building projects that require major financial commitments.*

1. Forecast/projection method
2. Flexible budgeting

   Flexible Budgeting: *A budgeting process that attempts to set expenditures based on a variable workload volume.*
3. Zero-based budgeting

   Zero-Based Budgeting: *A method that analyzes needs based on prioritizing of goals and objectives and not on past allocations.*

B. Operational budget preparation

1. Time frame
2. Forecasting stage
3. Scheduling stage
4. Synthesis of information

C. Review of budgeting procedures
Pro Forma Budget: *A budget based on the extrapolation of historical data.*

D. Monitoring and Feedback

II. THE CAPITAL BUDGET

A. Definition of capital
Capital Item: *A building project, piece of equipment, or instrument that meets specific institutional and regulatory guidelines of time, price, and purpose.*

B. Parts of a capital budget

C. Certificate of need
Certificate of Need (CON): *A document issued by a government regulatory body to authorize a capital project.*

D. Instrument/project capital proposal
1. Narrative tools
   a. Justification
   b. Prioritization
   c. Opportunity costs
      Opportunity Costs: *The value of what is given up in order to pursue another project.*
2. Quantitative tools
   a. payback period
      Payback Period: *The length of time it will take to recover the cash outlays for a project.*
   b. Average rate of return
      Average Rate of Return: *The average yield over the life of an investment.*
   c. Net present value
      Time Value of Money: *The future value of a dollar compared with today.*
   d. Internal rate of return
      Net Present Value (NPV): *The worth of future earnings at today's rates.*
      Internal Rate of Return: *The ratio of cash flow and cost-of-capital factors to the amount of investment required.*
   e. Required rate of return
      Required Rate of Return: *A bottom-line level of income required by a company before any project is considered.*

E. Financing a project
1. Acquisition options
2. Depreciation
   Depreciation: *The monetary value by which assets diminish with time and usage.*
   a. Salvage value
      Salvage Value: *The value of an item at the time of resale, trade-in, or disposal.*
   b. Allowance calculation methods
      Straight-Line Depreciation: *A method based on the time element of depreciation.*
      Unit of Output: *A method of determining the depreciation allowance based on unit output.*
      Accelerated Depreciation: *Methods allowed by regulatory agencies to encourage investments.*

F. Capital budget proposal

The Operational Budget

The term "budget" has many everyday applications: family budget, capital budget, tight budget, and so on. In accounting, **budgeting** applies to the process planning, forecasting, controlling, and monitoring the financial resources of the organization. The **operational budget** deals with the process of planning for the laboratory as an ongoing business concern, accounting for every-day needs and expenditures. It represents the financial parameters of the laboratory's goals for the coming year. The **capital budget** covers specific equipment acquisitions and building projects that require major financial commitments.

Preparation of the operational budget is covered here in four sections: (1) types of operational budgets, (2) stages in preparing the budget, (3) budgeting techniques and methods, and (4) use of the budget to monitor and provide feedback on the laboratory's success in meeting assigned financial objectives.

Types of Operational Budgets

Although the methods and techniques are quite similar, different terms apply to the budgeting process for government and private organizations. Government agencies and other public institutions refer to an *appropriations budget,* because expenditures must be approved and allocated (i.e., appropriated) by a governing body, such as the legislature or board of directors. In the private sector, the number of administrative groups involved in approval is limited to the organization itself, and the term is simply "the budget."

Forecast/Projection Method

Within this framework, different budgeting strategies have been proposed to meet the rapidly changing, dynamic nature of business organizations. However, all types of budgets continue to depend on the tools and techniques used in the *forecast/projection method.* Under this method a budget is prepared based on a forecast of what is expected to occur during the next period. This process makes projections of the increases or decreases that will occur on each line item in the budget based on historical information and adjustment for anticipated changes, such as inflation or nature of the business. Two other strategies, flexible and zero-based budgeting, are briefly defined next.

Flexible Budgeting

Many attempts have been made to arrive at a system of **flexible budgeting.** This system tries to set expenditures based on a variable workload volume. For example, at a certain patient census, the hospital should have a specific number of employees. When the number of patients increases, more staff is hired; when the census drops, employees are laid off. In practice, this has been difficult to implement because of recruitment and retention problems. Even supplies must be ordered in advance to ensure adequate levels. For this reason, a budget similar to the forecast method is prepared and then closely monitored to ensure that projections are on target.

Zero-Based Budgeting

Zero-based budgeting analyzes needs based on prioritizing of goals and objectives, not on past allocations. This procedure has had some success in setting priorities of large governmental and educational institutions. However, even in those cases some method of predicting how much an activity will cost is necessary, and historical data are the most dependable source of information.

For example, the laboratory may have a specific plan to examine each year which services should be performed in-house and which should be sent to reference laboratories. This would be much more than simply going down the test menu. Zero-based budgeting starts with the assumption that a service is *not* necessary, with extensive documentation required to explain why it must be performed in-house and not dropped in favor of a more productive option.

Operational Budget Preparation

Four issues must be addressed in preparing an operational budget: time frame, forecasting methods, scheduling, and format synthesis.

Time Frame

Budgets can be prepared to cover several time frames. The annual budget, which covers 1 year or budget cycle, is the main working guideline for management. Budgets are also frequently prepared to cover other periods, for example, a 5-year plan. Obviously the further a budget attempts to project, the more likely it will be incorrect. Long-term budgeting, however, is a tremendous help to the manager in planning the direction and long-term needs of the laboratory.

The time frame of the budget can also involve different dates. A budget cycle developed on a fiscal year may cover any 12-month period. For example, health care institutions experience their busiest, or peak, season during the first quarter of the year, so they may find it advantageous to postpone tax and budget preparation until a later date. They may, for example, select a fiscal year covering July 1 to June 30 for this purpose. Governmental agencies now tend to discourage the use of fiscal years; however, once established, change in the fiscal year requires special permission from taxing and regulatory authorities. A calendar year budget is the normal January 1 to December 31 schedule.

Forecasting Stage

Although most projections of future business activity are based on the extrapolation of historical data, several factors must be considered in all forecasts:

- Shifts in patient mix or volume
- Changes in medical staff composition
- Changes in business parameters such as inflation and reimbursement rates
- Expansion or cutbacks in services offered by the hospital or laboratory
- Population fluctuations brought about by changes in the local economy

If these factors are incorporated into forecasts based on historical information, a more realistic and predictable budget can be prepared.

Scheduling Stage

The budget preparation schedule varies from facility to facility. The document must go through several drafts, numerous meeting and negotiation sessions, and many revisions. For this reason, most institutions start the process about 6 months before the beginning of the new budget year. For example, if the hospital's budget cycle is based on a calendar year, the initial paperwork is delivered to the department manager during the first week in June.

The deadlines may be rotated by asking the manager to prepare the first draft of the revenue or volume section first because the rest of the budget depends on these figures. After a reliable revenue or volume projection is made, the rest of the budget can be completed based on this information. The labor hours budget is usually the next step because it is the largest cost item and the one most crucial to the operation of the facility.

Synthesis of Information

How the financial information is organized is very important. It must be presented logically, in a way that is useful to the manager and the organization. Figure 16 —1 (at the end of the chapter) provides an illustration of one type of budget report used in a hospital-based laboratory. Notice that each section lists the actual amount, the budget goal, and the variance in both dollars and percentage. This is given for both the current month and a year-to-date tally. The number for the same period a year ago is also provided for comparison purposes.

To provide this information in an orderly manner, the budget report is usually organized into three major parts:

- Revenue and volume figures
- Itemized cost categories
- FTEs and labor hours

The current, budgeted, year-to-date, and variance results for each of these parts are also listed.

Review of Budgeting Procedures

This section summarizes the budgeting procedures covered in the preceding chapters on revenue, salaries and wages, and costs. There are three methods of obtaining future budgeting figures, based on revenue or volume projections: actual costs, ratios, and percentage calculations. These figures are then used to prepare the **pro forma budget,** that is, the budget extrapolated from historical data. The pro forma calculations are used to determine the budget level for all other items.

The following steps and techniques are available for budget preparations:

1. The first step in any budget process is to develop a prediction of future volume. Once this is done, percentage and ratios calculations can be performed to project future economic activity. This forecast is usually done by applying a growth factor to the volume generated in the past. The growth factor includes expected increases in volume and changes in services or patient base.
2. A ratio can be calculated between the cost item and revenue or volume. An example is using the projection of testing volume as an indicator of volume along with currently available financial data. This information is then used to calculate an index for cost of supplies for the coming year. This is obtained by dividing supply expense by the number of procedures performed. The resulting factor may then be used to obtain the cost of supplies in the next budget cycle once an estimate of patient days has been determined. The ratio is set up as follows:

$$\text{Supply expense/test} = \frac{\text{current supply expense}}{\text{laboratory tests performed}}$$

3. Some budget items have predetermined costs. Instrument leases and service agreements are examples of items with fixed known costs for the coming year.
4. Expense items can be compared to the revenues of the department and a percentage calculated to project future relationships. For example, the cost of supplies may represent 17 percent of the revenues of the laboratory; this information can be used to project costs in the coming budget year.

Figure 16 —2 presents an example of a pro forma budget prepared using these four steps and based on the percentage-of-revenue method.

Monitoring and Feedback

The major objective in preparing a budget is management control of the financial resources of the organization. For this purpose the budget reports also include performance indexes (see Fig. 16 – 1 at the end of the chapter) tied to baseline statistics of patient days or testing volume.

Much attention is given to the achievement of budget goals, and comparing actual results with budget projections is an important method of control. The columns listing variance between actual costs and budget goals, in both dollars and percentage, highlights their importance. Other information, particularly the inclusion of the previous year's results for the same period on the report, is also helpful in comparing how well cost and revenue goals are being achieved.

ACTUAL CURRENT YEAR—TO—DATE DATA

Revenue	$2,450,000
Test Performed:	235,577
Revenue/Test =	$10.40

EXPENSES

Salaries and Wages	$ 820,750	(33.50% of Revenue)
Supplies	441,000	(18.00% of Revenue)
Reference Services	196,000	(8.00% of Revenue)
Instrument Leases	23,000	(0.94% of Revenue)
Maintenance Contracts	20,000	(0.82% of Revenue)
Education/Travel	2,500	(0.10% of Revenue)
TOTAL EXPENSES	$1,503,250	

****

PROJECTED BUDGET for NEXT YEAR

Predicted Growth Factor = 4%

Test Volume = 235,577 **x** 1.04 = 245,000

Revenue = 245,000 **x** $10.40 = $2,548,000

EXPENSES (expense item **x** % of revenue)

Salaries and Wages	$ 853,580	(33.50% of Revenue)
Supplies	458,640	(18.00% of Revenue)
Reference Services	203,840	(8.00% of Revenue)
Instrument Leases	23,951	(0.94% of Revenue)
Maintenance Contracts	20,894	(0.82% of Revenue)
Education/Travel	2,548	(0.10% of Revenue)
TOTAL EXPENSES	$1,563,453	

FIGURE 16 —2 . Example of pro forma Laboratory Budget

The Capital Budget

Capital budgeting is the process used by organizations to plan, evaluate, and choose between future investment opportunities. Specifically, this is the mechanism whereby the laboratory selects and authorizes the purchase of major equipment and building projects; these commitments often represent hundreds of thousands of dollars. Stringent rules of analysis are required when dealing with this level of expenditure; frequently, the budgeting of such items covers a multiple-year planning schedule. Both the capital and the operational budget enable the laboratory to determine revenue needs and manage its financial resources.

The four issues that must be addressed in preparing the capital budget are definition of capital, parts and formats of a capital budget, certificate-of-need requirements, and tools for analyzing and making purchasing and project decisions.

Definition of Capital

"Capital" is a term with many definitions. In one case it can refer to the monetary needs of the institution, as in "we must raise the needed capital." In accounting language it has a more narrow denotation. **Capital items** are purchases or projects that meet specific guidelines of *time, price,* and *purpose.* The ultimate financing plan (purchase, lease, or rental agreement) also determines how a project is budgeted. The influence of the payment program on classifying items in either the capital or operational budget is further reviewed in a later section on the budgeting considerations of purchase options.

Time criteria: The time frame of capital items is 1 year. If a product provides service for more than 1 year, it meets this criterion; if less, it is usually expensed during the year of acquisition.

Price criteria: The dollar value of a project also determines whether it is budgeted as a capital item or expensed. The cutoff amount varies widely and depends on the accounting policy of the business. For example, a new heating block costing $200 would meet the other two criteria for capital items, but because of the low cost and the paper work requirements, it would probably be handled as a supply expense for the year of purchase.

Purpose criteria: Entirely *new* instruments, furniture, or building projects are normally classified as capital projects under federal tax rules. If it is a repair or a replacement of part of existing equipment or structures, it is included in the operational budget.

Using these three criteria, an instrument purchase or building project can be classified as either a capital or an expense item and budgeted accordingly, depending on the standards applied and weight assigned by the laboratory to each factor.

Parts of a Capital Budget

Capital budgets are divided into two parts according to the amount of the expenditure. Projects costing less than a set limit need minimal paperwork, whereas those above this amount require extensive in-depth analysis. A common division point is $10,000.

Those projects meeting the minimal criteria frequently require only written justification describing the purpose, function, goals, and prioritization. Larger items need more extensive financial analysis, using the methods covered in this chapter.

Certificate of Need

In addition to preparing a capital budget for the institution's own use, federal and state regulations require health care facilities to submit capital plans on certain projects for approval and to obtain a **certificate-of-need (CON)** authorization before proceeding. This process is required for projects, equipment, or buildings above an established monetary level. Most states have set this limit at $150,000, following federal guidelines. A CON must also be obtained before new services such as oncology or obstetrics can be offered. This program was established in an attempt to control spiraling medical costs and to avoid duplication of services and the overbuilding of hospital beds.

Although the laboratory may not be directly involved in a CON process, the purposed instrumentation and building specifications for laboratory services are an integral part of the application.

Instrument/Project Capital Proposal

Two types of analysis are used in evaluating capital expenditures: (1) a narrative description, or *justification* of the need and intended use, and (2) quantitative techniques to determine the financial feasibility of the project. All capital projects must complete the justification section of the report. Those projects exceeding the set minimal dollar amount must also perform the financial feasibility studies.

For example, a capital proposal for a small chemistry analyzer costing around $8000 may need only the narrative justification; an analyzer costing more than $10,000 requires a financial feasibility study as well. Figure 16 — 3 provides an illustration of a capital budget proposal using the techniques described in this section.

Narrative Tools

Narrative tools include a written justification of the project and a prioritization of the competing proposals. These two concepts should be explained as completely as possible and then supported with a quantitative financial analysis.

Justification

In detailing the rationale for requesting an instrument or building program, the manager must explain why the project is needed, how it will benefit the laboratory, and why it should be considered over competing projects. Proposals can be justified by being grouped into one of four categories:

1. Necessary to maintain present service levels
2. Will provide significant savings over current methods
3. Will enhance or improve current programs
4. Will offer new procedures or services

As in any formal presentation, the more information the manager can provide to support a proposal, the better the chance of success. Statistics that demonstrate potential in cash flow or physician-to-patient satisfaction enhance the presentation. Increases in testing volume, reduction in reagent costs, and faster turnaround time are also factors that are certain to make an impression.

Prioritization

An additional step needed in the justification process is to prioritize the project, both in the time frame and in relation to other requests. Many capital budget forms have a scale to rank priority; others request a detailed narrative explanation of the acquisition and/or completion timetable.

PRIORITY: URGENT! Immediately needed to replace current instrument has constant downtime problems and limited capabilities.

TYPE OF PROJECT: Laboratory Instrument

NAME OF PROJECT: Automated Coagulation Timer

PURPOSE: Replace current model with a more reliable and technologically advanced instrument.

VENDOR: LSC Manufacturer

PRODUCT NAME AND ORDER INFORMATION:

PERFECT TECHNOLOGY	Automated Coagulation Timer Model: ACT2025 Catalog Number: LSC 2007

JUSTIFICATION:

The instrument will both significantly reduce turnaround time and enable the laboratory to automate frequently ordered tests now performed by time consuming manual methods.

The current instrument is more than 5 years old. Constant breakdowns have been responsible for extensive delays in the reporting of results. This has caused complaints from the medical staff and delays in the surgical schedule. The repair expenses for the current instrument were $7,500, and four major overnight repair problems occurred during the past year.

This new model will cut turnaround time in half and allow us to offer additional tests faster. The current instrument performs two procedures: PT and APTT. The new model will allow us to automate two additional tests, FIBROGEN, THROMBIN TIMES, and D-DIMERs reducing the turnaround time from 45 to 10 minutes. Also attached is a memo from Dr. Smith, chief of medical staff, requesting us to offer these services on a timely basis.

Operational expenses will be reduced drastically because the new instrument will use 80% fewer reagents and on-line refrigeration will eliminate any loss due to

PURCHASE PRICE:	$44,000
TRADE-IN CREDIT:	2,000
NET PURCHASE PRICE:	$42,000

ESTIMATED TESTING VOLUME: 20,000 tests a year

INCOME PER TEST: $12.50

ANNUAL INCOME GENERATED: $250,000

LIFE EXPECTANCY: 3 years (based on depreciation allowance provided by the hospital comptroller)

SALVAGE VALUE: The manufacturer estimates a trade-in value of $4000.

ACQUISITION OPTIONS: The manufacturer offers both lease and reagent rental plans. Details are attached.

FINANCIAL RATIOS:

Payback Period: 2 months
Average Rate of Return: 595%
Net Present Value: $558,000 (Cost of Capital estimate: 10%)

CONCLUSION: This project will not only improve the technological performance of the laboratory but also is a very attractive financial investment for the hospital.

FIGURE 16 —3 . Example of a Capital Budget Proposal

Examples of effective terminology include terms like "immediate," "urgent," "will replace a troublesome instrument that is on its last legs," or "anticipated need before the end of the year." Departments may submit several proposals; but they must be ranked according to their priority. A sound case must also be made so that the project receives a high priority ranking among requests from other departments.

Opportunity Costs

In any investment or acquisition decision, an important consideration is what other options are available and why this particular plan is better. **Opportunity cost** is the value of what is given up to pursue another project. In agreeing to buy a new chemistry analyzer this year and forgo upgrading the equipment in Radiology, Administration must see some potentially beneficial tradeoffs in service and money. Social as well as financial goals must be resolved. Few specific quantitative methods are available for this evaluation other than comparing the associated revenue and costs of each project. However, the impact of opportunity costs must be part of the overall decision making process.

Quantitative Tools

The quantitative techniques available to evaluate investment opportunities vary from simple profit-and-loss projections to sophisticated models that take into account taxation, inflation rate, economic forecasts, and revenue and cost predictions. Laboratory managers should be familiar with the techniques most frequently used and be able to apply them in support of their proposal. The most common methods used in health care facilities include payback period, average rate of return, and net present value. For-profit businesses and some health care organizations may want to apply a required rate-of-return standard to the capital proposal.

Payback Period

The **payback period** determines how long it will take to recover cash outlays. This procedure's value as an investment index has received severe criticism because it does not take into account any other monetary factors. Taken by itself, this point is true. However, the payback period is almost always required and is useful in that it demonstrates how long the company's money is in jeopardy.

Many investors and lenders perform this calculation to determine the length of time needed to recover their investment. Banks use a slightly modified form of this method to decide whether the customer can afford a new auto or home. A similar ratio is obtained by dividing the price of the home or car by the income of the borrower. For example, if a house costs $75,000 and the family's income is $30,000, it will take 2 ½ years at the current salary level to "pay back" the loan. Businesses use this same formula to assist in determining the affordability of a project.

$$\text{Payback period} = \frac{P}{I}$$

where P = purchase price of project
I = annual income generated

For example, a new chemistry profile instrument costs $110,000 and will produce an annual income of $380,000.

$$\text{Payback period} = \frac{\$110.000}{\$380{,}000/\text{yr}} = 0.29 \times 1\ \text{year}_{(12\text{months/yr})} = 3.5\ \text{months}$$

Also, by the nature of the business, laboratory instruments need a relatively shorter payback period because of the rapid technological obsolescence in this field.

Average Rate of Return

The average rate of return (ARR) is a straightforward calculation of the attractiveness of the average yield that will be earned over the life of an investment. If the chemistry instrument described has a life expectancy of 5 years, the **average rate of return** can be determined as follows

$$\text{Average rate of return} = \frac{I}{P}$$

$$= \frac{\$380{,}000}{\$110{,}000} = 3.46 \times 100 = 346\%$$

Net Present Value

To perform a net present value calculation it is important to understand the **time value of money**. This is most easily done by considering an offer from a colleague to borrow $1000, to be paid back in 1 year. If your money is in a savings account that pays 5 percent interest, it soon becomes obvious that the $1000 you lent today will actually be worth $1050 next year. You will be losing $50 in the transaction, plus the risk of losing your money. You may want to ask your friend to make up the difference.

The same thing happens if you buy a u.s. savings bond at a face value of $100, redeemable in 10 years. You pay $50 today on the basis of an agreement that says you will receive $100 at some time in the future. These two instances demonstrate that $1 today is worth more than $1 tomorrow. When inflation and interest rates are taken into account, the difference becomes even more pronounced.

Consider, for example, a major remodeling and instrumentation upgrade project that will offer more advanced and faster microbiology services, cost $1 million, and generate $300,000 a year over the next 5 years before it needs replacing. It may seem that the laboratory is making a nice profit of $500,000. However, the initial outlay of $1 million must be paid up front, and the payback period is 3.3 years; so, the $300,000 to be received over the next 5 years must be discounted to account for the time value of money.

The formula that provides this information is called the **net present value** (NPV). The calculation determines the current value of an investment taking into account the following two factors: the impact of interest and inflation on earnings and the anticipated revenue that will be received over a period of years. Although the calculations involved in this formula may appear cumbersome, there are tables and charts that have already factored in these figures, much like mortgage interest tables. Most business calculators are programmed to handle this calculation once the basic figures have been input.

$$PV = \sum_{t=1}^{n} Ct \frac{1}{(1+i)^t}$$

n = # of periods
Ct = cash flow received in period t
i = rate of discount
PV = present value

$$NPV = \left[\sum_{t=1}^{n} \frac{ACE}{(1+K)^1} + \frac{ACE}{(1+K)^2} + \ldots + \frac{ACE}{(1+K)^t} \right]$$

minus cost of renovation

Table 16 — 1 illustrates the impact of this calculation on a $500,000 microbiology project.

Year	Project Annual Cash Flow	Present Value (PV)*
1	$ 200,000	$181,818
2	210,000	173,554
3	225,000	169,046
4	240,000	163,923
4	253,000	157,093
Total	$1,128,000	$845,434

*Cost of capital is 10%

NPV = $845,434 (PV) — $5000,000 (cost of renovations) = $345,434

TABLE 16 — 1 . NPV Calculation for Renovation of Microbiology

Internal Rate of Return

The **internal rate of return,** also referred to as the *time-adjusted return method*, incorporates both cash flow and cost of capital factors and compares them to the amount of investment required. This equation is closely related to the net present value in formulation and complication. It is a useful tool in evaluating capital options, and business calculators have been programmed to perform this task with only three inputs: projected cash flow, initial cost of the project, and the expected life of the venture (years).

Required Rate of Return

Most for-profit enterprises have established a bottom-line level of income, or **required rate of return**, which must be achieved before any project will be considered. If the venture cannot be shown to benefit the company economically in cost savings, efficiency enhancement, or cash flow, it is rejected outright.

The counter to this requirement, particularly in health care organizations, is to make an extensive service enhancement justification that supports proceeding with the project even if it does not satisfy the required rate of return. Such justification may come by showing that the new project or laboratory instrument will reduce the length of stay of the patient or that the project is needed to support expanded services like a new operating room or cancer treatment center. This related or "fall-out" advantage should then be included in the capital proposal.

Financing a Project

After the financial proposal has been evaluated and a decision has been made to proceed, several alternatives are available to finance the project. If the plan involves building or remodeling, the company may either pay with current resources or borrow the needed funds.

With laboratory instruments, three options are available for consideration: outright purchase, leasing, and reagent rental plans. Depending on the financial terms, the costs may be either processed as an expense item in the operations budget or counted as a capital expenditure.

This section reviews two aspects of financing a project: acquisition options and depreciation. How these two factors affect the proposal greatly influences the decision the laboratory makes in how to purchase or finance the project.

Acquisition Options

If an item is purchased outright, it is considered a capital outlay and the expenses are written off through the process of depreciation. If the laboratory takes advantage of the many instrument or reagent rental plans, the costs may be included in the supply portion of the operational budget.

Lease agreements can be either a supply expense or a depreciable cost, depending on the terms of the contract. If the lease can be canceled at any time without further commitment by the firm, it is called an *operating lease,* and the costs are included in the supply part of the operational budget. A lease that cannot be canceled or includes an option to purchase is called a *capital lease* and is included in the capital budget.

Depreciation

The concept of depreciation takes into account the facts that capital projects are used over an extended period and that the value of these assets diminishes with time and use. This can be illustrated by the purchase of an automobile. As soon as the car is driven off the lot, its value drops significantly because it is no longer a "new" car. As the car ages, its value further declines with model year and mileage. The older the vehicle and the more miles it has been driven, the less it is worth. This process, called **depreciation,** is an important concept in accrual accounting methods (see Chapter 13).

The way depreciation is determined and recorded has a direct impact on the financial status of a company. In a for-profit business, the depreciation allowed in a year has a direct influence on the amount of taxes owed. Depreciation also plays a big role in determining the profit or loss of an enterprise. This is important in both for-profit and not-for-profit organizations because this information is used by lending and funding agencies. For these reasons, the company may be allowed a wide latitude in selecting the initial method to determine depreciation. Once this decision is made, however, it cannot be changed without special permission from lenders and government taxing authorities.

Depreciation is a factor in making other management decisions. Some institutions fund depreciation by putting aside a certain amount of money to cover replacement costs. Depreciation also provides a guideline in planning a replacement schedule for equipment, buildings, and other physical assets.

Two key points need to be clarified concerning how depreciation allowances are determined: final salvage value and methods for calculating depreciation allowances.

Salvage Value

In the automobile example, the car continues to decrease in value until it is traded in or sold to a junkyard. Either way, it has a residual value at the time of disposal. This can be the trade-in credit, the replacement cost, or the $50 obtained from the junkyard. This **salvage value** must be considered in determining the depreciation of an item. Salvage value is defined as the value of an item at the time of resale, trade-in, or disposal.

Allowance Calculation Methods

Because depreciation is a function of both time and usage, two main methods of calculating the depreciation amount have been developed: *straight-line* and *unit of output.* There are other methods; however, they must be specifically approved by taxing authorities and are normally allowed only when the government wishes to encourage investment in capital projects by special legislation.

Straight-line depreciation is the method based on the time element. As a product grows older, its value decreases and maintenance costs increase. This method can be used for all capital items, but it is usually used to establish depreciation rates for buildings and other structures with an extended life expectancy (i.e., greater than 10 years). Hence:

$$\text{Annual depreciation} = \frac{\text{cost of project} - \text{salvage value}}{\text{life expectancy}}$$

For example, an independent laboratory constructs a new building for a total cost of $500,000 ($50,000 for the land and $450,000 for the facility and site improvements). At current estimates, the building is expected to be used for 20 years, with a salvage value of *$45,000. Note:* Land is considered to last forever and is never depreciated.

$$\text{Annual depreciation} = \frac{\$500{,}000 - (\$50{,}000 + \$45{,}000)}{20\text{ yr}}$$

$$= \frac{\$500{,}000 - \$95{,}000}{20\text{ yr}}$$

$$= \$20{,}250/\text{yr}$$

Unit of output considers the fact that equipment deteriorates based on the rate of use as well as time. This procedure can also be used for most capital projects but is more commonly applied to equipment that has a measurable usage rate, such as mileage or units of production. The Internal Revenue Service (IRS) mileage allowance is an example of this principle.

$$\text{Unit depreciation} = \frac{\text{purchase price} - \text{salvage value}}{\text{estimated number of units produced over the life of the investment}}$$

For example, a hematology analyzer is purchased for $115,000 and is expected to perform 32,000 CBCs a year. The instrument will be traded in for a $35,000 credit after 3 years.

$$\text{Unit depreciation} = \frac{\$115{,}000 - \$35{,}000}{32{,}000 \times 3\text{ yr}}$$

$$= \frac{\$80{,}000}{96{,}000} = \$0.833 \text{ per CBC}$$

Accelerated depreciation methods can be used to take advantage of tax loopholes and manipulate the reporting of financial performance, as allowed by taxing and lending authorities. These may benefit the company over the short term by increasing costs to offset large profits or reduce the amount of the taxes owed. The double declining balance (DDB) and sums-of-year digits (SYD) methods are the most common acceleration techniques. Both methods can be computed using special tables or programmable calculators. Calculation factors and allowance amounts change frequently, depending on the rules and regulations established by the taxing authority.

Capital Budget Proposal

The capital budget process culminates in the preparation and submission of a capital budget proposal. The exact format and order in which information is presented vary depending on the accounting preference of the organization. Figure 16 – 3(above) provides an illustration of one model, proposing the purchase of an automated coagulation instrument. Near the top, the name and type of project must be identified, followed by the narrative justification and the financial analysis.

The capital budget proposal ends the chapter on *The Laboratory Budget*. The next chapter looks at the development of *Laboratory Information Systems*.

FIGURE 16 — 1 *pages 1 and 2*.
Laboratory Operational Report (Budget)

Next two pages

CODE	DESCRIPTION	CURRENT MONTH ACTUAL	BUDGET	VARIANCE $	VARIANCE %	PREVIOUS YEAR ACTUAL
10000	PATIENT DAYS	6,120	6,230	-110	-1.8	6,206
	PROCEDURES	34,519	35,600	-1,081	-3.0	35,479
	STATISTICS/ PATIENT DAY	5.64	5.71			5.71
10100	REVENUE					
10110	INPATIENT	673,929	694,805	-20,876	-3.0	689,213
10020	OUTPATIENT	180,262	184,655	-4,393	-2.4	182,333
	TOTAL	854,191	879,460	-25,269	-2.9	871,546
19000	EXPENSES					
19100	SALARIES & WAGES	74,887	70,055	4,832	6.9	70,625
19200	SUPPLIES	49,212	50,132	-920	1.8	47,044
10300	REFERENCE LABS	40,606	38,705	-1,901	-4.9	38,348
10400	SERVICE CONTRACTS	2,576	2,576	0	0	2,490
10500	TRAVEL	0	300	300	100	250
10600	SUBSCRIPTION	1,296	1,300	4	0	1,150
10700	OTHER	9,390	11,100	1,710	15.4	10,552
	TOTAL	177,967	174,168	-3,799	2.2	170,459
	GROSS MARGIN	676,224	705,292	-29,068	-4.12	701,087
	PER STAT					
	INPATIENT REVENUE	19.52	19.52	0	0	19.42
	OUTPATIENT REVENUE	5.22	5.19	-.03	0	5.14
	TOTAL REVENUE	24.74	24.71	-.03	0	24.56
	SALARIES & WAGES	2.16	1.97	-.19	-9.6	1.99
	SUPPLIES	1.43	1.41	-.02	-1.8	1.33
	REFERENCE LABS	1.18	1.09	-.09	-8.3	1.08
	SERVICE CONTRACTS	.07	.07	0	0	.07
	TRAVEL	0	.01	.01	100	.01
	SUBSCRIPTION	.04	.04	0	0	.03
	OTHER	.27	.31	.04	12.9	.30
	TOTAL EXPENSES	5.16	4.90	-.25	5.1	4.81
	LABOR HR	7.176	7.107	-69	0	7.147
	AVG HR RATE	10.38	10.42	.04	0	9.89
	HR/STAT	.20	.19	-.01	0	.20
	FTEs	41.4	41.0	-.04	0	41.2

FIGURE 16 — 1. Laboratory Operational Report (Budget)
Page 1 of 2

CODE	DESCRIPTION	YEAR TO DATE ACTUAL	BUDGET	VARIANCE $	VARIANCE %	PREVIOUS YEAR TO DATE ACTUAL
10000	PATIENT DAYS	18,420	18,721	-301	-1.6	18,128
	PROCEDURES	106,559	106,700	-141	-.1	104,910
	STATISTICS/ PATIENT DAY	5.79	5.71			5.79
10100	REVENUE					
10110	INPATIENT	2,082,163	2,087,329	-5,166	-.2	2,044,696
10020	OUTPATIENT	555,493	553,396	2,097	.4	546,581
	TOTAL	2,637,656	2,640,725	-3,069	-.1	2,591,277
19000	EXPENSES					
19100	SALARIES & WAGES	221,566	219,112	-2,454	-1.1	214,532
19200	SUPPLIES	155,514	150,257	-5,257	-3.5	146,666
10300	REFERENCE LABS	118,304	120,945	2,641	-2.2	118,421
10400	SERVICE CONTRACTS	7,728	7,728	0	0	7,470
10500	TRAVEL	459	450	-9	-2.0	413
10600	SUBSCRIPTION	3,921	3,900	-21	-.5	3,455
10700	OTHER	29,170	34,065	4,895	14.4	32,656
	TOTAL	536,662	536,457	-205	0	523,613
	GROSS MARGIN	2,100,994	2,104,268	3,274	.2	2,067,664
	PER STAT					
	INPATIENT REVENUE	19.54	19.52	-.02	-.1	19.49
	OUTPATIENT REVENUE	5.21	5.18	-.03	.6	5.21
	TOTAL REVENUE	24.75	24.70	-.05	-.2	24.70
	SALARIES & WAGES	2.08	2.05	-.03	-1.5	2.05
	SUPPLIES	1.46	1.41	-.05	-3.5	1.40
	REFERENCE LABS	1.11	1.14	-.03	-2.6	1.13
	SERVICE CONTRACTS	.07	.07	0	0	.07
	TRAVEL	0	0	0	0	0
	SUBSCRIPTION	.04	.04	0	0	.03
	OTHER	.27	.32	.05	15.6	.31
	TOTAL EXPENSES	5.03	5.03	0	0	4.99
	LABOR HR	21,284	21,028	256	1.2	21,648
	AVG HR RATE	10.41	10.42	.01	.1	9.91
	HR/STAT	.20	.20	0	0	.21
	FTEs	41.5	41.0	.5	1.2	41.7

FIGURE 16 — 1. Laboratory Operational Report (Budget)
Page 2 of 2

— Case Study —

Chapter Sixteen: The Laboratory Budget

"We need a new instrument for drug testing," announced the chemistry supervisor to the laboratory director as they were heading off to lunch. "The one we have is not only out of date, it's broken down constantly, and the doctors are asking us to do more toxicology and therapeutic drug workups on a STAT basis. They don't have time to do these on the second and third shift with the slow manual procedures we now do."

"I know," responded the laboratory director. "I just came out of a meeting with the pathologists and we need to make this a priority. This is also a good time. The new budget is just now being worked up. Why don't you start getting the information on the instruments available and we'll sit down and work up a capital proposal."

"No problem," answered the chemistry supervisor. "I've already been doing that, and I saw most of them at the convention last month. I have even received price proposals on all of them."

"Great ... let's do it tomorrow after the morning workload has been completed. Getting it in early will show administration that we really need it," suggested the laboratory director.

"I should be in your office around ten o'clock," agreed the chemistry supervisor as they entered the cafeteria.

Chapter Sections for Review

- The Capital Budget
  - Narrative Tools
    - + Payback
    - + Average Rate of Return
    - + Net Present Value
  - Capital Budget Proposal

Questions for Discussion

1. Use the following information to calculate the payback period, ARR, and NPV for the instrument selected.

Name of instrument selected:	TOX STAT
Purchase price	$ 55,000
Estimated testing volume:	23,000
Net income per test:	$14.00
Average annual income generated:	$322,000
Life expectancy:	3 years
Salvage value estimate:	$ 7,000
Cost of capital over life expectancy:	8%
Acquisition options:	Manufacturer offers both lease and reagent rental plans

2. Prepare a capital budget proposal using Figure 16 — 3 as an example.

SOLUTIONS

Payback period = $55,000 / $322,000 = 0.17/year   62 days or 2 months

AAR = $322,000 = 5.85 *x* 100 = 585%

NPV = [*note: This example is intended to be illustrative. If a programmable calculator or NPV chars is available, more precise calculations may be determined*.]

Year	Projected Net Cash Flow		Cost of Capital 8%		PV of Cash Flow
1	$322,000	*x*	(1--.08) .92	=	$296,240
2	$322,000	*x*	(1--.16) .84	=	$270,480
3	$322,000	*x*	(1--.24) .76	=	$244,720
Total *(cash flow)*	$966,000		*(Present value of cash flow)*	=	$811,440

Cost of Project $55,000
NPV of Project $756,440 [$811,440 — $55,000]
[Present value of cash flow *minus* initial outlay expenses]

[17]

Laboratory Information Systems

— Chapter Seventeen —

The term "laboratory information system" (LIS) has become almost synonymous with the process of computerizing the laboratory. However, this analogy is only partially true. Information systems organize and incorporate every aspect of the laboratory's operations into a unified network. They are designed to meet the complete information needs of the entire organization. This concept encompasses the systems theory of organizations and their continual cycle of intake of resources, internal processing of these resources, and returning the products and services to the external users (see Chapter 2).

Computers and their associated paraphernalia must be viewed from the perspective of their capabilities, limitations, and potential contribution to the delivery of laboratory services. They are a tool of management, not an end in themselves. Without human instructions they are merely bunches of plastic and wire. With human interaction, they can carry the operations of a laboratory beyond the boundaries of our current understanding.

As with all tools, however, how computers are used determines their potential. If we took the time to provide each other with the laboriously detailed instructions required to get the computer to perform even the most elementary task, almost anyone could seem as smart as these machines. The possibilities are in the person, not in the piece of equipment.

This chapter introduces the concept of computers as management tools, to be used within the context of a complete laboratory information system. An overview of information systems, major computer components, and systems analysis provides the reader with a basic understanding of the application of computer technology to laboratory information problems. The chapter begins by explaining the terms "data" and "information," which are used frequently throughout the chapter, and concludes with a discussion on the selection and implementation of a laboratory information system.

OBJECTIVES

After completion of this chapter, the reader will be able to demonstrate accomplishment of the following objectives.

1. Explain the characteristics and activities of an information system.
2. Describe the major components of a computer-based information system.
3. Recognize the features and purpose of computer networks.
4. Define the goals and objectives of a laboratory information system.
5. Describe the process of systems analysis and design of computer components in a laboratory information system.
6. Identify the four types of flow charts.
7. Develop a plan for the selection and installation of a laboratory information system.

Chapter Highlights and Glossary of Key Terms

I. DATA AND INFORMATION

***Data**: Raw elements, or single facts, that by themselves have no meaning, but when organized and evaluated together have the potential to reveal information.*

***Information**: Data that have been processed, sorted, and presented in such a manner that it increases the knowledge of the user.*

II. INFORMATION SYSTEMS

***Information System:** A collection of interlinked and dependent parts that are organized to collect and input data, process the data into information, output the information to users, and provide feedback to the system with the goal of meeting the complete informational needs of the organization.*

III. COMPUTER-BASED INFORMATION SYSTEMS

***Computer-Based Information System (CBIS):** An information system that uses the components and technology of computers.*

A. Components of computer-based information systems

1. Hardware

***Computer Hardware**:* The *physical (i.e., plastic and wire) parts of a computer.*

***Input Devices**: Mechanisms whereby the computer receives data; these include keyboards, bar-code readers, computer links, and data converters.*

Central Processing Unit (CPU): The *electronic portion of a computer; includes the controlling unit and the quantitative analysis and data processing unit (i.e., arithmetic logic unit).*

***Output Devices:** Mechanisms such as printers and screens that allow the computer to disseminate information and communicate with its users.*

***I/O Devices:** Input-output devices.*

a. Central processing unit

b. Computer memory and data storage

***Main Memory:** The primary storage space inside the CPU designed for holding data and instructions while they are actively processed.*

***Peripheral Storage Devices:** The secondary, or remote, storage devices such as CDs, flash drives MDI cards; used to store data not being actively processed by the CPU.*

***Read-Only Memory (ROM):** Part of the memory that is permanently protected from being modified, erased, or written over.*

***Random-Access Memory (RAM):** Part of the memory (main and peripheral) that is not protected from alteration.*

***Database:** In general, refers to all the data stored in both the main memory and peripheral storage devices; in particular, refers to a specific collection of related computer files.*

c. Data storage devices

***Hard Disk:** A disk stored inside the CPU; consists of a magnetic-coated metal plate used for the main operating programs of the computer.*

***Floppy Disk:** A removable flexible plastic disk with a magnetic coating, used to store information external to the CPU; also known as a diskette.*

***Flash Disk**: "A storage module made of flash memory chips. Flash disks have no mechanical platters or access arms, but the term 'disk' is used because data is accessed as if it were a disk. The disk storage structure is emulated."*

***Optical Disk:** Laser-read compact disk (CD); may be either CD-ROM (read-only memory) or CD-RAM (random-access memory).*

***Disk Drive:** The mechanical machinery and electronic unit that allows data and information to be extracted and entered on disks by the computer; may contain either a magnetic scanner or a laser reader*

2. Software

Software: *The instructions (i.e., program) given to the computer to perform its tasks.*

Applications Software: *Programs designed to meet specific needs of the users, such as word processing, payroll, or blood bank inventory management.*

Systems Software: *Programs designed to control and run the operating systems of the computer including communications, application software and database management.*

Middleware: *A software program which connects independent operating systems, allowing them to communicate and exchange information*

a. Software Verification and Validation

b. Computer languages

Machine Language: *The binary-coded language used directly by the computer.*

Programming Language: *A language used to write software for the computer; allows the program to be written in English-like symbols using rules (i.e., syntax) that are more easily understood by human beings than is machine language.*

c. CPU machine language and binary codes

Bytes: *The storage units of a computer, comparable to words in a human language.*

Bits: *Subunits of bytes, comparable to letters in an alphabetic human language; represent one position on a computer chip or a single digit in machine language.*

B. Computer networks

Local-Area Network (LAN): *A computer network that connects computers and their equipment in a confined area, usually a building or a place in which the users are in close geographical proximity to each other (e.g., a multi-facility medical center complex) .*

Wide-Area Network (WAN): *A computer network that connects computers and their equipment over a large, disbursed geographical area such as a state, nation, or the whole world, usually through the facilities of common carriers, such as telephone lines or satellite channels.*

1. Host-based laboratory information system (LIS)

Host-Based Laboratory Information System: *A local-area network interfaced with a central controlling CPU whose program determines how data are received, processed, and disseminated.*

2. Client-server LIS

Client-Server Laboratory Information System: *An open system that allows users to tap into the LIS with their independent computer systems, extract only the information they want, and present it in the format they wish on their own computer screen or printer.*

IV. THE LABORATORY INFORMATION SYSTEM

Laboratory Information System: *A complete network of computer components designed to incorporate all aspects of the informational needs of the laboratory and its customers from the intake of requests for services and the processing of work flow to the delivery of results.*

A. Planning for computerization

B. Systems analysis and design: laboratory needs assessment

Systems Analysis and Design: *The formal process of studying a problem and creating a solution.*

1. LIS computer hardware

Systems Hardware Diagram: *A document that diagrams the computer hardware components of an information system.*

2. LIS computer software

3. Autoverification

4. Flow charts

Systems Flow Chart: *A pictorial depiction of the system as a complete*

whole, showing only subsystems or major elements.
Procedural Flow Chart: *A graphic presentation of an individual task, operation, or data flow within the system.*
Logic Flow Chart: *An in-depth analysis of the sequencing of logical or mathematical steps in a specific order of events.*
Deployment Flow Diagram: *A flow chart that spreads out the format horizontally to depict the action and decision points in a separate column for each area.*

C. Selecting a laboratory information system
D. Installing the laboratory information system

Data and Information

The terms "data" and "information" are frequently used interchangeably in everyday language, but there is an important difference between these two words when they are applied to computers.

- **Data** are the raw elements, or facts, that have little meaning by themselves, but when organized and evaluated together have the potential to reveal information.
- **Information** is data that have been processed, sorted, and presented in a manner that increases the knowledge of the user.

A random quality control result is an example of a data point. Individually, the value is only part of the QC data and is basically meaningless by itself. However, when placed with other QC results and statistically evaluated, it helps provide crucial insights into the performance parameters of a procedure; in other words, it provides information that can ultimately lead to knowledge.

The US Food and Drug Administration provide a glossary of terms for computerized systems which is: "*This document is intended to serve as a glossary of terminology applicable to software development and computerized systems in FDA regulated industries. It will facilitate consistency in describing the requirements of the law and regulations applicable to such products and systems. It is also a resource for investigators who conduct inspections and investigations involving software and computerized systems.*"

Computers, with their speed and ability to process gigantic volumes of data, make it possible to turn data into information with remarkable efficiency. The data transformation process, or DTP (data → processing → information), goes through five steps.

1. The individual data points must be captured and verified.
2. The data must be sorted and arranged into a system that enables the data to be classified and summarized.
3. The data must be processed and manipulated (i.e., calculations must be performed) to arrive at the needed information.
4. The information must be readily available for recall by an efficient retrieval and reproducing system.
5. The information must be disseminated.

The ultimate aim of data processing is to provide relevant information to the designated user.

Information Systems

Like all systems, information systems, whether computerized or manual, have three characteristics in common (see Chapter 2 for additional information on general systems theory).

- Orderly grouping and interdependence of the parts.
- Centralized organization and control process.
- A common goal or mission

An information system pathway (ISP) functions in much the same way as the data transformation pathway, as shown in Figure 17 – 1.

This figure is intended to illustrate the progressional relationship and identical pathways that these three systems follow; and the primary role the CPU plays in any computer based information system.

- Information System Pathway (ISP)
- Data transformation Process (DTP)
- Computer-based Information System (CBIS)

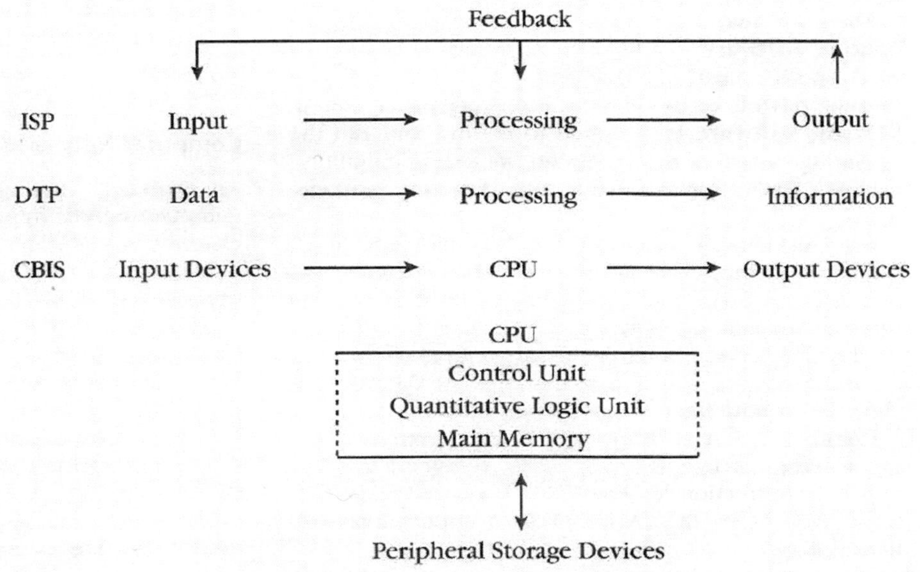

Figure 17 – 1. Centro Processing Unit (CPU) and Computer–based information System (CBIS)

1. The raw data *inputs* are collected from many sources, including laboratory instruments, manual results and data entry, the hospital's main computer system interface, and accounting and billing functions.
2. The data is then *processed* into usable information. The data are stored in the database and then manipulated as instructed; that is, certain calculations are performed, the results organized, and the data turned into information.
3. The information is delivered as *output* to users, usually in the form of printouts or screen displays, for operational purposes and decision making.

4. Users then use the output as a *feedback* mechanism to make corrections and adjustments in the input and processing functions.

Thus, an **information system** may be defined as a collection of interlinked and dependent parts that are organized to collect and input data, process the data into information, output the information to users, and provide feedback to the system with the goal of meeting the complete informational needs of the organization. These activities may be done manually (Varnadoe, 1979) but are usually performed with the help of computers.

An information system designed for the laboratory must follow the work flow of the laboratory in receiving inputs such as test requests and support services from
outside sources, through the processing of these requests and resources in the laboratory, to the final delivery of its services to its clients (Figure 17 – 2 and Chapter 2). Feedback from this output is then returned by the external users to the laboratory, where the process begins again.

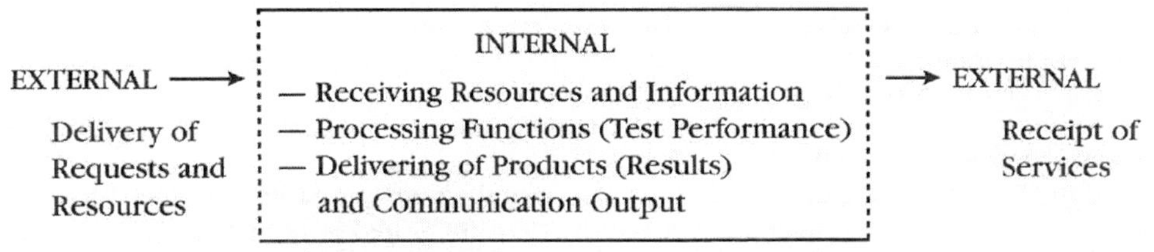

FIGURE 17 — 2. Communication and Systems Model (hospital-based laboratory)

An understanding of how the laboratory functions as a system — receiving, processing, and issuing activities — is the foundation for the analysis and design of data and information flow (i.e., systems analysis) into a complete laboratory information system.

Computer-Based Information Systems

A **computer-based information system (CBIS)** is one that uses the components and technology of computers to operate an information system. Because of their ability to store and rapidly process huge amounts of data computers have, in practical terms, become synonymous with information systems. Analyzing the organization's information needs, designing and selecting the specific components and configuration of the computer to be used, and installing the system are all parts of the process of computerization.

A key factor in the design of a CBIS is the selection and arrangement of the components of the computer. For this reason and to provide an overview of how the parts of an information system fit together, a short review of the major components of a computer system begins this section.

This review provides a brief description of the components of a computer-based information system and the software used to instruct and operate the system. The reader is referred to the many books and references available on this subject for a complete description of the elements and terminology of computer technology. [Alan Freedman and Franklin R. Elevitch and Raymond D. Aller are recommended. See also the bibliography for additional sources.]

Components of Computer-Based Information Systems

The two basic components of any computer system are the *hardware* and the *software.* Together these two components combine to form the basic elements and design of a computer system. Adding to and supporting the computer are the programmers and operators who use, design, and run the system.

Following is additional information about the terminology and main features of both the hardware and software components of a computer and a brief look at another important factor in a CBIS design, its network system.

Hardware

Computers range in size from small laptop models use d by individuals for personal projects to mainframes, which are capable of operating the space program. **Computer hardware** constitutes the physical (i.e., plastic and wire) parts of the computer. Figure 17 – $1_{\text{(above)}}$ offers a schematic of a computer-based information system, which includes the following hardware.

1. **Input devices**, which are the mechanisms that enable the computer to receive data. These are the keyboards, bar-code readers, scanners, computer links, and data converters.
2. The **central processing unit (CPU)**, which is the heart and brain of the computer. The CPU may be a stand-alone mainframe unit located in a central location with links to remote terminals or the tiny microchips, which are inside the single-unit desktop computers. The CPU processes data, performs calculations, and stores the information for retrieval.
3. The **output devices**, such as printers and screens, which allow the computer to disseminate information and communicate with its users.

Whereas most users are usually familiar with the readily visible input-output (I/O) devices of a computer (e.g., keyboards, printers, and screens), a closer look at the CPU, its memory functions, machine language, and data storage mechanisms may be needed to understand how these key components interact and operate to form the primary elements of any computer system.

Central Processing Unit

The CPU is the component of the computer that processes the data. The CPU includes the electronic elements used for controlling the system, quantitative analysis and data processing (i.e., arithmetic logic unit), and internal memory data storage compartments. These functions may be contained in a single unit, such as a desktop or personal computer, or the storage functions may be handled by ancillary mechanisms such as the abundant assortment of disks, drives, and remote internet servers, which then interfaces with a central CPU on an as needed basis.

The CPU executes instructions for processing data by collating, grouping, transforming, interpreting, and performing calculations on the data received. In performing these tasks, the CPU follows the instructions given by the program software, which is usually stored in the computer's main memory.

Carried forward from the review of information systems, Figure 17 – $1_{\text{(above)}}$ shows the primary role the CPU plays in any computer-based information system.

Computer Memory and Data Storage

With the introduction of the microchip, the biggest and most expensive limiting factor of a computer has become the availability and accessibility of memory storage space. Memory is the most expensive aspect of computer design. It is the major factor in the processing speed of the unit: each time a computer must pause and connect with a peripheral data storage source, there is a delay in processing speed. Available memory is determined by the space allocated within the CPU to data storage and retrieval (i.e., main memory) and the remoteness of peripheral storage devices.

Following are several terms and concepts associated with computer memory and data storage that directly influence the physical size, processing speed, and price of a computer system.

- **Main memory:** Main memory, or primary storage, is the space inside the CPU (imprinted circuits and the hard disk) designed for holding data and instructions while they are being actively processed.
- **Peripheral,** or secondary, **storage devices**: these are devices such as disks and drives that are used to store data not being actively processed by the CPU.
- **Read-only memory (ROM) :** Read-only memory is part of the memory that is permanently protected from being modified, erased, or written over. ROM is usually used to protect system control programs from unauthorized changes or patented products such as computer games and commercial programs. ROM is "nonvolatile," which means it will not be lost if the power or system is turned off.
- **Random-access memory (RAM) :** Random-access memory is the part of the memory (main and peripheral) that is not protected from alteration. RAM is used to temporarily store data for further manipulation or reference by the CPU. RAM is "volatile" in the sense that it must be protected from loss (i.e., the file must be "saved") in case the computer loses power or is turned off.
- **Database:** In general, the term "database" applies to all the data stored in both the main memory and peripheral storage devices. In its most limited technical use, however, it refers to a specific collection of related computer files.

Data Storage Devices

Many methods of storing data have been used during the evolution of computer technology. The earlier methods include the now obsolete computer punch cards, reels of magnetic tape, and even ordinary cassette cartridges. Current data storage devices include including various types of disks and external drives.

Computer memory mechanisms are made up of the internal (i.e., primary) space inside the CPU allocated to the main memory and of peripheral (i.e., secondary) storage devices. Internal data storage consists of the imprinted circuits of silicon chips and the hard disk. Additional peripheral devices are designed and connected to handle the system's speed and database requirements.

Because of the dependence on the rapid accessibility to data and the expense associated with keeping and organizing these items, computer disks and drives capable of storing tremendous volumes of data in a small amount of space have been developed and are now the most common form of peripheral storage.

Computer disks come in various sizes and formats and are designed to meet a variety of needs. The terminology used to describe major types of disks and associated equipment are described in the following list.

- A **hard disk** is stored inside the CPU and consists of a magnetic-coated metal plate used for the main operating programs of the computer.
- A **floppy disk,** also known as a "diskette" (e.g., 3.5-inch), is a removable flexible plastic disk with a magnetic coating, used to store information external to the CPU. While these types of disks are not as "floppy" as older models (e.g., 5.25 inch) this term is still in use. They are being rapidly replaced with other formats able to store enormous amount of data in very small places. However, they are still in use, mainly because of limita-

tions/familiarity of individuals for acquiring new technology. Often new items, such as **flash disks** and **memory cards** may be included in this category

- An **optical disk** is the same laser-read compact disk (CD) used to record music. They may be further classified as either CD-ROM (i.e., read-only memory, in which the memory database is protected against overwriting), or CD-RAM, which allows for the random access of memory and may permit data to be added or manipulated.
- A **disk drive** is the mechanical machinery and electronic unit that allows data and information to be extracted and entered on disks (external or internal) by the computer. Depending on the type of disk being used, such drives may contain either a magnetic scanner or a laser reader.

Software

Software consists of the instructions given to the computer — its program. The terms "software," "programs," and "instructions" are often used synonymously in computer terminology. The purpose and intended applications are the overriding factors in selecting a computer program. Prepackaged computer programs can be bought and installed in the computer, or programs can be customized to meet specific needs.

There are two broad categories of software. **Applications software** consists of programs designed to meet specific needs of the users, such as word processing, payroll, or blood bank inventory management. **Systems software** is designed to control and run the operating system of the computer, including communications, application software, and database management.

Software choices and design control the flow of information to the terminals, the way data are collected from input sources such as laboratory instruments and other computers, the way the information is displayed on the CRT screen, printout formats, and even the way the user accesses, enters, and modifies the database; in short, everything the computer does.

Computer software is prepared by programmers using a computer language especially designed to communicate instructions to the CPU. These languages offer a wide range of options in both applications and terminology.

Another term, use for software which is now commonly available to connect to independent systems, is **Middleware**. Described by Kenneth C. Laudon and Jane P. Laudon: *"Middleware is software that connects two otherwise separate applications, enabling them to communicate with each other and to exchange data." (p. 212)*

An example of middleware may be a program which allows the laboratory to use a separate system for microbiology or blood bank then the one used in the rest of the laboratory. The middleware program would interface and incorporate the two systems together without the users having to access or utilize several different links or access points, or having to go to an entirely different computer station.

Software Verification and Validation

Daniel F. Cowan states that: "*Validation of the laboratory information system is the continuing process of proving the system fit for its intended use, initially and over time.*" (p. 43) Software validation is one of the AABB 13 guidelines for installing computer systems (see last section of this chapter for an example of software validation in the blood bank).

The laboratory end used is almost always dependent on what is called "black box" testing with selects a task (external perspective) or end-function and sees how/if the system performs the task (e.g., does it call-up, or print out the report I need when I hit this button). "White box" testing (internal perspective) which checks and examines each software step/circuit against manufacturing functional specifications, is usually left for the vendor.

The U.S. Department of Health and Human Services, Food and Drug Administration have issued General Principles of Software Validation, which ... *"is based on generally recognized software validation principles and, therefore, can be applied to any software."* ... ***"Software verification** provides objective evidence that the design outputs of a particular phase of the software development life cycle meet all of the specified requirements for that phase."*

The guidelines apply to all software purchased or used by the government, which encompasses most computer software:

- Software used as a component, part, or accessory of a medical device;
- Software that is itself a medical device (e.g., blood establishment software);
- Software used in the production of a device (e.g., programmable logic controllers in manufacturing equipment); and
- Software used in implementation of the device manufacturer's quality system (e.g., software that records and maintains the device history record).

Also from the FDA are **General Principles of Software Validation; Final Guidance for Industry and FDA Staff:**

> The software requirements specification document should contain a written definition of the software functions. It is not possible to validate software without predetermined and documented software requirements. Typical software requirements specify the following:
>
> - All software system inputs;
> - All software system outputs;
> - All functions that the software system will perform;
> - All performance requirements that the software will meet, (e.g., data throughput, reliability, and timing);
> - The definition of all external and user interfaces, as well as any internal software-to-system interfaces;
> - How users will interact with the system;
> - What constitutes an error and how errors should be handled;
> - Required response times;
> - The intended operating environment for the software, if this is a design constraint (e.g., hardware platform, operating system);
> - All ranges, limits, defaults, and specific values that the software will accept; and
> - All safety related requirements, specifications, features, or functions that will be implemented in software.
>
> http://www.fda.gov/cdrh/comp/guidance/938.html
> General Principles of Software Validation; Final Guidance for Industry and FDA Staff Document issued on: January 11, 2002
> [connected July 13, 2007]

Computer Languages

A variety of languages are available for programming a computer. Some, such as FORTRAN, are designed for engineering and scientific applications. Others, like COBOL and $C^{++,}$ are best suited for business situations. MS-DOS is one language developed for personal computers (PCs). MUMPS is designed especially for medical applications.

CAP check in their report if Laboratory Information Systems utilize: Delpha, C++, C, ASP.net, Cobol, Java, PORT, 4D, HTML (a internet code language)

All computer programming languages originate in binary-coded **machine language,** which is used by the CPU. **Programming languages,** however, allow computer instructions to be written in alphanumeric symbols using rules (i.e., syntax) that are more easily understood by human beings. Current programming languages are constantly being revised and updated, and new languages are being introduced as the frontiers of computer technology continue to expand. But the systems software must always translate the program into the binary codes of machine language, which is the only language the CPU understands.

CPU Machine Language and Binary Codes

Machine language is stored in **bytes,** which are units comparable to words in a human language. Just as words are made up of letters from the alphabet, a byte is composed of subunits called **bits** (from binary *digit).* A bit represents one position on a computer chip; a byte contains eight bits in computer machine language.

The storage capacity of a computer is indicated by the number of bytes available; these are usually expressed in kilobytes (KB) (units of a thousand bytes) and megabytes (MB) (units of a million bytes), now we are well into the GB (units in the billion). For example, if the computer lists a capacity of 200 GB, it has the ability to store and process 200 billion bytes of data at one time without accessing another sources.

Bits are binary digits, either $0_{(zero)}$ or 1, which are the numeric counterparts of *on* or *off* status to the semiconductor materials and switches that are used to make processors. A group of O'*s* and I'*s* form a machine language coding for each number, letter, or symbol. The binary-coded machine language tells the CPU which semiconductor circuit to turn off or on to code the digital message. The order of O'*s* and I'*s* defining these characters forms a byte. For example, a byte with a binary code of 00101001 may represent the capitol letter *A* to the CPU.

Computer Networks

An especially limiting and defining characteristic of a computer-based information system is the network channel. A computer network may be very simple, or it may be an extremely complicated system. For the purposes of a laboratory information system, a network is "*a computer configuration that is designed to have many users simultaneously share programs and files.*" (Elevitch & Aller, p. 104). It is "*an interconnected system of communications links and transmission lines that provides multiple transmissions between computers, and providers and receivers of information.*" (Elevitch & Aller, p. 284)

There are two broad categories of computer networks: **local-area networks (LANs)** and **wide-area networks (WANs) .** LANs connect computers and their equipment within a confined area, usually a building or a place in which the users are in close geographical proximity to each other (e.g., a multi-facility medical center complex). WANs, by contrast, may cover and transmit data around the world by connecting a widely disbursed geographical network of computers through the facilities of common carriers, such as telephone lines or satellite channels.

Also popular now are wireless systems (e.g., Wi-Fi®); appearing to soon replace all the need for stringing wires around, or even between, buildings and towns. They have truly brought the world of portability to computerization. Laudon and Laudon point out: *"health care professionals can use wireless handheld to enter and view medical record, including diagnostic information in real time. They can review data immediately and update patient records while making their rounds."* (p. 329)

There are also many commercial networks, such as America Online® (AOL) and Google® that connect through the Internet (a sort of "network of networks"). Home or business computer users can connect to the Internet through these commercial networks and gain access to a wide variety of information sources, products, and services, or even communicate with other users through electronic mail (e-mail) and bulletin boards. **PubMed** is a network that allows medical literature research through the National Network of Libraries of Medicine.

The computer network, in practice, comprises the extent and complexity of the hardware and software required to meet the informational needs of the users of the information. For example, a simple network may be a small desktop computer interacting with a computerized laboratory instrument to capture QC data or provide patient demographics. Or it may be a large university medical center or commercial laboratory based LIS receiving input from hundreds of instruments and providing information to thousands of users, with both input and output sites spread across a wide geographic area.

To meet the diversity of needs present in health care situations, two types of laboratory information system networks are now possible: host-based and client-servers.

Host-Based LIS

Traditionally, particularly in a computer system dedicated to a single organization, the network has consisted of a LAN *closed* loop of remote terminals feeding into and out of a common CPU. This type of system developed for both technical and economic reasons. In this type of network, appropriately called a closed or **host based laboratory information system** network, how data are received, processed, and disseminated is determined solely by the program controlling the system.

Although participation in the design process of a host-based system is encouraged, users are in actuality, bound to the order, or format, of how information appears on the screen and is printed out. No spontaneous individual preference for how information is presented can be allowed in a host-based LIS because all terminals are interfaced and controlled by the CPU in the same way.

A common characteristic of a host-based LIS, for example, is that the ancillary screen/keyboard stations, such as those at bench workstations or physician office terminals, do not have a disk drive, requiring the user to rely totally on the host CPU.

Client-Server LIS

As computer and communication technology has advanced, another network channel has developed. This network is called **client-server laboratory information system** computing, because it is *open:* it allows users to tap into the LIS with their independent computer systems and extract only the information they want and present it in the format they wish on their own computer screen or printer (see Skjei; Bukstel; and Mendyk).

In true client-server computing, users in a physician's office can obtain information from the LIS on their own operational system, and chemistry techs can use their workstation computer to check procedure manuals, obtain results from a reference laboratory, connect with a vendor to troubleshoot an instrument, write and send a message, or run a quality management program, all independent of the host LIS. One obvious advantage of a client-server system is the elimination of excess screens and printers now cluttering the lab, each tied to its own host system.

Some of the features of client-server computing are as follows (Skjei, p. 48).

- **Scalability:** The hardware and software systems can support a small or large number of users.
- **Openness:** Users can work independently of the host system to run programs or design output format.
- **System management complexity:** Client-server systems can handle the interface and problem solving required of this type of network.
- **User empowerment:** This is the ultimate value of these combined features.

Let us now see how all these elements combine into a unified laboratory information system.

The Laboratory Information System

Building on the concepts of information systems and CBIS covered previously, a **laboratory information system** is a network of computer components (software, mainframe, and peripheral communication devices) that incorporates all aspects of the informational needs of the laboratory and its customers, from the intake of requests for services to the processing of work flow and the delivery of results.

The LIS enables managers to perform their management functions more efficiently. The LIS can provide information covering a wide range of topics.

- *Patient parameters,* including identification and status (admission, transfer, discharge, and so on)
- *Test information,* including requisition, stage of completion (ordered, dispatched, collected, in the lab, pending), and results
- *Work lists* (e.g., phlebotomy, manual result entry, instrument load lists, and overdue tests)
- *Test result records,* including current and cumulative patient reports, as well as associated normal and critical ranges
- *Master test list*
- *Financial functions*
- *Productivity and workload monitoring*
- *Quality management,* including operational quality assurance and improvement (QA&A), continuous performance improvement (CPI) parameters, procedure quality control (QC), and preventive maintenance schedules
- *Special processing requirements* (microbiology, blood bank, pathology, special chemistry, and so on)
- *Interface with other computer systems,* including host, reference laboratory, and so on

The reader may note that other terms have also been suggested to describe a computer system which incorporates all aspects of the laboratory's management needs. These include: "**LIMS**" for *Laboratory Information Management System* [Christine Paszka and Elizabeth Turner); and "**LBMS**" Laboratory Business Management System [Dennis Winsten].

Planning for Computerization

> *"Statistics indicate that nearly 60% of LIMS fail. Reasons for failure include that the system does not work as advertised, the users are not comfortable with the system, the vendor will not support and/or help maintain the system once it is installed, and the lab had not allocated enough resources to the project." [Paszka and Turner, p. 93]*

Elevitch and Aller estimate that it takes a minimum of 24 months to install a laboratory information system. Ideally, the first 18 months are invested in the following.

1. Assessing the informational needs of the laboratory
2. Conducting a systems analysis of the information and work flow of the laboratory
3. Selecting and purchasing a LIS, complete with program options and necessary hardware and software

Once it is installed and operational, the LIS serves as the primary link to other complementary computer systems, such as the hospital information system (HIS); ultimately, it is integrated into the clinical health information network (CHIN), providing for the needs of both patients and health care providers.

Systems Analysis and Design: Laboratory Needs Assessment

Systems analysis and design in general is the formal process of studying a problem and creating a solution (Freedman). In this particular instance, it is used to identify the informational needs of the laboratory and design the computer system, including both hardware and software that will meet the goals and objectives established for the system.

The process starts with a study of the organization's objectives and proceeds through the following phases to a determination of how the information system can meet these objectives (Dologite and Mockler, p. 394; Stair, p. 422):

- *Collect data and information* needed to conduct the systems analysis study. *Analyze* the laboratory's current computing status and informational needs and prepare a feasibility report.
- *Establish system specifications* using diagramming, flow charting, and other systems analysis techniques.
- *Determine hardware and software requirements* needed to meet the goals and specifications of the LIS.

According to Elevitch and Aller, this phase of planning covers four categories: database and applications software, operating systems, hardware, and, when applicable, interfaces. Following is a systems analysis and design approach that groups these four topics into the tools for evaluating and designing both the hardware and software components of a laboratory information system. A review of flow-charting techniques, one of the major tools of systems analysts, is also included.

LIS Computer Hardware

Determining the computer hardware components of an information system involves establishing the specifications of the CPU that will meet the computing and data processing requirements of the LIS and the ancillary devices that are needed at every communication and interface point.

CPU specifications include the computing *speed* of the control and logic unit and the primary data storage *capacity* necessary to meet the data processing needs of the LIS workload. CPU computing speed and primary storage *capacity* are directly related to the price of the unit.

Elevitch and Aller recommend forecasting the processing and storage needs of the laboratory for at least 5 years. They also caution that "the most generous estimates fall short of capacity within 3 to 5 years. Hardware and software must be modular and expandable to accommodate growth in the network" (p. 93). Determining the specifications for the CPU requires a realistic and accurate projection of the current and future workload and service needs of the laboratory during the expected life of the computer hardware.

The number and configuration of the peripheral I/O devices are determined by the needs and preferences of the users and by the interface requirements of laboratory instruments and computer networks. This includes an assessment of the types, location, and quality of screens (color and display quality), printers (ink jet, laser, and so on), keyboards, bar-code readers, and data converters needed at every I/O interface.

The main technique for determining the makeup and configuration of the ancillary devices is to prepare a **systems hardware diagram** of the sites at which these items are needed. Figure 17 – 3 shows a diagram of an LIS I/O network. Detailed diagrams may also be prepared of each workstation and interface link, specifying exactly the kinds of devices that will be used. The worksheet for selecting the hardware components of the LIS is created by combining CPU and I/O device specifications.

LIS Computer Software

Software design determines how the system works: how data will be entered into the computer, how data will be presented on screen displays and as hard-copy printouts, how abnormals will be flagged, when and what kind of reports will be available, how much patient information will appear on the screen and on work lists, and how long a patient's record will be retained in active computer databases. In fact, every aspect of the operations of the laboratory will be directly influenced by software decisions.

Although it is possible to hire a programmer to write a program directly, most software decisions now entail selecting from the features offered in an LIS package purchased from a commercial vendor. These decisions involve the specifications for database and applications software and operating systems.

Elevitch and Aller suggest that the systems analyst prepare a list of the operational steps that will be affected by the LIS, including printout format and displays, manual data entry screens, and laboratory test definitions and codes for each section. Specific operational items listed by the authors include the following steps.

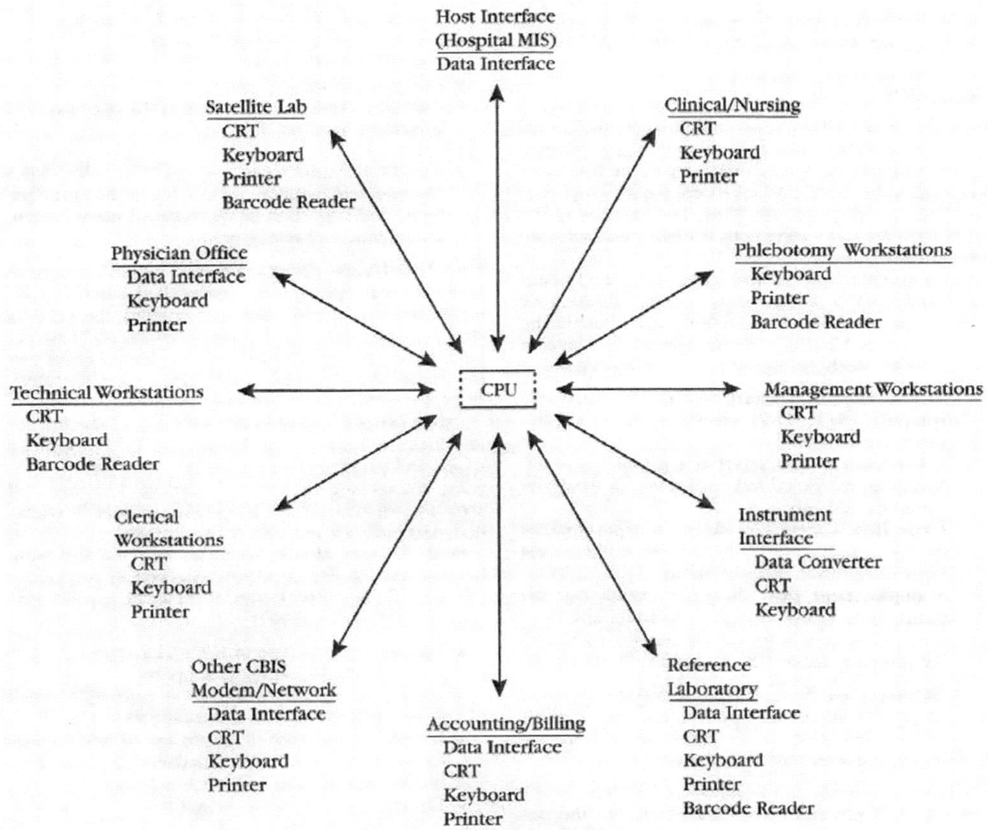

FIGURE 17 — 3. Diagram of Laboratory Information System Hardware

- Patient identification
- Admission, transfer, and discharge
- Master test list
- Orders

- Specimen collection
- Accession numbers
- Work list
- Results entry and verification
- Quality control
- Special microbiology requirements
- Special blood bank requirements
- Inquiry, reports, and lists
- Pathology and cytology

Operating systems include security and access control, file maintenance, disk pack maintenance, and system utilities (e.g., program loading, crash recovery, disk copying, usage monitoring, and problem diagnosis).

Autoverification

> Orchard Harvest LIS improves workflow efficiency and reduces errors by offering advanced customizable rules to aid in decision making for auto-approval of patient results, reflexing additional testing, automatic comments, clinical follow-up recommendations, and order splitting.
> http://www.orchardsoft.com/product/harvestlis.html
> [connected July 13, 2007]

This promotional claim by one provider of LIS brings to the forefront the issue of **Autoverification**; or as CAP describes in its Laboratory General Checklist (04-05-2006):

> Autoverification is the process by which patient results are generated from interfaced instruments and sent to the LIS, where they are compared against laboratory-defined acceptance parameters. If the results fall within these defined parameters, the results are automatically released to patient reporting formats without any additional laboratory staff intervention. Any data that fall outside the defined parameters is reviewed by laboratory staff prior to reporting.

This issue is both touted as a great time saving factor, and fraught with cries of potential harm to the patient with the release of erroneous results. Most agencies have not yet issued specific guidelines; but as the reader will note that most LIS are expected to have this feature. However, the criteria for Autoverification are being addressed as the following two citations will attest.

Stefanie McFadden listed several essential parameters for Autoverification in a column in Advance for Administrators of the Laboratory (November 2006).

- Reference ranges;
- Critical values for IP and OP
- Delta checks
- Relationship of parameters (e.g., H and H, Bun/Creatine)
- Dilution needs or manual processes
- Laboratory review policies
- Pathology review policies
- Specify units or physicians.

Below is a synopsis of the concerns of Autoverification found in the CAP General checklist.

- Quality control acceptable
- Range of acceptable values
- Checked for flags and warnings
- Delta checks
- Rapid suspension in case of an instrument problem

Flow Charts

No matter how well designed and packaged the LIS selected, the laboratory will need to go through a systematic evaluation of each operational step of the laboratory and identify the specific informational requirements necessary to meet its objectives. Flow charts are one of the major tools for conducting both hardware and software assessments.

There are four types of flow charts, each used to analyze and track a distinct organizational function or system. The basic design of all flow charts follows the format illustrated in Figure 17 – 4. Figure 17 – 5 gives a sample of the symbols used in preparing flow charts.

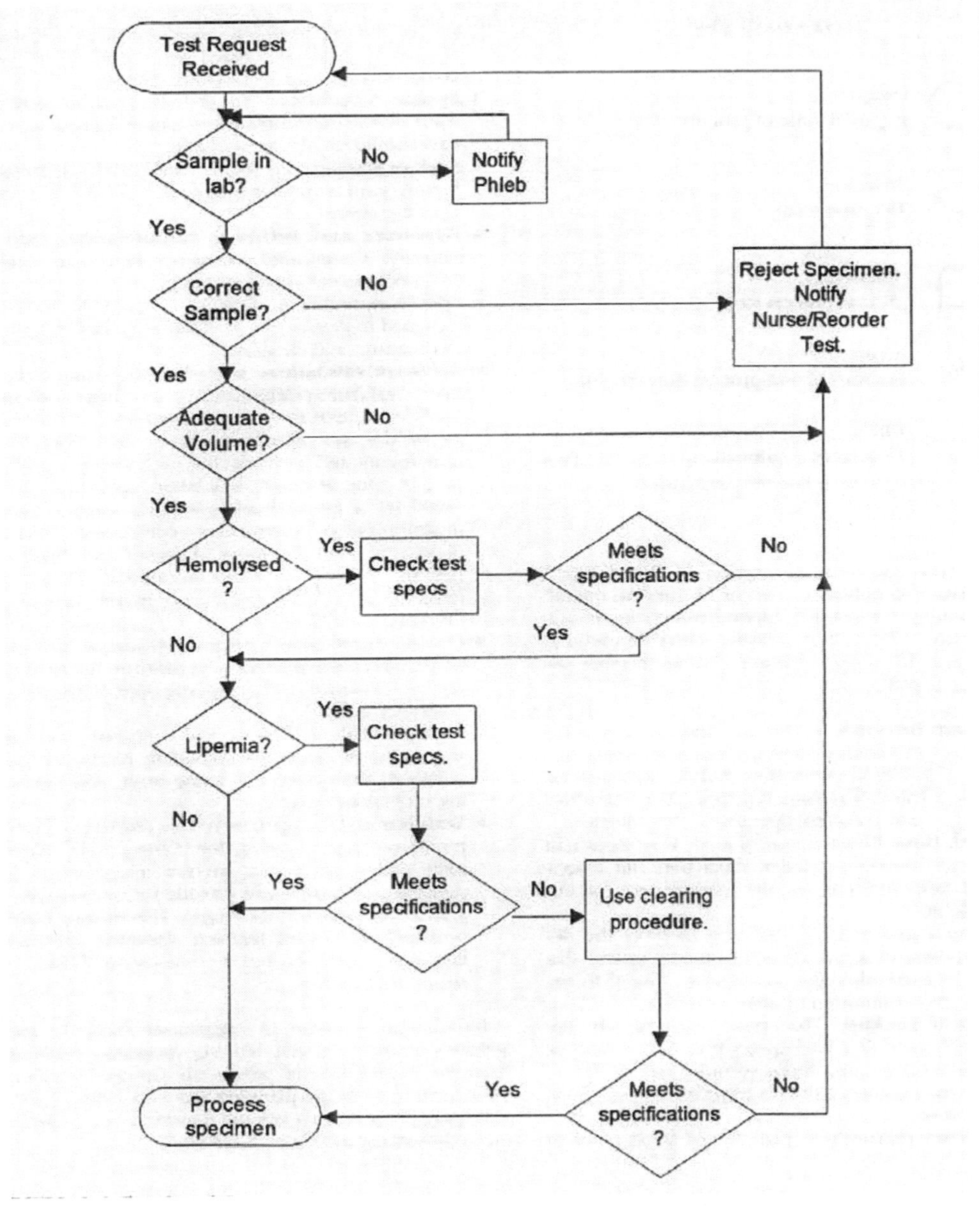

FIGURE 17 — 4. Flow Chart of Chemistry Specimen Evaluation
Prepared by Myra Kilker, MT(ASCP)

1. The **systems flow chart** depicts the system as a complete whole. Only subsystems or major elements are shown.
2. A **procedural flow chart** is a graphic presentation of an individual task, operation, or data flow within the system.
3. **Logic flow charts** provide an in-depth analysis of the sequencing of logical or mathematical steps in a specific order of events.
4. A **deployment flow diagram** spreads out the format horizontally to depict the action and decision points in a separate column for each area (i.e., Nursing, Laboratory, Chemistry, Phlebotomy).

To develop these flow charts and design a program for a computer information system, the analyst must make a complete study of the laboratory and all the contact points that interact with it, including the following.

- Current methods and workflow procedures
- Staff and procedure manuals internal to the department
- Other departments, staff, and database sources that make contact with the laboratory

Nurses, physicians, patients, salespeople, professional journals and textbooks, and support services such as material management should be consulted for insight into factors that are important to the efficient operation of a medical laboratory.

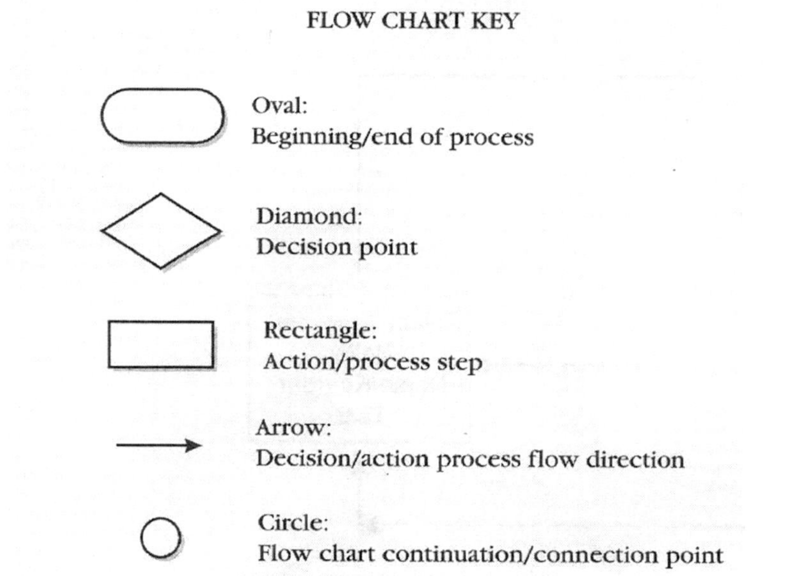

FIGURE 16-7. Flow chart symbol key.

FIGURE 17 —5. Flow Chart Symbol Key
http://www.wiley.com/college/busin/icmis/oakman/outline/chap05/slides/symbols.htm
[connected July 14, 2007]

Below are three websites which give instructional assistance in preparing flow charts [connected July 14, 2007]:

- http://deming.eng.clemson.edu/pub/tutorials/qctools/flowm.htm
- http://www.deneba.com/community/howto/flowcharts/default.html
- http://www.skymark.com/resources/tools/flowchart.asp

Selecting a Laboratory Information System

A survey by Aller and Weilert in 1994 lists 55 vendors with 65 laboratory information systems operational in at least one site. This list includes only vendors that provide total systems, not companies that provide only specialized software, such as for surgical pathology or the blood bank. This vast array of competitors vying for the laboratory's business may appear overwhelming but may be decreased by scrupulous questioning and maintaining a constant perspective of the purpose of the LIS and the priorities of the laboratory:

In the November 2006 issue of CAP Today thirty-seven (37) Laboratory Information Systems were included on the list. The following system features were cataloged (listed as percentage of live installs or based on availability).

- Chemistry and hematology
- Bar-coded collection labels
- Handheld devices for bedside-positive patient ID
- NCCLS POCT-1A standard interface for POCT devices
- Microbiology
- Blood bank donor and transfusion
- Surgical pathology/cytology
- HIS or EMR interface: A/D/T
- HIS or EMR interface: order entry
- HIS or EMR interface: results reporting
- HIS or EMR interface: package results into PDF format
- Ad hoc reporting
- Rules-based system
- Management and statistical reporting
- Outreach and commercial laboratory
- Compliance checking
- Billing and accounts receivable
- Materials management and inventory
- Test partition/remote faxing and printing
- Physician office outreach
- HIPAA-standard transaction formats
- Web-based remote inquiry of reports/Web access for order entry
- Specimen management and tracking

Other items not specifically included in the list but important to the selection decision are CPU processing speed and primary storage capacity, user-friendly software, networking capability, record of hardware and software reliability, voice recognition system for dictation, and patient record retention capacity.

Some laboratorians recommend that the following features should also be closely checked as part of the LIS selection process (Jeffrey E. Kinkead, written personal communication).

- The number and type of HIS and instrument interfaces the vendor presently supports.
- The variety of cumulative report types and format flexibility and the ease of customization.
- The ability and ease of calling up ad hoc reports: for example, a list of all pediatric patients who had blood lead levels above 30 *u*g/dL.
- The ease of retrieval of purged patient information (e.g., CDs, remote storage, or microfiche).
- A graphical user interface (GUI) Support of point-of-care testing.
- Ability to meet CLIA'88 specifications.
- Some type of e-mail or message system.

The selection process requires intensive investigation and understanding of the needs of the laboratory and the suitability of the commercial LIS systems. Vendor demonstrations, site assessments, reference checks, and visits to laboratories using the system under consideration provide crucial insight into the usefulness of a particular LIS package.

Installing the Laboratory Information System

No matter how smooth the planning process, the installation of either a complete laboratory information system (LIS) or a department-specific program, such as for Microbiology or the blood bank, is a management challenge; this is especially true for a laboratory being computerized for the first time. Bringing any computer on line is a major change for both the laboratory and its clients, requiring close cooperation and patience in solving problems.

Experienced laboratorians frequently cite the importance of following the vendor's installation checklist religiously, allowing enough time to complete each step in an orderly fashion. Someone who is computer-literate and fully familiar with both laboratory procedures and the host system must be readily available.

Until recently there were no specific guidelines or regulatory requirements for laboratory computer systems, other than that they maintain the technical and records integrity of the testing process. However, in 1988 and 1989 the Food and Drug Administration issued directives on the computerization of blood bank services. The American Association of Blood Banks (AABB) has also published a set of 13 standard operating procedures for installing blood bank computer systems (Steane). These guidelines may be useful to laboratorians installing computer systems in other departments as well.

- **System integration:** This step involves the actual process of installing or upgrading a computer system as part of the work flow. AABB suggestions include a conversion team, timetable plan, work flow analysis, and computer operational procedures.
- **Work flow:** Identification of work flow steps that directly involve computer interaction and associated task functions are the main aspects of this guideline.
- **Manual procedures:** This area involves the development of a manual or alternative system that can be used when the computer is "down" to ensure the continuation of service.
- **System backup:** This point recommends the maintenance of a backup copy of information or records (programs, donor records, and so on) in case the primary computer records become lost or unusable.
- **Disaster recovery:** A plan should be in place to get the system back into operation after a major disruption, such as caused by a fire, storm, or computer hardware or software damage.
- **System shutdown:** An orderly plan to notify users of routine maintenance and downloading of data should be readily available.
- **System start-up:** Procedures are needed detailing how to load computer programs and boot and reboot the system.
- **Hardware and software maintenance:** Provisions for routine and emergency repairs to computer equipment must be arranged.
- **System security:** An ongoing program should be designed to ensure the confidentiality and integrity of programs and database.
- **Software validation:** According to AABB guidelines, "validation demonstrates, at a high level of confidence, that the software performs according to vendor specifications, meets laboratory requirements and is ready for use" (Steane, 1991, p. 23). One software validation approach provided by a blood bank computer vendor uses digital-to-video conversion components (i.e., making a video recording of screen and data input) that support an audio description of what is happening on the screen and in the program (Varnadoe, 1995, p. 7).

- **Quality assurance:** A program should be in place to systematically monitor and measure the quality and performance of the ongoing operations of the computer system.
- **Change control:** Orderly and continual planning should be in place for upgrading hardware and software, identifying and fixing bugs, and repairing broken equipment.
- **Training and competency:** This crucial guideline points out that planning for training must begin long before installation, involve intensive pre-installation education, and provide for ongoing programs for updates and changes. This training must be based on specific learning objectives, completion of set schedules, and documentation of demonstrated competency.

By adhering to these 13 suggestions, following the vendor's instructions and training programs, learning from the experiences of fellow laboratorians, and including all users in the planning and installation phase, managers can achieve a smooth transition to a computerized laboratory information system.

Laboratory Information Systems is the last chapter in Part III: Management of Financial Resources. Part IV: Management of Operations begins with *Policy and Procedure Manuals.*

— Case Study —

Chapter Seventeen: Laboratory Information Systems

"I can't believe we cannot get a simple report on how many units of blood the patient has had in the past few hours, without spending all day on the phone to the blood bank and nursing stations," exclaimed a frustrated hematology tech.

"How am I supposed to respond to these Delta checks on hemoglobins if I have to call everybody in the hospital just to find out some simple information? With computers all over the laboratory, why can't I just hit a key to find out this important information! I hope the new update fixes this problem."

Chapter Sections for Review

- Computer Networks
    - Local-Area Networks
    - Wide-Area Networks
    - Host-based LIS
    - Client-Server LIS
- Flow chart

Questions for Discussion

1. Does this kind of problem sound familiar in your laboratory? Why does it exist, and what kind of solutions may help resolve the tech's need for information? Is it a hardware, software, or network problem, or a combination of each? What kind of LIS (Host/Client-Server) would be best in this type of situation?
2. What type of flow chart may best illustrate the current process and be used in a system analysis of the situation?
3. Think about the LIS where you work. What do you like about it? What things do you dislike or feel could be done better? If you have worked with several LISs, compare them, and identify what you like and dislike about each system. How would you change your current LIS given the lessons learned in this chapter (e.g., hardware, software, network)?
4. Think about a process that needs upgrading on your LIS, or a problem in the laboratory that you would like to see improved. Prepare a flowchart of the process using the example presented in the book.

PART 3: BIBLIOGRAPHY

This book is presented as a 2nd edition, revision, update, additional text content, and sequential of: Varnadoe, Lionel A; Medical Laboratory Management and Supervision: *Operations, Review, and Study Guide*; F. A. Davis Company, Philadelphia; 1996. Following is the initial bibliography (p. 206) plus additional current citations.

Aller, RD, and Weilert, M: Survey of US vendors. CAP Today, Nov 1994.

Beck, DR: Basic Hospital Financial Management, ed 2. Aspen Publications, Rockville, MD, 1992.

Bukstel, E: Application of a laboratory results reporting system in a CHIN American Clinical Laboratory, 13:26 1994.

Burch, JG, and Strater, FR: Information Systems: Theory and Practice. Hamilton Publishing Company, Santa Barbara, CA, 1974.

Center for Biologic Evaluation and Research: Recommendations for implementation of computerization in blood establishment (letter). US Department of Health & Human Services, Food and Drug Administration, Bethesda, MD, April 6,1988.

Center for Biologic Evaluation and Research: Requirements for computerization of blood establishments (letter). US Department of Health & Human Services,

College of American Pathologists: Manual for Workload Recording Methods. Author, Northfield, IL, 1989.

Cowan, Daniel F., editor; *Informatics for the Clinical Laboratory A Practical Guide*; Springer-Verlag, New York; 2003

Dept of health New York State
http://www.health.state.ny.us/nysdoh/hospital/drg/
[Connected July 12, 2007]

Dologite, DG, and Mockler, RJ: Using Computers, ed 2. Prentice-Hall, Englewood Cliffs, N], 1989.

Elevitch, FR, and Aller, RD: The ABCs of LIS: Computerizing Your Laboratory Information System. ASCP Press, Chicago, 1989.

FDA Glossary of Computerized System and Software Development
GLOSSARY OF COMPUTERIZED SYSTEM AND SOFTWARE DEVELOPMENT TERMINOLOGY
http://www.fda.gov/ora/inspect_ref/igs/gloss.html
[connected July 13, 2007]

Fess, PE, and Warren, CS: Accounting Principles, ed 16. South-Western Publishing, Cincinnati, 1989.

Food and Drug Administration, Bethesda, MD, September 8, 1989.

Frings, Christopher S.; Workload Assessment; Medical Laboratory Observer, May, 2005
http://www.findarticles.com/p/articles/mi_m3230/is_5_37/ai_n13784487

[connected July 12, 2007] {**Warning**, experienced a persistent commercial advertising pop-up on this site}

Freedman, A: The Computer Glossary, ed 7. American Management Association, New York, 1995.

Gendler, SM: LIS expert systems: Feature evaluation. American Clinical Laboratory, 14:12, 1995.

General Principles of Software Validation; Final Guidance for Industry and FDA Staff – Document issued on: January 11, 2002
http://www.fda.gov/cdrh/comp/guidance/938.html
[connected July 13, 2007]

Hilker, WR, and Gee, EP: The MBA Toolkit. Chilton, Radnor, PA, 1985

Horngren, CT: Accounting for Management Control, ed 8. Prentice Hall, Englewood Cliffs, N], 1989.

Laboratory General Checklist 04 06 2006
Commission on Laboratory Accreditation
College of American Pathologists
http://www.cap.org/apps/docs/laboratory_accreditation/checklists/laboratory_general_april2006.pdf

The Laboratory Management Index Program (LMIP)
http://www.cap.org/apps/docs/lmip/lmip.html
[connected July 12, 2007]

LMIP® Standardized Billable Test Counts (SBT)
http://www.cap.org/apps/cap.portal?_nfpb=true&cntvwrPtlt_actionOverride=%2Fportlets%2FcontentViewer%2Fshow&_windowLabel=cntvwrPtlt&_state=maximized&_pageLabel=cntvwr&cntvwrPtlt%7BactionForm.contentReference%7D=lmip%2Funitcount.html
[connected July 12, 20077]

List of DRG Relative Weight
http://www.med.cmu.ac.th/hospital/drg/DRG.htm
[Connected July 12, 2007]

McFadden, Stefanie; *Decision Time*; in Advance for Administrators of the Laboratory; Vol.15 No. II, November 2006; p. 70

Mendyk, RW: A blueprint for implementing an open physician/laboratory interface system. American Clinical Laboratory, 13:27, 1994.

National Committee for Clinical Laboratory Standards: Cost Accounting in the Clinical Laboratory. Proposed guidelines, Villanova, PA, 1990.

Neumann, BR, Suver, JD, and Zelman, W: Financial Management: Concepts and Applications for Healthcare Providers, ed 2. Kendall Hunt, Dubuque, IA, 1991.

NPV; some websites concerning NPV for those who may be inclined.
Investopedia®
http://www.investopedia.com/terms/n/npv.asp

[connected April 18, 2007]

From Wikipedia, the free encyclopedia
http://en.wikipedia.org/wiki/Net_present_value#Formula
[connected April 18, 2007]

(CCH) Business Owner's Tookit™
http://www.toolkit.cch.com/text/P06_6530.asp
[connected April 18, 2007]

Sattler,], and Smith, A: A Practical Guide to Financial Management of the Clinical Laboratory, ed 2. Medical Economics Books, Oradell, N], 1986.

Skjei, E: Client/server computing breaks into the lab. CAP Today, 8:1, 1994.

Stair, RM: Principles of Information Systems. Boyd & Fraser, Boston, 1992.

Steane, S: Guidelines for preparing standard operating procedures for blood blank computer systems. American Association of Blood Banks, Information Systems Committee, Washington, DC, 1991.

Travers, EM, et al: Cost Accounting in the Clinical Laboratory. Publication GPII-P. National Committee for Clinical Laboratory Standards, Villanova, PA, 1991.

Varnadoe, LA: A personal management information system. Laboratory Medicine, 9:25, 1978.

Varnadoe, LA: Blood bank computer guidelines as easy as A(A)B(B).Advance for Medical Laboratory Professionals, 7:9, 1995.

Ward, WJ: Healthcare Budgeting and Financial Management for Non Financial Managers. Auburn House Greenwood Group Publications, Westport, CT, 1993.

Medical Laboratory Management and Supervision

Part 4: Management of Operations

[18]

Policy and Procedure Manuals

— Chapter Eighteen —

Preparing and writing the laboratory's policy and procedure manuals encompass all the elements of the management process including the planning, organizing, directing, and controlling functions. Procedure manuals involve a great deal of planning and organizing in their preparation and form the foundation for directing and controlling the activities of the laboratory. The manuals contain instructions, explanations, and criteria for behavior and performance expectations.

This chapter discusses the types of procedure manuals needed to operate a laboratory, meet the requirements of licensing and accreditation agencies, and review recommended formats for ensuring that manuals contain essential information

OBJECTIVES

After completion of this chapter, the reader will be able to demonstrate accomplishment of the following objectives.

1. Explain the needs and purpose of laboratory policies and procedures.
2. Write a general department policy.
3. Prepare a technical procedure according to the guidelines issued by the Clinical and Laboratory Standards Institute.

Chapter Highlights and Glossary of Key Terms

I. OVERVIEW

Policy: *A statement or memo that outlines the institution's position on an administrative or operational issue.*

Procedure: *An instructional document that provides explanations and step-by-step directions on how to perform a task, test, or process.*

Policy Manual: *A manual that contains policies that apply to the general and overall operations of the institution.*

Procedure Manual: *A manual containing procedures that apply to specific work tasks and duties.*

II. OBJECTIVES OF POLICY AND PROCEDURE MANUALS

A. Policy manuals

B. Procedure manuals

III. TYPES OF POLICY AND PROCEDURE MANUALS

A. External manuals

Specimen Collection Manual- *A manual, or section of the laboratory service manual, that contains detailed instructions for patients and health care providers for collecting, labeling, storing, rejecting, transporting, and delivering specimens to the laboratory.*

Laboratory Service Manual: *A manual designed for users of the laboratory; covers policies and procedures concerning operational factors such as business hours, services provided, specimen submission requirements, and billing practices.*

B. Internal manuals
   1. Administrative manuals
   2. Technical manuals
      Technical Manual: *A procedure manual that contains information and step-by-step step instructions for operating instruments and performing individual tests, tasks, and duties.*
   3. *Safety manuals*
   4. *Quality management manuals*

IV. WRITING POLICY AND PROCEDURE MANUALS
   A. Policy manual format
   B. Procedure manual Format

Overview

A **policy** is a statement or memo that outlines the institution's position on an administrative or operational issue. A **procedure** is an instructional document that provides explanations and step-by-step directions on how to perform a task, test, or process. **Policy manu**als are collections of statements and memos that outline the position of the institution on a wide range of administrative and operational issues. **Procedure manuals,** in contrast, provide detailed information about subjects only alluded to in memos, performance evaluations, training sessions, and the day-to-day verbal and written interchange between laboratorians and their clients. These documents are the resource that allows other communication efforts to be brief, referring the person to a specific manual for further information. To meet these goals, manuals must be complete, clear in instruction and explanation, and organized to allow easy and timely location of needed information.

Policy and procedure manuals should also be dynamic documents with up-to-date, pertinent, and accurate information. In the past, this was often an extremely difficult, time-consuming task of low priority. It was usually left for times when the laboratory was preparing for inspection by an outside agency or, at best, for an annual review. With the increased availability of word processors, which allow for quick and easy updates, this excuse is rapidly becoming obsolete. The time and effort expended in writing a memo announcing a change in a policy or procedure, with corrections left for the annual review, can now be used to directly update the primary document.

Following is a review of the basic purposes and objectives of policy and procedure manuals, along with the types of manuals designed to meet these objectives.

Objectives of Policy and Procedure Manuals

The primary objective of policy and procedure manuals is to ensure effective *communication* between the members of the organization. The manuals must attempt to remove any ambiguities and allow uniform and consistent application of the laboratory's policies and procedures. To accomplish this goal, they must be living documents continually adjusting to the rapidly changing circumstances generated by the social, technological, and legal environment in which the laboratory operates.

Several broad agenda issues should be built into policy and procedure manuals: fair and consistent treatment of all employees, standardized performance and behavior expectations, and information about the dayto-day operation of the laboratory. From this foundation arise the supporting roles and documents found in the laboratory. The following examples are only a small sample of activities that are tied directly to the contents of policy and procedure manuals.

- Responsibility and control
- Performance appraisals
- Completion of tasks and duties
- Quality standards and monitoring indexes . Job descriptions
- Work flow and job analysis
- Productivity measurement
- Financial accountability

All organizations, including the laboratory, normally have two types of manuals. The first usually contains the policies that apply to the general and overall operations of the institution such as administration and employment policy manuals. Procedure manuals contain detailed instructions about specific work areas and tasks.

Policy Manuals

A policy can range from a simple statement about the intent and philosophy of a company to a detailed plan of implementation. For example, a policy on discrimination may be a short and direct statement:

All persons and employees are entitled to equal employment opportunity and treatment regardless of race, color, religion, sex, martial status, national origin, age, or handicap.

A policy may also be a more extensive document listing strategies on how minorities will be recruited as potential employees. They normally, however, contain only a couple of paragraphs, with sufficient explanation to establish intent of the policy, leaving the details for the procedure manual.

A hospital has general policies that are relevant to the whole institution as well as department policies that address issues specific to each area. Below are some of the general topics which may be commonly found in policy manuals.

- Administrative organization
- Employment and personnel policies such as hiring practices, grievance procedures, benefits, attendance and tardiness rules, and statements concerning discrimination, drug screening, and termination
- Adherence and enforcement of safety and health procedures
- Disaster plans
- Confidentiality and release of patient information
- Security and access to facilities
- Solicitation on the premises

At the laboratory level, the policy manual refers to topics that may have particular relevance to the area, as well as contain specific departmental policies. Examples of laboratory policies may include the following.

- Dress codes
- Food and smoking rules
- Telephone use
- Specific statements about enforcement of safety rules
- Laboratory organization and reporting relationships
- Writing, review, and authorization of procedures
- Absences and late-arrival notification

- Vacation and holiday requests
- Supply requisition
- Reporting and releasing of test results

CONFIDENTIALITY AND RELEASE OF PATIENT INFORMATION

1. ALL patient information is to be held in strict confidence and released only to hospital personnel and physicians who are directly involved in the care of the patient, with access limited to only the information that is needed to deliver this care; that is, on a need-to-know basis. Staff is also cautioned about discussing a patient's care in a public area, such as the cafeteria, hallway, or elevator, where confidentiality may be compromised.

2. Request for information from sources outside the hospital (news media, insurance, law enforcement agencies, other healthcare providers, etc.) should be referred to the Medical Records Department for proper authorization. A daily report on each patient's status is available to the public through the main switchboard as permitted by the patient and their physician.

3. Questions from patients or their family about their care or testing results should be referred to their attending physician.

4. Results may be issued ONLY to the patient directly by the department giving the care (Laboratory, Radiology, etc.) upon specific authorization of the attending physician. Patients may obtain copies of their medical records through their physician or from the Medical Records Department by completing and signing a release form.

5. All problems or special requests not covered above should be referred to the Medical Records Department, Administration, or the House Supervisor for resolution.

Violation of this policy is a serious infraction of both the hospital's responsibility and the patient's trust and may result in the immediate dismissal of the employee.

Policy Approval

Medical Records: Date:

Administration: Date:

Medical Staff President: Date:

Effective Date; October 31, 2xxx
Review Due Date; September 30, 2xxx

FIGURE 18 —1. Example of a General Policy

An example of a policy that applies to both the hospital and the laboratory is one that covers the confidentiality and release of test results for patients. This policy is illustrated in Figure 18 – 1.

Procedure Manuals

Procedures are often referred to as SOP, a term adopted from the military, meaning "standard operating procedure." Technical manuals that contain procedures for performing tests, operating instruments, or processing quality control information are examples of procedure manuals found in the laboratory.

Standardization of the way that tasks and tests are performed is one of the primary objectives of procedure manuals. The justification for this emphasis is that it ensures that all work is performed to the criteria set by the laboratory and assists in troubleshooting when problems occur.

But standardization is also criticized for stifling creativity, discouraging innovation, and reducing everything to its lowest common denominator instead of encouraging personal and professional growth. This criticism is especially aimed at procedures that are lengthy, nonspecific, ambiguous, condescending to the users, and largely trivial. The balance between these viewpoints is to have manuals that are concise, contain information pertaining only to the task being performed, and are targeted toward the skill, knowledge level, and needs of the intended users.

Laboratory procedure manuals represent a major investment of time and effort and are in constant need of revision because of the continually evolving work situation. A variety of manuals must be maintained. The next section reviews the types of manuals that are designed to address the specific needs of the laboratory and the people using its services.

Types of Policy and Procedure Manuals

Policy and procedure manuals can be divided into two broad groups: those that are designed for the internal use of the laboratory and those directed at the users of laboratory services, including nurses, physicians, and patients. Internal manuals include safety, quality monitoring, technical procedures, and administrative matters.

The best examples of external manuals are the laboratory service manual for nurses and the instructional booklets or sheets given to patients about preparation for testing. A list of the more common laboratory manuals and brief descriptions of their intended purpose follow.

External Manuals

A procedure manual that is designed for external use is the **specimen collection manual**. This is required by inspection agencies to be distributed to all areas in which specimens are collected for submission to the laboratory, specifically, all nursing units, physicians' offices, and satellite collection sites. The specimen collection manual may be a separate document, or it may be incorporated into a service manual.

Factors that affect the users of laboratory services are discussed in the **laboratory service manual**. These may include policy statements concerning the hours of operation for outpatients, collection and courier pickup schedules, insurance and other billing practices, who may order tests and receive reports, and general business items such as telephone numbers and location of facilities.

The laboratory service manual may be an all-encompassing document designed to meet a wide range of user needs, or it may be customized for a specific market segment such as hospital nursing units or physicians' offices. In all cases the service manual contains information on the general policies of the laboratory; information on how to fill out request forms or order tests through the computer system; detailed instructions to both the nurse and the patient for collecting, labeling, storing, transporting, and delivering specimens; and specimen rejection criteria. It usually contains a list of tests and services offered by the laboratory.

Internal Manuals

Internal manuals are intended for use by the members of the laboratory. Inspection agencies require that certain information be readily available to the staff, but they usually give the laboratory significant leeway in how it wishes to organize the material to meet these requirements. For example, there may be several individual manuals or the information may be placed in a single, all encompassing document. Some topics, such as quality and safety subjects, frequently have their own manuals to emphasize the importance and priority given them, even though pertinent information may be duplicated in other places. Following is a list of common manuals found in the laboratory and a short description of each.

Administrative Manuals

The administrative manual addresses policies that apply to the entire laboratory. Included here are subjects such as work schedules, vacation and holiday staffing, dress codes, telephone use, call-ins and other requests for changes in the schedule, and supervisory delegation and responsibility. This is also the place in which many laboratories maintain their disaster plans and their procedures for purchasing and ordering supplies.

Technical Manuals

Technical manuals are probably the most familiar to professional staff members. **Technical manuals** contain information and step-by-step instructions for operating instruments and performing individual tests, tasks, and duties. They are commonly organized according to discipline, with sections such as Hematology, Microbiology, and Phlebotomy having their own individualized manuals.

Instructions in technical manuals should be comprehensive. They should include, among other things, procedures for calibration, specimen collection, quality control, safety, actual test performance, troubleshooting, and reporting results.

Safety Manuals

Although important instructions about handling reagents should be included in each procedure, most precautions are universal in nature, and general safety rules apply in all settings in which specimens and hazardous material are processed. In the interest of both ease of access and regulatory requirements, instructions for handling dangerous substances and biological samples are frequently organized in one document, with additional references made to specific procedural precautions in other manuals. The type of information contained in the safety manual is covered in Chapter 20.

Quality Management Manuals

The overall policies, procedures, and rules for ensuring the quality of laboratory services are contained in this manual. Although specific quality control instructions are included as part of each procedure, the quality management manual addresses issues of specimen acceptability, administrative and technical review of quality data, coordination and integration with the institutional quality plan, and the assignment of authority and responsibility for ensuring that quality standards and goals are achieved. This material is presented in Chapter 21.

Writing Policy and Procedure Manuals

Policy and procedure manuals should be written in a way that enables easy consultation and retrieval of information. Consistency in design allows the users to become familiar with the location of needed .information and serves as a checklist for all pertinent directions.

The emphasis of any policy or procedure should be on the user of the manual, not just on having a pretty document to show an inspector. The format and style selected by the laboratory should consider the following factors:

- Skill and technical ability of the users
- The manual's use as a ready resource for checking performance criteria
- Performance and behavior expectations of the laboratory

With these general guidelines in mind, the preparation and writing of policy and procedures can begin.

Policy Manual Format

Policies, by their nature, are not as specific or detailed as procedures. For this reason they are usually organized by topic and composed according to standard writing styles. Many dictionaries and writing textbooks have a style section that recommends formats for business as well as for everyday communications. These normally suggest that information be presented using an outline model, with subject headings highlighting the relationship of the material. This book is an example of the way policy manuals are written and organized with topic and subject headings.

A policy can range from a one-sentence statement to a more extensive discussion of a topic. If you include too much detail, however, it becomes a procedure. An example of a policy on the dress code for clerical and administrative staff may be the simple statement: "All clerical and administrative staff will present a professional appearance at all times." Then again, it may provide a complete list of acceptable and unacceptable personal grooming items, including shoes, clothes, jewelry, hair styles, cosmetics, and even fragrances.

Procedure Manual Format

Procedures, in contrast to policies, are detailed and comprehensive documents. Regulatory agencies have specific guidelines governing the information that must be provided, and many have recommendations about the format that should be followed in preparing procedures.

The laboratory must adhere to the rules and guidelines of a variety of agencies governing the hospital and the laboratory itself. Among these are the Joint Commission on Accreditation of Healthcare Organizations (JCAHO), the College of American Pathologists (CAP), the American Association of Blood Banks (AABB), as well as the numerous federal and state licensing agencies (e.g., CLIA'88 and OSHA). Fortunately for the laboratory, most of these organizations either accept or defer to the format proposed by the Clinical and Laboratory Standards Institute (CLSI, formerly NCCLS) *Procedure Manual guideline* (GP2-A5).

All regulatory agencies require that the laboratory maintain specific procedures relating to the work done in its facility. This usually means that photocopies from reference books, package inserts, or manufacturers' instruction sheets are not acceptable as a procedure if they do not actually describe the work being done. Package inserts and manufacturers' manuals are acceptable under CLSI guidelines if they are followed in practice and documented accordingly; however, some agencies may require procedures to be prepared and typed as individual documents. In all cases these sources can be transposed, referred to in the procedures, and cited as references, but the procedure must be tailored to the specific methodology being performed in the laboratory.

Many manufacturers provide customized procedures for their products. While this may relieve supervisors of the drudgery of typing up a procedure, it does not remove their responsibility for its accuracy and applicability to the setting and the way tests are performed in their laboratory.

Whatever format is chosen, it should be consistent throughout the laboratory. The following items are often found in the laboratory's technical procedure manual and are consistent with the requirements and recommendations of JCAHO, CAP, AABB, CLSI, and CLIA'88:

1. Name of test, procedure, task, or duty.
2. Effective date and any subsequent changes.
3. Short summary of the main elements of the procedure, or a list of items that may frequently be checked or looked up: wavelength, specimen or reagent volumes, calculations, and so on.
4. Brief discussion of the principle of the test, with key points that may be of use to the analyst.
5. Specimen requirements, patient preparations, and rejection criteria.
6. Instrumentation, equipment, and glassware requirements and care.
7. Reagents and their preparation.
8. Calibration and control material requirements and preparation.
9. Calibration procedure, including linearity and test limitations.
10. Quality control procedures, including run acceptance and rejection protocol.
11. Primary problem detection, such as interfering substances or special testing situations (temperature, light, specimen handling, and so on).
12. Actual testing procedure, with detailed, step-by-step instructions.
13. Calculation and interpretation of results.
14. Results reporting parameters and instructions.
15. Normal or reference ranges, along with critical or panic levels.
16. Procedure notes concerning important aspects of the tests.
17. Troubleshooting suggestions.
18. Lists of references and sources for additional information.
19. Authorization and schedule for review. This section should include the signatures and dates of all individuals reviewing the procedure. Specifically, it should list persons to contact with problems, questions, or suggestions for improvements.

Many procedures do not require every one of these items, particularly those not covered in the technical manual. However, the principles and completeness of the previous suggestions serve as a guideline for writing any policy or procedure. When using this list, remember that it is meant as only one possible model. Procedures must be customized to meet the individual needs of the laboratory and the user. Figure 18 – 2 which follows, uses this model in a procedure for confirming the presence of bilirubin in urine.

Confirmation Test for Bilirubin in Urine Using BEYER® ICTOTEST® Reagent Tablets for Urinalysis

Effective Date: December 31, 2xxx
Review Due Date: November 30, 2xxx
Contact: Urinalysis Supervisor

KEY POINT SUMMARY:

Use 10 drops *of fresh* urine as sample.
Read after 60 seconds.
Check package insert for example of color reactions and additional instructions.
Test used to confirm positive urine bilirubin because of color inference.

PRINCIPLE OF TEST SUMMARY:

The reaction is based on the coupling of a unique solid diazonium salt with bilirubin in an acid medium to give the blue or purple color.

SPECIMEN REQUIREMENTS:

Specimen Collection and Preparation
Bilirubin is rapidly decomposed once excreted, particularly in the presence of light or heat. Urine preservatives do not prevent this composition. Consequently, it is import that ICOTEST® Reagent Tablets be used with a fresh specimen [1 hour*]. If this is not possible, the urine should be refrigerated immediately and tested as soon as possible.

Reject any specimen that does not meet the above criteria unless testing is approved by the supervisor.

SUPPLIES AND EQUIPMENT:

1. Distilled water
2. Disposable pipettes or droppers

REAGENTS:

BAYER® ICTOTEST® Product No. 2591

No special preparation or calibration is needed. Reagent container should be recapped promptly and tightly after use. PROTECT AGAINST EXPOSURE TO LIGHT, HEAT, AND AMBIENT MOISTURE

CONTROL MATERIAL:

Quality control tests on both the POSITIVE and NEGATIVE urine controls are to be included in the daily quality control (QC) urinalysis procedures and when a new bottle of reagents is placed in use. The results are to be recorded on the daily urinalysis QC log.

TESTING PRECAUTIONS:

AVOID contact of reagent tablet with skin.

Extremely high dosages of certain medications or their metabolites, such as Pyridium®, chlorpromazine, and Lodine® (etodolac), may cause false positives or atypical bright red or orange colors.

NOT FOR INTERNAL USE

TESTING PROCEDURE:

1. Place a square of the absorbent test mat supplied with ICTOTEST@ onto a paper towel. Place *10 drops of urine* onto the center of the test mat.
2. Shake one ICTOTEST@ reagent tablet into the bottle cap and transfer the tablet to the center of the moistened mat. Do not handle tablet with the fingers. Recap the bottle promptly.
3. Place *one drop of water* onto the tablet. Wait 5 *seconds,* then place a *second drop of water* onto the tablet so that the water runs off the tablet onto the mat.
4. Observe and read the color of the mat around the tablet at *60 seconds.*

INTERPRETATION AND REPORTING OF RESULTS:

POSITIVE: *Blue or purple* color develops on the mat within 60 seconds. See package insert for examples of positive tests.

NEGATIVE: No blue or purple color develops on the mat within 60 seconds. Pink or red color should be ignored.

Results should be reported by entering them into the computer as soon as the test is completed.

REFERENCE VALUES:

Bilirubin is not normally found in the urine in concentration sufficient to give a positive result with this procedure.

There are no critical or special reporting levels for this procedure.

PROCEDURE NOTES AND TROUBLESHOOTING SUGGESTIONS

ICTOTEST® reagent tablets will detect as little as 0.05 to 0.1 mg bilirubin/dL in urine.

If procedure fails QC criteria or if difficulties are encountered in the testing process, check the following parameters:

1. Check reagent tablet for signs of deterioration. A tan-to-brown discoloration of the tablet may denote deterioration. If signs of reagent tablet deterioration are present, discard and retest with a new unopened bottle.
2. Confirm that product is within the expiration date shown on the label. If product has expired, discard and use in-date material.
3. Check performance of reagents with QC controls. If results are not acceptable, discard and use fresh reagents.
4. Consult supervisor if these steps do not correct the problem.
5. Document problems and action taken in QC log.

REFERENCES AND SOURCES FOR ADDITIONAL INFORMATION

Package insert; BAYER® ICTOTEST® Reagent Tablets for Urinalysis; Bayer HealthCare, LLC., Elkhart, IL, Rev. 5/06.

*UTMB POINT OF CARE TESTING PROCEDURES
http://www.utmb.edu/poc/SOP/sop2004/Dec2004/SOPUA%2012-04.pdf

Brunzel, Nancy; Fundamentals of Urine and Body Fluid Analysis, 2ed; Elsevier Health Sciences (Sanders), 2004

REVIEW

Prepared by: Urinalysis Supervisor
Contact: Urinalysis Supervisor

Procedure Approval:

Section Supervisor	Date:
Laboratory Supervisor:	Date:
Pathologist:	Date

Effective Date: December 31, 2xxx
Review Due Date: November 30, 2xxx

BAYER® ICTOTEST® is a registered trademark of Bayer HealthCare, LLC.
Pyridium® is a registered trademark of Warner–Chilcott Company.
Lodine® is a registered trademark of Wyeth

FIGURE 18 — 2. Example of a Technical Procedure

The example of a technical procedure ends *Policy and Procedures*. *Staffing and Scheduling* is next.

— Case Study —

Chapter Eighteen: Policy and Procedure Manuals

"Where is the buffer to dilute the specimen?" asked Tom loudly.

"What buffer? What test are you doing? I thought you were doing that STAT mono for the ER we missed," answered Mary.

"I am," responded Tom. "It says right here in the procedure manual that the specimen is to be diluted with the buffer before being run."

"Let me see," said Mary, puzzled, taking the procedure manual from Tom.

"Oh, we haven't used that method for some time," laughed Mary. "We have been checking out different kits. You need to use the package insert, until the new procedure gets typed up. Look . . . there is a note on the bulletin board from Jane [the section supervisor]."

"I would," answered Tom, "if I could find it. Bur it's not in the box with the reagents, and I can't find it anywhere."

"Look in the new kit package that just came in a few days ago. I think Jane took that package insert to write up a new procedure, but she must have left for vacation before she had a chance," suggested Mary, handing Tom the new kit.

"Oh, no . . . it looks like someone has already borrowed the insert from this box also. They must not have been able to find the old one either, but I can't see where they would have left it," announced a frustrated Tom. "What do we do now?"

"I guess you'll have to let Betty [the laboratory manager] know, and call the manufacturer for a new one. They should be able to Fax it or tell us how to access it over the internet," advised Mary.

"ER, on line two," announced the laboratory secretary over the intercom. "They want to know the results of Mono. The patient is complaining and wants to go home. They said they've been waiting over 2 hours already for the results."

Chapter Sections for Review

- Overview
- Procedure Manual Format
- Figure 18 – 2

Questions for Discussion

1. Is using package inserts to perform tests allowed under regulatory and accreditation rules?
2. How could this problem have been prevented? Should the laboratory have a policy or place for saving package inserts? What about the actions of the section supervisor?
3. Write a procedure, following the model presented in Figure 18 – 2, for any laboratory test that interests the student or reader.

[19]

Staffing and Scheduling

— Chapter Nineteen —

Preparing a schedule is one of the most prominent duties of a laboratory manager. The posted schedule represents in many ways the operational plan for the immediate future. It encompasses the work on job design and analysis, the labor budget, and the prediction of current testing volume. Although the staffing process is a long-tem effort reflected in job descriptions and the budgeting process, the release of the schedule represents the application of the plan to the everyday operations of the laboratory.

This chapter examines the staffing and scheduling of laboratory personnel by first looking at the staffing levels of the department and then reviewing traditional and alternative mechanisms for preparing a schedule.

Objectives

After completion of this chapter, the reader will be able to demonstrate accomplishment of the following objectives.

1. Distinguish between the staffing and scheduling processes.
2. Select an effective staffing and scheduling strategy for the laboratory.
3. Establish staffing levels for the laboratory.
4. Prepare a periodic staffing schedule.

Chapter Highlights and Glossary of Key Terms

I. THE STAFFING PROCESS

Staffing: *The setting of long-term goals and objectives for the number and types of personnel needed to meet the labor requirements of the laboratory.*

A. Types of personnel needed
B. Staffing levels
C. Performance training
D. Workload projections

II. THE SCHEDULING PROCESS

Scheduling: Matching the people presently working in the laboratory with current workload requirements.

A. Issues and factors influencing schedule decisions
B. Availability of staff
C. Type and volume of work performed
D. The workplace
E. Work schedule

8/80 Hour Rule: *A special provision to the wage and hour law that allows health care employees to work extended periods of time outside the 40-hour rule, and sets overtime*

pay when they exceed 80 hours in a 2-week calendar period or work more than 8 hours in a single day.
40-Hour rule: *Wage and hour laws that require employers to pay overtime to employees who work more than 40 hours in a 7-day calendar period.*
1. Traditional work schedules
2. Alternative work schedules
    a. The compressed work cycle
    b. Flexible working hours
    c. Job sharing
    d. Other alternative and innovative work schedules

III. STEPS IN MAKING A SCHEDULE
- A. Types of Schedules
- B. Staffing Levels
- C. Staffing pool
- D. Schedule terminology and keys
- E. Time frame
- F. Skeleton stage
  Skeleton Schedule: *The first working draft of a schedule that posts only weekends and requested time off.*
- G. Routine stage
- H. Filling in the gaps
- I. Computer programs and posting

IV. GENERAL COMMENTS ON STAFFING AND SCHEDULING
- A. Floaters
  Floater: *A person who is able to work in many sections of the lab and is assigned according to fluctuating daily and hourly workload needs.*
- B. Professional extenders
  Professional extenders: *Technical and clerical assistants who do tasks traditionally performed by a professional.*
- C. Management of work flow
  1. The three Ws: what, where, and when
  2. Micromanagement of work flow
     a. Workload priority
     b. Bulk or bottleneck management
- D. Management of absenteeism
  1. Absenteeism defined and measured
     Absence: *Occurrence of an unscheduled absence.*
     Absenteeism: *A failure to meet the standard for attendance set by the laboratory.*
  2. Absenteeism management plan

The Staffing Process

In its technical sense, staffing is the process of determining personnel and job needs, recruiting qualified staff, matching them with the appropriate job, and training them to perform the work assigned. From this definition it is apparent that the staffing of the laboratory is the realization of the human resource component of the planning management function conducted to develop the labor budget and the organizational tasks of jobs design. These two topics, job design and descriptions and salary and wage management, are covered in corresponding chapters on Job Design and Job Descriptions, and Salary and Wage Management. Sections relevant to staffing and scheduling in the laboratory are reviewed here.

Staffing establishes how many and what types of personnel are needed, whereas scheduling determines the names of the persons who will work at these times. For example, staffing levels may dictate that five techs, three phlebotomists, and two clerks are needed to operate the laboratory on a Saturday evening, and scheduling is the posting of the specific names of the individuals assigned to work this shift.

In its everyday use staffing means ensuring that the laboratory has the appropriate personnel to deliver a timely, high-quality service that meets the needs of its patients. To accomplish this goal, staffing must address the following issues.

1. Set the types of personnel needed by the laboratory (e.g., clerks, phlebotomists, technicians, technologists, specialists, supervisors).
2. Determine the number and placement of each type needed.
3. Ensure that the staff is suitably trained to perform its duties (orientation, continuing education, competency assessment, employee development).
4. Project long-term variations in personnel needs caused by such factors as changes in workload, tests mix, methodology, and extent of automation.

These factors, of course, must be accomplished within the fiscal restraints and requirements of the entire economic enterprise. For this reason, the staffing function is an integral part of the process for the planning and development of the laboratory budget.

Types of Personnel Needed

The types of personnel needed to staff a laboratory depend on the following factors.

- The technological and analytical complexity of the procedures being performed.
- The amount of supervision and support available to the persons actually performing the tests.
- Testing volume or workload
- Analytical throughput or turnaround time expectations.
- Equipment, instrumentation, and computer technology available (i.e., testing methodology).

How these factors are combined is crucial in determining the appropriate personnel mix. A highly sophisticated reference laboratory that offers specialized procedures performed mostly by graduate-level clinical scientists may need only minimally trained assistants working with them, whereas a high-volume hospital laboratory performing a wide range of procedures requiring rapid turnaround needs a technical staff made up almost entirely of highly trained professional laboratorians. In the first case, each step of the analytical process can be double-checked, but the hospital laboratory has no opportunity for a supervisor to recheck each result before release.

From this example, plainly no set rules determine the specific combination of types of laboratory personnel needed in a particular setting. The overriding principle, however, remains the interest of the patients and the quality of care they receive. In applying this principle to the laboratory, the guideline that becomes evident is the technical expertise of the staff and the amount of supervision it requires. The information in this section is intended to enable managers to evaluate and develop an appropriate staffing mix for their particular laboratory situation.

Staffing Levels

The primary determinant in the staffing decision is the level of service expected from each unit and the resulting workload. The weekday day shift, for example, may be expected to perform all services offered by the section and needs the specialized personnel to accomplish this mission.

If, however, only routine procedures are performed during weekends, evenings, or night shifts, then technologists with general laboratory skills may be appropriate. Technical skills, matched with workload, set the types and numbers of personnel needed during each staffing period.

To be effective, the staffing function should support the scheduling process and help to avoid the gaps in personnel that could cause a scheduling crisis and possible disruption of service. This situation may result with there are insufficient numbers of personnel for a shift or section or when the only person who can perform a certain test is out sick or on vacation.

Performance Training

An important aspect of staffing is to make certain that employees are properly trained to perform their assignments. Training personnel to staff the laboratory begins with their arrival (orientation) and follows through with the employee development programs run by the laboratory to ensure competency, availability of future staff, and the continual growth of both the laboratory and its employees. Management has a distinct responsibility to properly educate and train the staff for the tasks and duties it is expected to perform (see also chapters on *Human Resource Management* and *Training the Laboratory Professional*).

Workload Projections

Accuracy in workload projections is an obvious factor in establishing a stable labor force and an effective staffing plan. Anticipating needs and matching the right people with the workload are goals of staffing plans. Data on which to prepare the workload projections may come from three sources.

1. Historical records, such as productivity and financial data, which form the basis for current staffing requirements and the preparation of the schedule for the immediate period.
2. Analysis of future trends, based on an examination of past and current testing volumes to detect tests that are gaining in popularity, becoming obsolete, or giving way to alternative methodology.
3. Analysis of foreseeable changes resulting from the introduction of new procedures, discontinuance of old tests, acquisition of new instruments, changes in medical staff, and availability of new services such as an outpatient center or open heart surgery.

Such information helps to predict current and future needs and prepare the staffing budget, personnel position control records, and the schedule.

The Scheduling Process

Preparing the schedule can be both routine and challenging. It is routine in the sense that it is a regular task that follows set patterns. The challenge of scheduling is to find someone to fill in the gaps caused by previously known and unexpected absences.

Scheduling is matching the people now working in the laboratory with current workload requirements. During the staffing process managers are allowed to take time to plan and organize, but in scheduling the manager must ensure that someone is in the laboratory to process the specimens when they arrive. Hence, scheduling is a major part of the *directing* and *controlling* management functions.

The section that follows will review the process of preparing a schedule by discussing the issues and factors that influence scheduling decisions, and by examining examples of both traditional and alternative work schedules.

Issues and factors Influencing Schedule Decisions

Many factors must be considered in preparing a schedule. These are the same issues reviewed in the staffing section but must be dealt with on an immediate basis. They also fall into three broad categories that must be coordinated and reflected in the final schedule: availability of staff; type and volume of work; and, the workplace itself.

Availability of Staff

The availability of staff is, of course, a major determinant and limitation. Not only the number of persons available but also the types and skills represented in the labor pool must be considered. These are some of the staff availability issues that define the scheduling options.

- The skills of each worker, whether generalist or specialist in one of two areas only.
- The paper qualifications of the employee (licensure and accreditation).
- The employees' flexibility in hours available to work. This issue is usually addressed with shift assignments for both full-time and part-time employees. In almost all cases, the best solution is a *regular* staff core supplemented with fill-in assignments. This allows for stability and continuity in both service and the personal lives of the staff. A less desirable solution is to *rotate* all personnel to evening and night shifts. This is usually not an acceptable solution because of the disruption it causes in the personal lives of the staff and the inconsistency in the delivery of laboratory services.
- The total number of persons available, including their employment status. The mix of full-time, part-time, on-call, and professional extenders (phlebotomists, clerical workers, laboratory aides, and so on) defines the resources available to the person preparing the schedule.

Type and Volume of Work Performed

The essence of scheduling is creating a match between the previously listed factors and the workload of the laboratory. Workload is usually determined by the patient base; such as emergency rooms, outpatients, surgery, and hospitalized patients.

The Workplace

The workplace involves instrumentation, methodology, organization, and facility layout; as well as support resources such as extent of automation, computerization, and the availability of support staff.

Work Schedules

For several reasons, including the requirements of wage and hour laws, the cultural influence of the 9-to-5 job, and the organizational ease of the division of 24; three 8-hours shifts have become the custom in most institutions that require around-the-clock staffing. An additional factor, because of the perceived uniqueness of their services, hospitals are allowed to use a specific **8/80-hour rule** as an exception to the **40-hour rule** overtime requirements of the wage and hour laws. This allows the facility to work its employees up to 10 days in a row without paying overtime as long as any one day does not exceed eight hours of duty. This allowance further strengthens the three 8-hour shift tradition.

With the advent of specialization in services that could not fit into the 9-to-5 mold and the increasing shortage of qualified personnel, the health care community has been forced to look for alternatives to the restraints of the 8-hour day, provide incentives to attract employees, and gain flexibility in scheduling options. This movement has seen the growing trend to adopt the 40-hour workweek over the 8/80, which has in turn allowed such innovations as the 10- and 12- hour workday.

Traditional Work Schedules

40-hour work week: 5 days on and 2 days off
8/80-hour work cycle: 10 days on and 4 days off during a 2-week calendar period.

Alternative Work Schedules

Compressed work cycle: An individual may work multishifts or extended time periods (10-, 12-, or 16-hour shifts) within a 40-hour calendar week.
Flexible working hours: Employees are responsible for a set amount of work but are allowed to establish their own hours around a core period.
Job Sharing: Two individuals share the responsibilities and benefits of a position usually filled by one worker.
Exempt and professional status: Employees are exempted by salary levels or professional classification from the overtime provision of wage and hour laws.
Work-at-home programs
Off-site testing and satellite laboratories
Freelance employment

Table 19 – 1. Types of Work Schedules

The following section reviews the advantages of traditional and alternative work schedules and discusses the mechanisms of preparing a schedule. Table 19 –1 provides a summary of the types of work schedules currently in use.

Traditional Work Schedules

The traditional work schedule can be most easily defined as a standard 8-hour shift, consisting of 5 days on and 2 days off within a calendar week. This time may comprise of 5 straight days of work with every weekend off, which is common in administrative and routine services areas; 5 days during 1 calendar week; or, in the case of the 8/80rules, 10 days in a 2-week period, which allows the employee to work weekends with scheduled days off during the corresponding time period. An interesting and important note to this definition is that there are no limits as to days of the week or hours. This means that many schedules in the laboratory do not necessarily fit the customary 9-to-5, Monday-to-Friday workweek of the business world.

The main advantage of the traditional 8-hour workday is that it presents a neat three-shift "package," which fits quite nicely in the 24-hour day. With the usual half-hour lunch break, which makes it an 8½-hour time frame, it allows for overlapping coverage. It also is aligned with the standard work philosophy of our society: 8 hours of duty, 5 days at work, with 2 days off. The disadvantage of this and any "standard" system is that it discourages and restricts flexibility and individualization. Very few people have life schedules which fit nicely into "standard" routines.

Another characteristic of the traditional work schedule is that it is usually covered with a regular core staff and supplemented with other personnel according to need. This offers the strong advantages of stability and continuity to both the services provided and the employees. The main disadvantage of this system is that it tends to build a staff whose identity and skills are tied to a particular work area or group and discourages interaction and cooperation between different sections of the laboratory. The inclusion of members from all areas of the laboratory in continuing education, problem-solving sessions, quality assessment committees, and other operational functions is a management strategy that can build identification with the laboratory as a whole.

Alternative Work Schedules

In the general business community, alternative work schedules have centered around three main modifications: the 4 – day workweek; flexible working hours; and, job sharing. In the health care industry, an additional adaptation has gained popularity: the clustered, or compressed, work cycle in which the employee may work 7 days on and 7 days off. These adjustments have been driven by the needs of the hospital to meet the changing nature of its patient population and to aid in the recruitment and retention of its workforce.

The Compressed Work Cycle

Creative scheduling programs allow employers to match production goals with reduced facility costs. In the 1970s, when faced with soaring energy costs, industrial managers found that the same production quantity could often be produced in 4 days rather than the customary 5 if the employees worked longer shifts, saving the company the costs of starting up and running the plant and machinery for an extra day. Employees also found the extra time off to be extremely attractive.

These changes, introduced in manufacturing plants and matched with the staffing and scheduling crisis caused by shortages of nursing personnel caused health care facilities to re-examine traditional staffing schedules. These programs were first developed in medical centers such as Baylor University Hospitals (*and frequently referred to as the Baylor plan*), where a large pool of qualified personnel seeking graduate degrees could work weekends and evenings but needed large blocks of time off during the week to attend to their studies. By working in concentrated blocks of time, such as 16-hour shift on the weekends, the students could make money and release the regular staff to cover the times when specialized skills were needed.

Below are some examples of compressed schedules.

- 10- to 12-hour shifts spread over 3 to 4 days.
- 7 days on, 7 days off.
- Five 8-hour days 1 week, and four 10-hour days the next.
- Intensive weekend coverage, during which the employee might work 16-hour days every weekend and the weekdays off.
- A variety of options in which employees may work double (16-hour) shifts during certain weekdays or seasonal periods in exchange for specific days off.

These programs have proven highly effective in staffing off-shifts such as evenings, nights, and weekends, when workload and methodology sophistication are greatly reduced but basic coverage must be maintained. They have also offered opportunities to persons with special need and scheduling problems. Full-time students, families who must coordinate child-care responsibilities, and persons seeking second jobs are the kinds of employees who have benefited from and been attracted to these schedules.

The major advantage of such options is that managers have been able to look at the scheduling function as a fluid process that matches staff with workload without the restrictions imposed under the traditional model.

Flexible Working Hours

Breaking the mold of the traditional workweek has led to other solutions to scheduling problems. One of the more promising has been *flextime*.

Under flextime, employees are required to be on the job during a core period, but they are allowed to establish their own arrival and departure times depending on their personnel needs and the demands of the workload. For example, a person may be assigned a core period of 10:00 AM to 2:00 PM, but when the employee works the other four hours of the shift is determined by how the employee views personal and work priorities.

A *deadline*, or completion goal, may in some cases be substituted for a core period. A project or specific volume of work may be due at 4:00 PM and employees may be given the latitude to schedule their work hours with this objective in mind. A key advantage of a flexible work schedule is that it recognizes the ability of workers to take responsibility for their own performance.

Another variation of flextime is a split shift approach, which allows the employee to work at different times of the day. This arrangement can offer benefits to the laboratory to meet workload peaks and to employees who may need to coordinate family responsibilities with a spouse or pursue a special interest or hobby. What makes split shifts work is the mutual benefit factor. However when split shift conditions have been forced on workers with only the needs of concentrated workload peaks in mind, they have been met with considerable resistance because of the disruptions they may cause in the employee's daily life.

Although flextime programs are gaining in popularity in other industries, they are still uncommon in health care settings and are particularly rare in the laboratory. However, because of the advantages to both the employer and the staff, they are bound to gain increasing acceptance. Some areas in which flextime and other compressed-scheduling options may be useful in the laboratory include:

- Tests that can be saved and batched together, e.g., thyroid profiles, infrequently run tests, and other special chemistry procedures; especially where saving and performing tests in batches are cost effective and patient care is not compromised.
- Preadmission and preoperative work, as that commonly performed in blood banks and on evening shifts.
- End-process procedures, like cytology screening and interpretation of electrophoresis patterns.
- Administrative tasks, such as policy and procedure writing, quality control records reviews, and preparing the schedule.

Job Sharing

Job sharing occurs when two or more persons are responsible for a job that is normally performed by a single employee. Critics of job sharing point out that this often just a cover for the growing practice of depriving workers of the benefits to which they would be entitled if they work full-time. Job sharing, however, is much more than two part-time employees doing the same kind of work.

Job sharing requires each employee to take full responsibility for the total job and all the duties that the position entails. They are accountable for coordination of their time and work so that there is a smooth transition of duties and the work is completed in the same manner that would be accomplished by a single employee. In a true job-sharing program the "dual unit" also shares the benefits due a full-time employee.

In managing a job-sharing unit, a laboratory supervisor would deal with the group as a single unit in all matters including scheduling and problem reporting. As an illustration for a job-sharing relationship, a Hematology schedule would reflect one position for a job-sharing team, and the details would be left to the persons sharing the job in the same manner as with an individual staff member.

<u>Other Alternative and Innovative Work Schedules</u>

Even more pressure will be exerted on manager to develop creative schedule solution in the future because of changes in technology, the nature of work, health care financing and delivery mechanisms, and lifestyles of the work force. Some of the more recent trends and adaptations affecting the laboratory include:

> **Exempt and professional status**: One major scheduling change allowed by professional standing is that staff can be classified as *exempt* payroll-status employees, which means they can be "exempted" from the restraints imposed by the overtime provisions of the wage and salary laws. These changes have not been welcomed in many professional situations, where staff is committed to specific working (punch-clock) times, or where personal time off is highly restrictive [see the chapter on *Human Resources: The Personnel Process* for more information on this topic].
>
> **Work at home**: In the laboratory community, cytotechnology is setting the pace in the work-at-home movement, although this practice is under regulatory and professional criticism over quality and working conditions. Data entry, transcription, and information analysis are further examples of work that can be done in the employees' home.
>
> **Off-site testing**: This includes not only satellite labs but point-of-care testing at the patient's bedside, which may be in another facility such as a nursing home or the patient's home. With the tremendous technological growth in this area and the use of remote data entry, technologists are no longer bound physically to the main laboratory.
>
> **Freelance employment**: The opportunity for laboratorians to work away from the traditional laboratory has exploded since the 1990s. Professional freelance work has become common in the economic environment of these decades, and it is only natural that it would find its way into health care. The laboratory especially has experienced this phenomenon with the advent of CLIA'88 and the opportunities to be technical consultants of laboratories in physician's offices. Agencies which specialize and coordinate "*Traveler Techs*," or place temporary (freelance professionals) staff now represent a major portion of recruitment advertisement in laboratory journals.

CLIA'88 has brought to many laboratorians the technical and marketing skills necessary to work independently and become successful consultants and has demonstrated to the medical community and industry the value of this profession's knowledge and expertise. This option is further spurred by the seasonal fluctuation in the workload of many laboratories and the increasing need for fill-in help. As the consultant pool increases, there will be a growing demand for people who can offer services that met the special needs of individual laboratories such as compliance with inspection agencies and development of marketing strategies.

Steps in Making a Schedule

Once decisions have been made about staffing and scheduling, the actual preparation of the work schedule is relatively straightforward.

There is a wide variety of scheduling software available which streamlines the process of making schedules. After basic personnel information is entered the system keeps track of past schedules and will prepare a preliminary model based on historical patterns. This then allows the manager to modify and adjust assignments as information on workload, time off requests, and personnel changes becomes available. Some software even permits employees to enter requests for schedule changes and time-off directly into the computer and allows the manager to review how these adjustments would impact the schedule and provide more timely approval or feedback to the staff. While these programs make much of the mundane tasks of filling in blanks with Xs and Os automatic, they do not provide an elixir for having to find enough staff to fill in the "*blank*" or "*help needed*" cues. For this reason, a basic understanding of the scheduling process is necessary and the major steps in preparing a schedule is presented in this section.

Table 19 – 2. SUMMARY OF STEPS IN PREPARING A SCHEDULE

1. Select type of schedule
2. Establish staffing level
3. Develop staffing personnel pool
4. Determine format, terminology, and schedule keys
5. Set posting time frame
6. Prepare skeleton stage
7. Complete routine scheduling stage
8. Fill in gaps
9. Post schedule

The following exercise goes through the various steps for preparing a schedule for the afternoon shift in a hospital laboratory [Table 19 – 2; (the final schedule is presented in Figure 19 – 2 at the end of the chapter)].

Types of Schedules

Schedules can assume any one of several formats depending of the needs and customs of the lab, but they usually fall into one of the following categories:

1. A format that simply lists *attendance*, showing who is working and who is off.
2. Work *assignments*, which give the station or section in which the laboratorian is to work on a particular day.
3. A *combination*, which lists both attendance and work assignment. This is accomplished frequently by modifying the attendance schedule with a code depicting the place the person is assigned to work.

Staffing Levels (example)

The staffing requirements for the shift example used in this exercises are as follows:

	Techs	Phlebs	Clerical
Weekdays	5	2	1
Weekends/holidays	4	2	0

The techs are all generalists, including both the assistant and the shift supervisor.

Staffing Pool

In this example, there are five full-time techs and three full-time phlebotomist assigned to the shift who routinely work every other weekend. Along with one full-time clerical worker who covers the weekdays. There are also three techs and two phlebotomists who usually work every other weekend in addition to several weekdays. The supervisor must compete with other sections for additional needed personnel from the part-time pool of employees on the laboratory roster.

Schedule Terminology and Keys

Acronyms, symbols, and marks used on a schedule vary according to the institution. Some laboratories use a letter to designate the work assignment: for example, **C** for chemistry, **H** for hematology, **B** for blood bank, and **U** for urinalysis (see Figures. 19 – 1(below) and 19 – 2[at the end of the chapter]). Other symbols may include:

V = Requested paid time off (vacation, holiday)
M = A day that employee must have off, usually a request to have their regular scheduled day off at this time rather than using any paid time off.
P = A preferred scheduled day off, but the employee will work if necessary.
X = Scheduled work day
O = Routine scheduled day off.

Time Frame

Schedules are frequently posted for either one (1) month or four (4) weeks. The 4-week format is easy to read and fill out because the weekends and the days of the week always follow the same pattern. Monthly schedules are also popular because they follow the calendar. Whatever the format selected, the final schedule should be posted at least two (2) weeks prior to the end of the current cycle to allow the staff time to plan accordingly.

Skelton Stage

The skeleton schedule (Figure 19 – 1) is a working draft that includes weekends and requested time off. It should be started as far in advance as feasible; even three (3) months ahead is not too soon. It can serve as a working document in which the supervisor notes any changes and requests that will influence the final schedule.

The skeleton stage process is as follows.

1. Fill out the form with dates (day or month and week) and names of staff members.
2. Mark required time off: vacations (V), must days (M), and so on.
3. Pencil in preferred time off (P).
4. Record routine weekend work and off-day patterns.
5. Post and update skeleton schedule so that employees can note time available and check for any oversights in requested time off.

By following this preliminary preparation procedure well in advance of the schedule deadline, the supervisor can spot problems areas early and begin to make plans to arrange for coverage.

Routine Stage

This phase normally follows a set pattern of making Xs and Os, as follows.

1. Fill in the off days (O) (see guideline suggestions later in this section).
2. Fill in the set workday schedule (X) of full-time and part-time employees.
3. Fill in part-time personnel who can work a variable schedule according to need.

4. Compare the schedule at this stage with the staffing requirements and identify any gaps in coverage.

Figure 19 – 1. 3:00 to 11:00 PM schedule: skeleton stage

July	3	4	5	6	7	8	9		10	11	12	13	14	15	16
Tech:	Su	M	Tu	W	Th	F	St	•	Su	M	Tu	W	Th	F	S
Full-time															
Smith (Sup)	O				O		X	•	X		O				O
Johns	O					O	X	•	X			P			O
Wilson	X			O			O	•	O					O	X
Casey	X	O					O	•	O	V	V	O	V	V	V
Adams	X		O				O	•	O				O		X
Part-time															
Horne	O						X	•	X						O
Rogers	O						X	•	X						V
Black	X		M	M			O	•	O	MT	MT				X
PT Lab Pool															
Hill												MT		MT	
Duval															X
Total Staff:	4	5	5	5	5	5	4		4	5	5	5	5	5	4
PHLEBS:															
Full-time															
Jones	X			O			O	•	O					O	X
Tomas	O				O		X	•	X		O				O
Small	X		M				O	•	O				O		X
Part-time															
Shell	O	O	O	O	O	O	X	•	X	O	O	O	O	O	O
Total Staff:	2	3	3	3	3	3	2		2	3	3	3	3	3	3
Clerical															
Murphy	O	X	X	X	X	X	O	•	O	X	X	X	X	X	O

KEY:

X = Scheduled to work
O = Scheduled off
V = Scheduled paid time off
MT = Mystery Tech (open, request to work)
M = Must (Requested regular day off)
P = Preferred day off (Requested day off)

Several additional guidelines have proven of value to supervisors in preparing the routine phase of the schedule.

- Follow a pattern of *4-day stretches* for traditional 40-hour or 8/80 schedules. For example, if a person works a weekend and has the following Monday off, he or she would automatically be off the previous Wednesday. The matching days are Wednesday – Monday, Thursday – Tuesday, and Friday – Wednesday. This rule helps to ensure equity in the number and frequency of days worked and time off. Exceptions (such as every Friday – Monday off) should be carefully considered and staff should understand the reasons special requests are being approved.
- Within the guidelines of the 4-day stretch, allow for personal preference as much as possible. Understandably, people like to have as much continuity in their schedule as possible, especially those who are committed to weekend hours. Have a set pattern of Thursday-Tuesday off, for example, enables employees to plan for their personal lives and also aids the supervisor in filling in the routine parts of the schedule.
- Make any modification in the normal routine patterns as far in advance as possible. Everyone understands the need for occasional modifications, and people are willing to cooperate when the reason for the change is explained and they are allowed as much flexibility as possible in helping to meet scheduling needs.

At this point in the preparation process, the schedule is nearing its final stage and has to be reviewed only to identify and staffing discrepancies and fill in vacant slots.

Filling in the Gaps

No matter how well the manager plans for staffing needs, unanticipated scheduling slots need to be filled. These can be caused by unexpected resignations, dismissals, last-minute request for time off, and illness. There should be, however, adequate full- and part-time staff to cover these occurrences, and with some creative shuffling of personnel, the laboratory always seems to meet its patients' needs.

A lack of management planning, however, magnifies this situation. Waiting until the last moment to deal with shortages is an obvious example of poor planning. If the laboratory is adequately staffed, most of the scheduling problems can be resolved quickly.

Some suggestions for completing the schedule and filling in the gaps include the following.

Check with *part-timers* to see if they can work any of the open days, or adjust the schedule of full-time employees to match staffing needs. These adjustments may be changes in preference, days off, or shift.

Seek *volunteers* who may be willing to work an unusual schedule for a short time or who will work an extra day. For example, if one person stays longer and another comes in earlier, a shift may be covered on a temporary basis. Soliciting volunteers is a matter of preference, however. Two common strategies are (1) letting each member of the staff know on an individual or collective basis of the time slots that need to be filled and (2) posting a notice on a bulletin board listing the times when assistance is needed.

Use *incentive pay programs* such as overtime and additional differential payment for working additional hours.. This can be both an incentive for staff looking for extra income, and as a tool to staff acute shortages. Heavy dependence on overtime for an extend period of time as a solution for routine scheduling problems is a sign of poor personnel and staff management. In most institutions overtime is viewed as an immediate solution to an urgent staffing problem, such as when many people call in sick at the same time. Overtime may also be necessary when there is an acute shortage of staff due to recruitment problems. Long time dependence on overtime strategies also wears out its welcome as an incentive for staff. The supervisor should keep in mind the availability of overtime as a tool to attract and reward people willing to work the extra time, but use this option with discretion while keeping the laboratory and hospital administration up to date on the situation.

Figure 19 – 2. 15:00 to 23:00 PM schedule: Combination

July	3	4	5	6	7	8	9		10	11	12	13	14	15	16
Tech:	Su	M	Tu	W	Th	F	St	•	Su	M	Tu	W	Th	F	S
Full-time															
Smith (Sup)	O	F	F	F	O	F	C	•	C	F	O	F	F	F	O
Johns	O	B	B	B	B	O	B	•	B	H	H	O	H	H	O
Wilson	U	C	C	O	O	C	O	•	O	B	B	B	B	O	B
Casey	H	O	U	U	U	U	O	•	O	V	V	O	V	V	V
Adams	B	H	O	H	F	H	O	•	O	U	F	U	O	U	U
Part-time															
Horne	O	O	H	C	O	O	H	•	H	O	O	O	U	B	O
Rogers	O	O	O	O	H	B	U	•	U	O	O	C	O	O	V
Black	C	U	O	O	O	O	O	•	O	C	C	O	O	O	C
PT Lab Pool															
Hill											U	H		C	
Duval															H
Total Staff:	4	5	5	5	5	5	4		4	5	5	5	5	5	4
PHLEBS:															
Full-time															
Jones	X	X	X	O	X	X	O	•	O	X	X	X	X	O	X
Tomas	O	X	X	X	O	X	X	•	X	X	O	X	X	X	O
Small	X	X	O	X	X	X	O	•	O	X	X	X	O	X	X
Part-time															
Shell	O	O	X	X	X	O	X	•	X	O	X	O	X	O	O
Total Staff:	2	3	3	3	3	3	2		2	3	3	3	3	3	2
Clerical															
Murphy	O	X	X	X	X	X	O	•	O	X	X	X	X	X	O

KEY:

X = Scheduled to work
O = Scheduled off
V = Scheduled paid time off
F = Float
H = Hematology
C = Chemistry
U = Urine/Micro
B = Blood Bank

Call in temporary or "*travelers*" staff. Temporary staffing agencies have gained popularity since the 1980s because of the shortage of nursing personnel, and have often provided solutions in laboratories until more permanent staffing can be recruited.

Force a *schedule change*. Forced or involuntary schedule changes are a last-ditch method for filling in gaps. Because of the major disruptions in the personal lives of the staff, this move must be considered only after all other efforts have failed. The ability of the manager to successfully implement this plan depends on the following crucial factors.

- The staff's understanding of the possibility, however remote, of the need for this policy because of the nature of the services provided. An explanation of the laboratory staffing policy should be spelled out *very early* in the employment process, certainly before a final offer is made, so that any problems or misunderstanding may be resolved.
- The reason and necessity for instigating this action must be clear to all involved.
- The burden should fall equally on all eligible employees and not be left for one section or shit to deal with alone. This can be an extremely stressful decision for supervisors, who are aware of the hardships this may cause a particular staff member. However, they must remain fair and objective and not make personal judgments on the impact a move will have on any one individual [remember this comment is made within the problems of a *forced* schedule change; of course where possible, every possible consideration should be made to accommodate individual needs, especially if there are several openings which need to be filled].
- There must be a highly visible all-out effort by administration to obtain the needed staff to alleviate the situation. Many personnel managers view placing help-wanted ads for professionals in local small-town newspapers as being futile; however, this is often the most conspicuous sign to the laboratory staff that management is doing everything possible to solve the staffing crisis.

Computer Programs and Posting

The final step is posting the schedule for the next period. Making the schedule available well ahead of the starting date enables both the employee and the supervisor the chance to find and correct any deficiencies.

Numerous computer programs are available for preparing a schedule. However, these programs' usefulness diminishes rapidly beyond the routine stage, and managers are left to their own creative devices in finding employees to cover the nonroutine openings that make each scheduling process a unique experience (Figure 19 – 2 [above] present a finished schedule ready for posting)..

General Comments on Staffing and Scheduling

This section offers some advice and comments on several important aspects of the staffing and scheduling process that do not fit into one of the previous categories

Floaters

A **floater** is a person who is able to work in many sections of the lab and is assigned according to fluctuating daily and hourly workload needs.

What could possible be wrong with this job? Isn't it a key strategy for meeting variable workload needs? Why don't laboratories use as many floaters as possible? Why do floaters almost always appear dissatisfied with their jobs? The answers to these questions lie in how floaters are treated with respect to other techs that are committed to a specific section or job assignment.

Historically as well as today, in industry and in health care, specialization has been the route most encouraged and immediately rewarded, particularly in the early stages of a professional career. This trend has caused generalist, in many instances, to feel like second-class citizens who are used and then passed on to someone else without receiving either monetary or professional recognition for their contributions. Every one likes to have a place to belong. No one minds helping out a coworker or another section once in a while; however, if this need is frequent or the employee feel they are not being dealt with fairly, they may become resentful and uncooperative.

The floater is often shifted to hot spots constantly, without being able to use the slack time to recuperate and renew professionally. Just when one area is caught up and the regular staff begins to relax, the floater is hurried off to another crisis. The communal feeling of teamwork and bonding that arise from identification with a job, accomplishment, and contribution are missing and many floaters may feel that they are being used rather than recognized and appreciated.

The persons most amenable to floater situations appear to be part-time and temporary personnel. The manager may find someone, however, whose personality fits the floater position perfectly or who likes the variety and challenge, similar to those who prefer to work unusual hours or schedule. Like all staffing and scheduling functions, the manager should match the person with the job as closely as possible.

The real solution to this valuable staffing options in the development of special recognition and pay programs that reward floaters and generalists for their broad range of skills and technical flexibility rather than reward only increased specialization.

Professional Extenders

Professional extenders are technical and clerical assistants who do tasks traditionally performed by a professional. As the demand for health care services exploded from the 1980s to today, physician assistants and nurse practitioners became more numerous and accepted. Nursing has developed many innovative approaches for transferring nonprofessional duties to support personnel.

In the laboratory, phlebotomists and clerical staff perform tasks that used to be performed mostly by techs. Technical and clerical assistants may be assigned to individual techs or sections to help with routine tasks and allow the skilled professionals to focus their time on more sophisticated tests and procedures.

Management of Work Flow

This topic is include here to remind the manager that there may be alternatives to meeting staffing and scheduling problems other than shifting people around. Part of the staffing and scheduling equation includes maintaining constant vigilance on the management of the work being done in the laboratory.

The Three Ws: What, Where, and When

What, where, and when are the key components of work-flow analysis.

1. *What* test should be done? This assessment requires constant review of the menu of services offered by the laboratory, including discontinuing out-of-date procedures and looking for opportunities to better meet the needs of patients.

2. *Where* should these tests be performed? This assessment involves not only deciding on the laboratory section best suited for the activities, but also the proper use of satellite stations and central testing facilities.
3. *When* should tests be performed? The answer to this question, like the previous two, sets the boundaries and limits of the laboratory's ability to adapt in a timely manner to both short- and long-term staffing changes. Options for consideration include use of reference laboratories (send-outs) to help in times of staffing shortages, batching infrequent or low-volume test to once or twice a day or week, and shifting workload to periods or shifts that may have slack time or may be underutilized.

Micromanagement of Work Flow

Micromanagement of work flow concerns the actual, live, ongoing processing of the work in the laboratory, much as a football coach changes strategies and personnel during a game as the play-byplay situation fluctuates. Another analogy is that Monday morning quarterbacking analysis may be fun or even useful in the long run; however, the coach must be there when the team is trying to make a first down if they want to win the game. The manager must be near enough to the bench to see the work in process and anticipate developing problems,. They must be assessable to make immediate adjustments to ensure success; not off in some distant office or meeting when disruptions in service occur.

Micromanagement is usually accomplished at the bench with the establishment and management of workflow through two kinds of prioritization: (1) ranking of workload by factors such as STATS, instrument availability, and turnaround times; and, (2) bulk or bottleneck management.

Workload Priority

The prioritization of workload is a system with which the laboratory is quite familiar. Performance of tests based on factors such as clinical urgency and patient throughput (outpatient, emergency room, and so on) is a tradition that should be clearly coded to make sure the laboratory personnel know the immediacy of each order. If the STAT system is properly managed — then everyone knows the priority assigned to each request.

A poorly defined and enforced priority system wreaks havoc and may simply result in a first-come, first-served order because everything is marked STAT — sort of a "routine STAT" approach.

In a well-managed priority system that operates properly, an effective strategy is "working off the top of the list," completing tests by priority [e.g., STATS, timed specimens, unit priority (OR, ICU, ER, Nursery, etc.)]

Bulk or Bottleneck Management

It is usually easy to detect where bottlenecks will occur because of their distinct character. Their main feature is that most, if not all, of the work must pass through a narrow point before reaching the internal production machinery of the organization, or they are a task which ties up the system.

These bottlenecks are most often individual specimens that require unusually large amounts of time, often holding up the completion of other samples: for example, a difficult phlebotomy, a DIFF with abnormal cells, or a blood bank antibody workup. A main bottleneck obstacle may also be caused by telephone calls, requiring extensive time to locate a nurse or doctor to report critical values or explain a problem with a sample. The strategy at the micro level is to get the bulk of the work out, leaving the items that take up a large amount of time to the end of the work cycle or assigning them to a workstation (tech/phlebotomist) dedicated to this tasks. This increases the odds that any test results of special interest to nursing or physicians will be completed and not left sitting while all the techs are busy working on one or two difficult samples.

Management of Absenteeism

From time to time everyone needs to be away from work unexpectedly. But it is sometimes difficult to define the point at which absenteeism is a problem, rather that part of the normal routine of human and business life. Overreaction places excessive stresses on the manager and workers, as well as making the manager appear hard-hearted and inhumane. However, under reacting may cause serious workplace disruption and may arouse resentment toward coworkers who are perceived as abusing the system. Both situations undermine the unit, cohesiveness, and effectiveness of the work group.

Mutual understanding and respect, along with fair and forthright communication about expectations and rules, are the basis of a sound policy of absenteeism management. An absenteeism management program contains several key elements: (1) a clearly defined policy on when absenteeism becomes a corporate problem; (2) measurable and objective criteria for monitoring attendance; and (3) a plan for following and correcting a problem at its earliest stage in a mature manner beneficial to both the individual and the organization.

Absenteeism Defined and Measured

Absence occurs any time a person is not at work when scheduled. The seriousness of absenteeism depends on its duration and frequency of occurrence. One possible definition of an absence may be an *occurrence of an unscheduled absence.* The concept of <u>occurrence</u> is the important defining point. An occurrence may be a single day or several weeks in duration. For example, a person may miss one day because of the flu or one month because of surgery; each occurrence constitutes one absence.

Purposely avoided from this definition is the reason for missing work. Employees must be considered responsible adults who are at work if possible and who are expected to manage their personal affairs to meet this obligation. It is the employee who decides whether the absence is justified. The supervisor in no way is expected to make a value judgment over the priority or appropriateness of one absence over another. Remember that it is the *frequency*, not the reason for a single event, which creates a concern over the ability of employees to meet their obligations to the organization.

Absenteeism is a failure to meet the standard for attendance set by the laboratory. On this point a wide range of opinions and controversy exist. But whatever attendance standard is adopted must be fair and workable in its application.

There must also be some flexibility in interpretation and management of the program, but the reasons for any variance must be open and clear to everyone. For example, a long-term employee with practically no history of absenteeism would justifiable be given more latitude than a person who continues to have periods of concentrated absences. An average of one unscheduled absence per month is generally considered excessive and usually triggers the absenteeism management plan.

Absenteeism Management Plan

Absenteeism must be handled in the same framework as all behavior and performance problems, following closely the corrective action policies of the institution (i.e., Corrective Action and Discipline Program as described in the Human Resource Management: The Personnel Process module). Identifying the existence of a possible problem at an early stage and attempting to resolve and correct it before it reaches a crisis for either the employee or the laboratory are important in all cases but especially crucial in an area that is often subjective and personal. Long before the formal intervention process begins, the manager should talk with the employee, inform him or her of the concern, and offer help in addressing any job-related factors that may alleviate the situation.

One clue is identifying and proposing job related assistance is the appearance of an absenteeism pattern —certain days of the week or month (e.g., Mondays, Fridays, day after payday, school holidays, and so on). The employee may not even be aware of the pattern and changes in scheduled days off, arrival and departure times, change to another shift, or even a leave of absence may offer some remedy.

The key is to show a concern and willingness to help within the restraints of the staffing needs of the laboratory. If this strategy does not bring the attendance of the employee in line with expectations, the manager is left with little alternative except to begin the formal corrective action policy of the institution. Any delay only increases the seriousness and unpleasantness of the problem for the employee, coworkers, the manager, and the organization.

These ideas on management of absenteeism, ends the chapter covering *Staffing and Scheduling*. Next: *Laboratory Safety*.

— Case Study —

Chapter Nineteen: Staffing and Scheduling

"June called in sick, again," announced the night tech to the laboratory manager as she walked into the laboratory. "Hematology is already behind. I couldn't reach Sue, and all of our night techs have early morning appointments, including myself. I can stay until eight o'clock, but that's only another half hour, then I have to go. We need someone else to call, more help, or something."

"I know," responded the laboratory manager. "Let me go check on hematology now, and see what we can do."

"Good morning," the laboratory manager said cautiously to the hematology staff.

"Another great day in the salt mines," joked one tech sharing the humor with her partner.

"I have to talk to you," said the hematology supervisor, pulling the laboratory manager quickly toward her office. "What happened when you talked to June? It doesn't seem to have done any good, whatever it was."

"Well, I really haven't had a chance to speak to her," answered the laboratory manager. "You know how busy I've been, and when I could have talked to her, she called in. You know she's had a lot of problems with child care, and her mother has been very sick."

"Well, it's too late now," the hematology supervisor responded, "I don't want her in my department anymore. We resent having to cover for her, all the time. We all have problems, but somebody has to show up to do the work. Anyway, even if she was here all the time, we need more help. Our workload has nearly doubled since they started doing open heart surgery, and the new outpatient clinic opened. Those two new hematology oncologists have just piled the work on with all their bone marrows. I must have some more help."

"I know … I have a meeting tomorrow with administration to talk about our staffing problems, but until then we have to make do," agreed the laboratory manager.

"Well, I need another tech right now, to help us 'make do' this morning," the hematology supervisor continued. "Don't even try chemistry or blood bank, I've already asked them. They are way behind in their work and are tired of always having to give us somebody. Susan and Mary said this is last day of the month, and they have to go over quality and instrument records, or they will have to come in both Saturday and Sunday. I do too, and there is no way I can come in this weekend."

"I'll have to talk to them. Maybe we can get someone to come in early form the evening shift," suggested the laboratory manager.

"I'm sure Bob [the evening shift supervisor] will love that," answered the hematology supervisor, as she hurried back to her department. "He has been trying to get someone to work overtime this weekend for a month now."

Chapter Section for Review

- The Staffing Process
  - Staffing Levels
  - Workload Projections
- Availability of Staff
- Filing the Gaps
- Management of Work Flow
- Management of Absenteeism

See also

- Chapter 14 — Salary and Wage Management
  - The Productivity Model
  - Productivity Standards

Questions for Discussions

1. What happened in this case? Did these staffing and scheduling problems just pop up, or do they appear to be caused by failure of management to address long-term issues?
2. What do think about June's absenteeism, and its impact on the laboratory? Has the manager handled this problem well? What suggestions would you recommend in managing absenteeism in this case? Is June entirely to blame?
3. Using the information below, calculate the number of FTEs used and productivity for the period. From your analysis of this data, what appears to be the major cause for the staffing problems? Use this information to prepare a staffing proposal to present to administration, using the example provide as a mode. What questions do you anticipate administration will be asking?

[same 3 month Period]	2004	2005	2006
Billable Procedures	171,123	205,991	216,291
Total Paid Hours	19,479	20,807	21,415
Total Worked Hours	14,563	16,093	15,788

Solution:

[same 3-month Period]	2004	2005	2006
Billable Procedures	171,123	205,991	216,291
Total Paid Hours	19,479	20,807	21,415

Total FTE*	34.5	40.0	41.2
Total Worked Hours	14,563	16,093	15,788
Worked FTE	28.0	30.9	30.4
Total Productivity	179,123 / 19, 479 = 9.2	205,991 / 20,807 = 9.9	216,291 / 21,415 = 10.1
Worked	179,123 / 14,563 = 12.3	205,991 / 16,093 = 12.8	216,291 / 15,788 = 13.7

* FTEs can be calculated directly by dividing the number of hours by 520 (2080 ÷ 4 [i.e., Number of hours a full-time employee works in a year {2080} ÷ 12 months/3-month period {4}])

NOTES:

1. Total and worked FTEs actually went up in 2005 to reflect the workload; however;
2. In 2006, while total FTEs went up, worked FTEs went down (i.e., the actual number of people who showed up in the lab to do the work). This example is intended to illustrate to the participant the impact a major difference in these two financial indices can have on the actual operations of a laboratory.

[20]

Laboratory Safety

— Chapter Twenty —

The safety of the laboratory as a place to work is an issue of concern to government and professional agencies, the organization itself, and, of course, the individual who is working there. Because of AIDS and hepatitis, OSHA, universal precautions, the proliferation of right-to-know laws, and the assessment of stiff penalties on employers who do not comply with these regulations, the topic of safety has attracted great interest, not only in health care and the laboratory but also in all places that people work in potentially hazardous situations. This interest has made the subject of laboratory safety (explanation, implementation, and enforcement) one of the most popular topics in professional journals and at conferences.

This chapter reviews the general nature of hazards in the workplace, discusses hazards that are common in many work settings, looks at the special problems facing the laboratory, and concludes with an overview of the safety management in the laboratory

Objectives

After completion of this chapter, the reader will be able to demonstrate accomplishment of the following objectives.

1. Recognize the nature of hazardous working conditions present in the modern work environment and the types of danger inherent to the medical laboratory.
2. Encourage a commitment on the part of both the organization and the employees for ensuring the safety of the workplace and compliance with safety rules and guide lines.
3. Evaluate OSHA standards as they relate to the specific requirements of the laboratory.
4. Prepare and implement a plan for the management of safety in the laboratory workplace.

Chapter Highlights and Glossary of Key Terms

I. HAZARDS OF THE WORKPLACE: A MATTER OF ATTITUDE
- A. The role of the individual
- B. The role of the employer

II. HAZARDS IN THE WORKPLACE
- A. Structural requirements
- B. Fire prevention
  - 1. Fire prevention plans
  - 2. Handling of flammable substances
  - 3. Fire-fighting strategies
    - a. Construction
    - b. Fire-fighting equipment
    - c. Training and practice
- C. Electrical safety
- D. Chemical safety

1. Right-to-know regulations
   Occupational Safety and Health Administration (OSHA): *The agency responsible for developing and enforcing regulations governing safety in the workplace.*
   Material Safety Data Sheets (MSDS): *A document required by OSHA detailing safety information about each hazardous substance.*
2. Physical and health hazards
   Personal Protection Equipment (PPE): *Equipment such as eyeglasses, gloves, aprons, or full protective suits necessary to eliminate any hazards after all structural safety features have been installed.*
   Time-Weighted Average (TWA): The *level of exposure to a specific chemical agent that a worker may experience during a normal 8-hour workday, or 40-hour week.*
   Short-Term Exposure Limit (STEL): The *maximum exposure a person may receive for a short period (less than* 15 *minutes).*
   Ceiling (C): The *level above which no exposure is permitted at any time.*
3. Protective measures
4. Waste disposal

E. Other safety concerns

III. OSHA PATHOGEN REGULATIONS

A. Definition of infectious materials
   Bloodborne Pathogens: *Any material that could possibly become contaminated with blood — must be treated as having the potential to carry a pathogen transmitted by blood.*

B. Exposure control plan

C. Methods of compliance
1. Universal precautions
   Universal Precautions: The *policy of treating all blood, tissue, body fluids, and other potentially threatening material (OPTM) as equally hazardous.*
2. Engineering and work practice controls
3. Personal protective equipment
4. Housekeeping techniques

D. Regulations regarding hepatitis B vaccination

E. Communication of hazard to employees
1. Labels and signs
2. Information and training

F. Record keeping

IV. MANAGEMENT OF LABORATORY SAFETY

A. Responsibility for safety
1. Safety committee
   Safety Committee: *A committee assigned to overall development and monitoring of the safety management program.*
2. Safety officer
   Safety Officer: The *person charged with the implementation and day-to-day management of the safety program.*

B. The safety management program
1. Policies and procedures
2. Communications
3. Disaster plan
4. Safety audits and inspections
5. Accident investigation and prevention.

Hazards of the Workplace: A Matter of Attitude

The hazards found in the workplace are no different from those of everyday life — just more concentrated in their potential to cause harm. All of the dangers and risks of life in general are present where we work-plus the special perils presented by the tasks and duties of the jobs we perform. These include such common items as moving parts (vehicles, machinery, and supplies), electric shocks, fire, structural failures, communicable diseases, and the physical limitations of our own bodies.

The point is, we must be constantly aware of the safety elements that surround us, take the steps that are conducive to a safe working environment, and ensure that the measures necessary to protect ourselves from any threats to our wellbeing are in place. Both the individual and the organization must accept responsibility for workplace safety.

The Role of the Individual

The individual must ultimately assume responsibility for his or her health and safety. This may sound contrary to what you may have been taught, but the employer can do only so much. Individuals who do not follow the rules or who use the equipment improperly suffer the injury. Everyone has a responsibility to ensure that the workplace is as free of danger as possible and that the worker is effectively protected from any hazards that remain. This responsibility is shared by society at large — government and professional agencies and the employer — but it is the employees who are the final arbitrators of acceptable risk and responsible for performing their work in a safe manner, using the safety equipment as trained and reporting any possible danger and safety violations to the proper authorities.

The Role of the Employer

PHYSICAL HAZARDS
Compressed gas
Explosives
Flammable: aerosol, gas, liquid, or solid
Organic peroxide
Oxidizer
Pyrophoric (i.e., capable of spontaneous ignition when exposed to air)
Reactive/unstable
Water-reactive
HEALTH HAZARDS
Toxic and highly toxic agents
Reproductive toxin
Carcinogen
Irritant
Tissue corrosive
Sensitizer
Liver, kidney, and nervous system toxin (hepatoxin, nephrotoxin, and neurotoxin)
Agents that act on or damage other body systems: amatopoietic, lungs, skin, eyes, or mucous membranes.

Table 20 — 1. OSHA: Physical and Health Hazards of Chemicals

The employer is obligated both morally and legally to see that employees have the training, support, equipment, workload, resources, environment, and oversight necessary to perform in a safe and secure manner. Many government and professional agencies provide guidelines and regulations regarding workplace health and safety.

Both workers and employers must be committed to enforcing workplace safety. Workers must recognize that safety rules and procedures are meant for their own protection and not just as an impediment to frustrate cherished work habits. And the employer should make the work environment as conducive to compliance as possible.

Hazards in the Workplace

Most of the hazards found in the laboratory are common to all work sites: fire hazards, faulty electrical equipment, poor ventilation, blocked entrances and exits, hazardous clutter, poor lifting and handling techniques, and unmet building safety requirements (Table 20 – 1). Laboratory workers must also deal with chemicals, compressed gas, infectious material, toxic waste, and potentially dangerous machinery — all hazards that are found at many industrial sites. Laboratory workers are also particularly vulnerable to pathogens in blood and body fluids.

Structural Requirements

The very first place in which safety factors should be considered is in the design and layout of the building and laboratory (see chapters covering these topics). Errors made at this stage of the management plan can be extremely costly to correct. National, state, and local fire and safety building codes dictate most basic facility design features.

These structural safety rules involve building materials, storm damage control, fire prevention and firefighting systems such as the location of sprinklers and fire extinguishers, entrance and exit routes, storage of flammable materials, blockage of hallways and doors, ventilation systems, and other factors that have a direct effect on the safety of the occupants. Even the number and location of parking spaces have safety implications. .

In addition to the general safety provision of building codes, the laboratory should be designed to minimize any exposure to hazardous material through its work-flow processes. Issues to be addressed through the floor plan layout and workspace design include the following.

- The separation of nontesting functions, such as clerical and administrative offices, from areas containing hazardous materials by means of structural barriers and control of traffic patterns.
- The delivery and storage of potentially hazardous chemicals, 'Such as flammables and corrosive materials. This includes how they are brought into the laboratory, where they are placed until they can be unpacked, and their final storage arrangements.
- The processing of specimens, from their collection and arrival in the laboratory to their final delivery to the testing site.
- The ventilation back-up plan. This factor is especially critical in sections such as Histology and Microbiology, where there may be unusually heavy concentrations of chemical and biological material. These two sections should have direct access to outside venting (windows and fans) in case of an emergency.
- The location, ease of use, and rapid availability of any special safety equipment such as fume hoods, decontamination facilities, and first-aid stations.

These and many other factors, including those that follow, must be made an integral part of the building and the layout plan of each area of the laboratory.

Fire Prevention

Fire prevention and safety can be divided into three topics: general fire prevention plans, storage and handling of flammable substances, and firefighting strategies.

Fire Prevention Plans

A fire has three ingredients: an ignition source, oxygen, and fuel. All building codes and fire prevention plans focus on preventing these three items from combining. The main fire prevention strategies include keeping flammable substances in separate rooms and storage cabinets; using fire-resistant building products, explosion-proof refrigerators, and hoods; and performing procedures that result in highly combustible reactions under water or in a vacuum chamber.

Handling of Flammable Substances

The most obvious method for preventing fire is to control the union of fuel and ignition sources. In the laboratory, especially in Histology and Special Chemistry, many procedures require the use of flammable chemicals such as methanol and xylene. This presents a problem both at the bench and in the bulk storage of these reagents.

Government and professional organizations have strict regulations concerning the volume of material allowed in a specified area, how it is used, and where it is stored. JCAHO, CAP, and most local fire ordinances comply with the guidelines recommended by the National Fire Prevention Association (NFPA). Following are a few key rules for handling flammable substances, most of which are significant enough to be made a part of CAP inspection checklists.

- For a laboratory or given area (per 5000 square feet of space), a maximum of 10 gallons of flammable liquids can be in use or stored in the open, outside of a safety room, cabinet, or safety can.
- For the same space restrictions, 60 gallons of flammable liquids can be stored in a safety cabinet. If a safety cabinet or room is not available, up to 25 gallons may be stored in NFPA-approved safety cans.
- Safety cans must be used for more than 1 pint of class A flammables (e.g., ether/isopentane), more than 1 quart of class B flammables (e.g., acetone, ethanol, methanol), and more than 1 gallon of most other flammables (e.g., xylene, mineral oil). If testing protocols require that the purity of the chemical be maintained by the use of glass bottles, then the chemical should be purchased in as small a unit quantity as practicable and stored in a safety cabinet when not in use.
- Flammable gas cylinders should be stored separately from other flammable material.
- Persons working with flammable material must be properly trained in handling, storage, processing, cleanup, and accident control. They must also have the appropriate equipment (ventilated hoods, transportation aids, and working space) to safely perform their duties.

This list is intended only as a brief introduction to the many factors that must be considered in handling flammable substances; requirements may vary widely, depending on local regulations and the work setting. Supervisors should ensure that they are familiar with the guidelines and rules that apply to the materials with which they are working, that their staff is properly trained in safety techniques, and that the rules are strictly enforced.

Many publications issued by regulatory agencies, local fire departments, and professional organizations such as CAP and JCAHO provide useful information on the topic of fire prevention and control. The material safety data sheets (MSDS) required to be provided with all hazardous material, no matter how small the risk, are also excellent sources of information.

Fire-Fighting Strategies

What will you do if the unthinkable happens? This question must be anticipated and planned for. Despite all precautions, fire remains a leading cause of death in the workplace.
Health care facilities are especially vulnerable because of the nature of the work and because of its clients. High concentrations of people in the hospital setting have limited ability to respond to a crisis, and a large number of procedures require the use of flammable materials. For these reasons, fire-fighting strategies should be developed on three fronts: construction, firefighting equipment, and training and practice.

Construction

The structure of a building, the materials used for construction, the layout plan for entrances and exits, and the storage of flammable materials are major deterrents to a fire. These factors are also crucial in the quick isolation and extinction of any fire and in the control of the number one cause of fire death: smoke inhalation.

Building codes generally require a fire-resistance rating of at least 2 hours for walls around high-risk areas, such as flammable materials storage rooms. Codes also require that highly explosive substances, such as ether and compressed flammable gas, be stored in a room with at least one outside wall and a direct vent.

A host of other building specifications governs the operation of elevators, smoke and fire alarms, traffic patterns, evacuation routes and plans, and the use of automatic self-closing doors designed to isolate and control air and smoke flow.

Fire-Fighting Equipment.

Many fire-fighting features are designed directly into the construction of the building. These require fire resistant building materials, automatic sprinklers, self closing doors, and fire hydrants. Most of the furniture and fixtures used in a hospital or laboratory must also meet strict fire- and smoke-retarding standards.

Other required fire-fighting and protective equipment are fire extinguishers, fire blankets, and bulk material such as sand or other highly absorbent substances that can be used for fire containment as well as spill control and neutralization. The number, kinds, and location of these items should be based on the work being done, not solely on the minimal requirements dictated by regulatory agencies.

Class	Fire Type/Category	Acceptable Extinguisher Material	Extinguisher Rating Required
A	Common combustible material: paper, wood	Water	A, B. C
B	Flammable liquids: gas, alcohol, solvents plastics (furniture)	Dry chemicals CO_2	B, C
C	Electrical: wiring, equipment	Dry chemicals, CO_2/foam	C
D	Combustible chemicals /metals: magnesium, sodium, titanium	Sand	D, or sand bucket

Table 20 — 2. Fire Type and Extinguisher Requirements

Fires and extinguishers are grouped into four classes, according to the nature and source of the fire and the type of material needed to extinguish it.

- *Class A* fires are the most common and are usually started by the ignition of such material as paper and wood. They can be extinguished with water.
- *Class B* fires consist of flammable liquids, such as alcohols, gases, and solvents. Class B extinguishers contain dry chemicals or $C0_2$ which smothers the fire by depriving it of oxygen.
- *Class* C fires are caused by electrical malfunctions. Class C extinguishers use dry chemicals or $C0_2$.
- *Class D* fires involve combustible chemicals or metals (e.g., sodium or magnesium) that need highly specialized extinguishers or bulk material such as sand for control.

Table 20 – $2_{(above)}$ summarizes the main features of the four classes of fires and extinguishers.

<u>Training and Practice</u>

The best-designed equipment and emergency plans are of no use if workers don't know what to do or how to use them. A deficiency in training could even aggravate a bad situation if workers panic because they are not aware of the help that may be right next to them.

Orientation and in-service training should cover all aspects of the fire plan, with individual hands-on training in the use of fire extinguishers, fire blankets, emergency eyewash and shower stations, and fire isolation techniques.

Frequent and comprehensive drills in identifying fires, sounding the alarm, fighting fires, and evacuating according to emergency plans, with training in assisting patients and injured coworkers, should be conducted. The educational sessions and fire drills should include, but not necessarily be limited to, the following points:

- Sounding the alarm and making sure help is on the way before taking any other action, particularly in situations in which the person may be working alone.
- Decision-making strategies about when to fight a fire and when to abandon the site by establishing smoke barriers (i.e., shutting windows and doors) until help arrives.
- Skill in using fire extinguishers and water-hydrant hoses.
- Techniques for when personal garments catch fire, specifically rolling on the floor to smother the flames.
- Use of fire blankets, both in assisting a person on fire to smother the flames and as a shield when making an escape.
- Evacuation plan from the work site, as well as from locations throughout the building.
- Any special fire prevention and fighting methods that pertain to specific tasks and workplaces

Managers must ensure that they and their staffs are well informed and prepared to handle any emergency that may arise.

Electrical Safety

Electrical equipment and wiring present two major hazards in the laboratory: (1) physical harm from shocks or burns when a person comes into contact with an electrical source; and (2) dangers from fire caused by heat and sparks generated by malfunctioning wiring or equipment. Even though these dangers are real, people often become lax when handling electrical devices because of constant contact and familiarity with the use of electricity. For these reasons, dealing with electrical problems requires constant vigilance.

Following are a few of the safeguards recommended by NFPA and adopted by CAP, JCAHO, and most fire districts.

- There should be no extension cords or outlet adapters.
- All equipment, including the coffee pots and microwaves in the break room, should be checked for compliance with electrical safety standards upon arrival or before being placed into use. Many laboratories obtain the advice of the engineering department before purchasing an instrument as part of the procurement procedure to make sure that any power needs and requirements are resolved before the equipment arrives.
- Electrical safety checks should be part of the laboratory preventive maintenance programs for each piece of equipment. This should entail examinations at least once a year for proper voltage and grounding, as well as for current leakage and broken, worn, or frayed ends on plug." and cords. These checks should review the power needs of the laboratory and make certain that there are adequate electrical receptacles.
- Circuit breakers should be conveniently located and labeled in case of a major water spill or other accident requiring that power be cut off immediately.
- Electrical equipment should not be used in areas with flammable materials because of sparks or ignitions, unless the equipment (hood motors and all electrical devices) have been checked and determined to meet the standards necessary to be certified as explosion-proof.
- Electrical safety should be part of the orientation and educational program of the laboratory. Procedures and directions for cleaning up water spills around instruments and rescuing a coworker who may have come in contact with a live wire or malfunctioning electrical equipment should be part of the training session. A list of recommended procedures for dealing with water spills and accidents involving electrical equipment is summarized in Table 20 – 2.

WATER SPILLS

1. All electrical apparatus affected by the water or wet spill should be unplugged or the power shut off at the circuit breaker if the person will be placed at risk by disconnecting a single piece of equipment.
2. After the power has been disconnected, the instrument and the spill should be cleaned up thoroughly and allowed to dry completely.
3. The instrument should be checked by the engineering staff before it is reconnected to a power source to make sure that operational and electrical parameters are all within safety standards.
4. Never operate an electrical device with wet hands or when it has come in contact with water or other liquid until it has been cleaned and checked to certify its safety.

ELECTRICAL ACCIDENTS

1. Never directly touch a person who is being shocked or is in contact with a live wire or piece of equipment; you may become part of the electrical circuit.
2. The victim should be immediately rescued by either unplugging the electrical source, if possible, or separating the victim form the wire or equipment by using a non-conducting item such as a glass pipette or wooden/plastic broom handle.
3. Do not attempt to move the person unless other dangers are present; protect the victim form clinical shock by keeping him or her covered with coats or blankets until help arrives.

Table 20 — 3. Water Spills and Electrical Accidents

Chemical Safety

Chemicals have proven their benefit to humanity throughout history. However, except for the obvious danger inherent in acids and alkalines, we have only recently become aware of their subtle potential to harm us and our environment. Government and professional agencies have taken aggressive steps to identify, and protect workers from, the hazards posed by long-term exposure to chemical substances. This movement has given rise to the strictly enforced rules implemented by OSHA and many state agencies concerning the right-to-know laws, exposure-limit standards and precautions, and waste disposal regulations.

Right-to-Know Regulations

Most laboratorians and employers are familiar with the initiatives of the U.S. Department of Labor **Occupational Safety and Health Administration (OSHA).** This federal agency was charged with protecting workers' health and well-being in the workplace, particularly in providing guidance and regulations concerning chemicals and infectious materials.

OSHA classifies chemical hazards into two groups: *physical* hazards and *health* hazards (Table 20 – 1$_{\text{[above, near beginning of chapter]}}$). OSHA requires both the manufacturer or supplier and the purchaser of hazardous chemicals to provide employees with information on exposure and safety precautions. The employer is also held responsible for the enforcement of safety rules in the workplace.

In-service and training sessions must be held at least annually to update employees on the proper procedures for handling hazardous chemicals in the workplace. A document detailing safety information about each hazardous substance must be available to employees at all times in an obvious and easily accessible location. These documents are called **material safety data sheets (MSDS).** The MSDS must be incorporated into the training program. Over-the-counter substances and substances that cause harm only if ingested in significant quantities, such as commercial cleaning agents (household bleach, ammonia, phenol solutions, and so on) and drain cleaners, are usually exempt.

MSDSs are not required for chemicals that are included in minimal concentrations in reagents used on many analyzers, providing the substances have proper warning labels and are packaged in safe containers. Many state and local agencies may have additional rules, and managers should obtain information that may apply to their situation, especially when using common chemicals in unusual ways or in large quantities.

The common format for the preparation of an MSDS lists each safety topic in separate sections, beginning with the product name, the manufacturer, important phone numbers to call for emergency information, the effective and review dates, and the signature of the person preparing the sheet. Each safety topic section usually consists of the following information.

- Identification of the hazardous material or compound ingredients with their common and technical names.
- The physical or chemical characteristics of the substance, such as boiling point, vapor pressure and density, solubility in water, specific gravity, evaporation rate, and water reactivity.
- Fire and the explosive nature of the chemical, flash point, flammable air concentration levels, and fire-fighting and extinguishing procedures.
- Reactivity, including stability, chemical incompatibility, dangerous decomposition products, and polymerization.
- Specific health hazard data, giving the primary route of contamination, health complaints and symptoms that may result from contact, medical conditions that may be aggravated, first-aid procedures, and specific health dangers that may arise from exposure: cancer, cell mutation, organ damage, and so on.
- Personal protection equipment, ventilation requirements, and other precautions. Protective equipment may include respirators, gloves, protective garments or suits, eyewear, and hoods or isolation chambers.

- The final part of the MSDS usually lists safe handling, storage, spill and leak control, and disposal methods.

Information required to prepare an MSDS is available from many government agencies, professional associations, consulting firms that specialize in hazardous substance control, and a wide variety of publications. The most readily available source of information for MSDS report forms is companies that supply the laboratory with reagents and chemicals. Most of these companies provide MSDS documents that meet OSHA requirements for their products.

Physical and Health Hazards

Table 20 – 1$_{\text{(above, near the beginning of the chapter)}}$ lists the potential physical and health hazards of chemical agents. The concentration level or length of exposure needed for a substance to cause harm is a crucial factor in determining the safety requirement for a given chemical. Several organizations issue guidelines and suggestions for identifying different types of chemical hazards.

OSHA classifies chemicals based on the potential for exposure and the time limits allowed at this exposure point. The American Conference of Governmental Industrial Hygienists (ACGIH) issues an annual report that classifies harmful chemicals according to the maximum threshold limit values (TLV) and Biological Exposure Indexes (BEI). These two indexes are particularly important for setting safety levels for exposure to possible carcinogens, such as formaldehyde and xylene.

The National Fire Prevention Association's system is the most widely used method for labeling potential hazards of chemicals and reagents. NFPA recommendations consist of a color-coded label, in the form of a triangle, a rectangle, or a combination of the two, with a danger rating number for each type of hazard. Color codes and rating keys used in the NFPA system are listed in Table 20 – 4. Under the NFPA system, xylene has a health threat rating of 2, a fire hazard rating of 3, and a reactivity or instability danger of O$_{\text{("zero")}}$.

Color-coded for danger rating:
Red = fire hazard
Blue = health hazard
Yellow = instability hazard
Danger rating key:
0 = none
1 = minor
2 = moderate
3 = severe
4 = extreme

Table 20 — 4. National Fire Prevention Association (NFPA) Labeling System

The hazardous materials identification system (HMIS) ratings of the National Paint and Coating Association commonly used for industrial compounds, is similar to the NFPA's (hazards are rated on a 0-to-4 scale, 4 being a "severe hazard"). It adds a personal protection equipment (PPE) code, ranging from A (use safety glasses) to K (use air line, hood or mask, gloves, full suit, and boots). The U.S. Department of Transportation also has a labeling system that uses a graphic symbol and bold letter warning (corrosive, flammable, and so on) on the outside of shipping containers.

For examples of the NFPA labeling system and rating for common chemicals see:
NM State Environmental Health and Safety
http://www.nmsu.edu/~safety/programs/chem_safety/hazcom_NFPA_labels.htm
– or – The ORCBS http://www.hazmat.msu.edu:591/nfpa/ [both connected June 10, 2007]

The threshold limit values (TLV) system designed by ACGIH, establishes three points that should be monitored to ensure a safe work environment:

- The **time-weighted average** (TWA) , defined as the level of exposure a worker may experience during a normal 8-hour workday or a 40-hour week.

- The **short-term exposure limit** (STEL) , which is the maximum concentration level a person may be exposed to for a short period (15 minutes at most).
- The **ceiling** (C) concentration, which is the level above which no exposure is permitted at any time.

In areas where hazardous chemicals are used, both the air and the breathing zone (i.e., a monitor attached to the person near the nose and mouth, usually around the collar) of each employee should be continually monitored to ensure that TLV levels are not exceeded.

Protective Measures

Four groups of protective measures can be taken to safeguard a person dealing with hazardous materials: the structural or building layout, protective barriers or shields, personal protection articles, and emergency and first-aid supplies.

The *structural features* of the area where the chemical is handled are crucial to the safety of the worker. They include the layout of counter and bench space and their relationship to storage, processing, and disposal centers. For example, chemicals, especially corrosive substances, should never be handled above waist level; this protects against any possibility of an accidental splash or spill resulting in injury to the eyes or face.

Adequate ventilation must also be ensured. This involves not only the necessary air flow and exchange but also the comfort of the person performing the tests. Most of the personal protective items (gloves, masks, garments, and so on) required to safely handle hazardous substances are bulky, hot, and uncomfortable. If the temperature of the room is not kept at a comfortable level, the worker may be tempted to take shortcuts or not use the protective items at all.

Physical barriers include the availability and use of glass or plastic shields, chemical hoods, and even walls to prevent exposure to a danger. In extreme situations, mechanical or automated handling and testing equipment may be necessary to ensure safety. Controlling the flow of traffic through an area and the isolation of testing sites are important factors to consider, especially in protecting unaware or casual visitors.

After structural and physical factors have been evaluated and improved to the extent possible, the next level of defense involves providing the worker with the *personal protection articles* necessary to eliminate any remaining hazards. Eyeglasses, face masks, gloves, aprons, full protective suits, or self-contained breathing respirators may be appropriate, depending on the type of danger a chemical element may pose during its use or in the cleanup of a spill. For most chemicals found in the routine laboratory, hand and eye protection is usually sufficient, but each situation must be evaluated on its own.

The laboratory must be prepared to deal with any accident or emergency that may occur. Each employee should be well trained in treating a personal accident and coming to the aid of a co-worker. The following *emergency equipment and supplies* should be standard in any area that contains potentially hazardous substances, along with easy-to-read instructions.

- Numerous and conveniently located facilities for hand and body hygiene.
- Immediate access to emergency eyewash and overhead showers.
- Neutralizing solutions suitable for eye and body care.
- Cleanup and confinement supplies and equipment.
- Fully stocked first-aid kits or close proximity to medical care.

Waste Disposal

Concerns over the dangers of chemical and biological waste, especially in the protection of the public and the environment, have proliferated the laws and regulations governing disposal of this material. The overriding principle for disposal of any such material should follow this precept:

> **Do not purchase or allow into your laboratory any substance for which a practical waste treatment and disposal option is not available.**

The most reliable source of information about acceptable disposal methods is usually the manufacturer or supplier of the product. Some chemical manufacturers are placing suggestions or warnings about the disposal of their products on the label along with other safety facts. The information may list cautions about environmental contamination resulting from incineration or flushing the material into the sewer system.

Processing hazardous waste should be included in chemical hygiene plans for the interim storage of the material and transportation to the final disposal site. Often placing the substance back into its original container provides a solution to these two problems.

A limited number of alternatives are available for the final disposal of chemical wastes. These options include incineration, landfill burial, flushing into the sewer system, and arranging for a licensed waste disposal firm to remove the waste. Many federal and local regulations govern each of these alternatives and will influence the final selection.

Recycling is rapidly gaining in popularity. Recycling of the xylene used in histology is one example of this approach. Histology is also leading the laboratory in finding less-toxic chemicals to use.

Other Safety Concerns

The laboratory shares many additional safety concerns with other organizations. Here is a short list and commentary on several areas not previously reviewed that should be included in the safety agenda of the laboratory manager:

- Employees should receive training in the *proper body mechanics* and availability of *lifting apparatuses* to avoid injuries to the back, knees, and so on. This is especially important when a person is working alone and may have to handle large or heavy items.
- The *safe operation of machinery and equipment* is crucial. This is certainly true when there is potential harm from moving parts such as belts, centrifuges, or gears; extreme temperature burns from heating or cooling elements; or cuts and puncture wounds from sharp objects like sampling probes, mechanical scissors, broken glassware, or veinpuncture needles.
- *Compressed gas* may pose a threat if tanks are not securely anchored during use or storage. If the container's valves are suddenly broken when dropped or knocked over, they may become an uncontrolled missile, capable of great physical damage.
- *Radioactive material* requires special training, monitoring, and safety equipment if used in quantities above the levels established by government agencies, specifically the requirements set by the Nuclear Regulatory Commission (NRC), which controls the possession, use, and transfer of licensed radionuclides. Most reagents used in wet lab procedures fall well below safety thresholds; however, regulations vary widely according to local ordinances, and the laboratory should be certain that it complies with all licensure and handling requirements. Professional laboratory organizations recommend that all persons who are continually exposed to any radioactive material be monitored because of the potential threat from long-term exposure.

OSHA Pathogen Regulations

Although other work situations may share some of the problems of handling biological specimens, not many places can compete with the unique flood of human blood, tissue, and body fluids concentrated in the medical laboratory. The special challenges presented by this aspect of laboratory work require precautionary procedures that begin with the first initial contact with the patient and continue through the final disposal of the specimen.

OSHA's bloodborne pathogen standards, effective as of July 1992, provide a detailed framework for reviewing the special problems of the laboratory in dealing with pathogens carried in blood, tissue, and body fluids (OSHA, 1991).

Definition of Infectious Materials

Infectious materials encompass the complete range of specimens processed by the laboratory. In fact, it would be difficult to think of a situation in the laboratory, outside of isolated clerical and administrative areas, that should not be considered biologically hazardous. Tissue, organs, semen, vaginal and mucous secretions, saliva, and any materials subject to contamination with blood are to be treated as if they contain **bloodborne pathogens.** This list includes body fluids such as pericardial, peritoneal, cerebrospinal, pleural, synovial, and amniotic fluids and exudates from wounds.

The only material that is not included in OSHA's definition is urine; however, because blood and blood elements are frequently found in urine specimens, it must also be considered a possible source of bloodborne pathogens. To be safe, and to meet the spirit as well as the letter of the law, all specimens and areas that may come into contact with bloodborne or other potentially infectious materials (OPIM) should be rigidly controlled.

Exposure Control Plan

Regulations require that all facilities processing specimens that contain the potential for bloodborne pathogens have an *exposure control plan* in place. This plan must be updated at least annually and whenever there are changes in the work situation. The plan must include policies and procedures to identify any potential hazards, inform the workers of the dangers, and provide protective measures that ensure a safe work environment. The exposure control plan must specifically address the following topics.

- Identify all jobs, tasks, procedures, and situations that may present a risk of exposure to bloodborne pathogens. Jobs are to be classified according to level of occupational exposure. The key here is to assess existing danger without regard to protective clothing or equipment.
- Establish methods that protect the worker and comply with OSHA regulations.
- Implement a hepatitis B vaccination and monitoring program.
- Inform, communicate, and warn employees of the hazards identified in the workplace and the proper use of protective clothing and equipment.
- Maintain and monitor records to prove compliance with regulations and ensure that safety procedures are enforced.

Methods of Compliance

Although OSHA calls this section "methods of compliance," it may more properly be titled *protective methods and procedures.* Compliance or protective methods are grouped into four areas: the adoption of a universal precautions policy, engineering and work practice controls, personal protective equipment, and housekeeping techniques.

Universal Precautions

Universal precautions are the policy of treating *all* blood, tissue, body fluids, and OPIM-not just those specimens collected from patients known to have infectious diseases-as equally threatening. This is a very commonsense approach. Despite the distinct difference between the real and immediate danger from a known carrier and the possible threat from the general specimen population, the existence and nature of the threat may not be known until after a specimen has been collected and processed. For these reasons, all protective procedures and methods should be applied universally in all situations with a potential for exposure to bloodborne pathogens and OPIM.

Engineering and Work Practice Controls

Engineering and work practice controls involve taking physical steps to isolate or remove any possible pathogen hazards from the workplace. Next is a list of the primary areas in which OSHA requires specific engineering action by employers.

- Hand-washing facilities must be immediately available in the workplace, and the employer is required to take all necessary steps to enforce hand washing policies. This includes appropriate hand care before and after contact with a patient, after handling any infectious material, and upon removal of protective apparel such as gloves, aprons, or other garments.
- Needles and other sharps must be handled with great care and caution. Recapping needles is not allowed unless absolutely necessary and then only with mechanical devices (e.g., forceps). All sharps must immediately be placed in puncture-resistant leak proof containers, labeled with a hazardous warning, and securely sealed prior to storage or disposal. If there is a possibility of the outside of the primary sharps container becoming contaminated, it must be placed into a secondary receptacle with instructions for decontamination if leakage occurs during shipment.
- Eating, drinking, smoking, and applying cosmetics must be banned in areas in which exposure to pathogenic material is possible. Food and drink must also be stored in separate areas and refrigerators from biological specimens.
- Procedures that minimize splashing, spraying, or generating aerosols must be adopted. This includes keeping all specimens in closed containers as much as possible during centrifugation and testing, as well as prohibiting mouth pipettes.
- Equipment and instruments that may become soiled with biological material must have warning labels attached stating the potential hazard and instructions for decontamination.

Personal Protective Equipment

If a potential for exposure to blood or OPIM remains after all possible engineering and work practice controls have been implemented and enforced, the employer is required to provide the worker with the personal protective equipment (PPE) necessary to provide complete protection from any remaining danger. Identifying the types and usage of PPE is an integral part of the exposure control plan and depends on the nature and extent of the possible danger. This decision about the kinds of PPE to be provided is crucial because it is the direct barrier between the hazardous agent and the last line of protection for the worker. Following are several comments on important aspects of these PPE items:

- Gloves are to be worn whenever there is even a remote possibility of the hands coming into contact with blood or OPIM. The gloves must be replaced between patients and when their protective integrity is compromised, that is, after gross contamination, extended wear, or any break or tear.

- Eye and face protection items include goggles, glasses, masks, hoods, and counter shields that provide barriers to splashes, splatters, sprays, or aerosols caused during the handling or processing of infectious materials.
- Protective body clothing (gowns, aprons, lab coats, surgical caps and scrubs, shoe covers, and disposable arm sleeves) must be worn when there is the threat of contamination to parts of the body or garments not covered by gloves or eye and face guards.

Government rules require that all protective items be supplied free of charge to the worker, including initial purchase, replacement, decontamination, laundry, and disposal.

Housekeeping Techniques

Employers must ensure that the work site is maintained in a clean and sanitary condition. OSHA provides guidelines for the cleaning and decontamination of work surfaces, protective coverings of counters and equipment, receptacles (reusable pails, cans, bins, and so on), broken glassware, and laundry and the processing of hazardous waste. These rules generally require the institution to have policies and procedures for the frequent and effective cleaning, decontamination, disposal, and replacement of any item or surface that may come in contact with blood or OPIM.

Housekeeping procedures are required to be detailed and specific, including the specific disinfectant or sterilization (chemical or physical) method to be used to render the surface or item no longer capable of transmitting infectious particles and thus safe for handling and disposal.

The collection, storage, and transportation of waste must follow the guidelines described previously for needles and other sharps. These rules state generally that waste must be placed immediately in a receptacle that can contain the item leak-, puncture-, and spill-proof, and so on), with a secondary cover if decontamination of the primary container ("double-bagging" or two-container system) is possible, and properly labeled with a warning and instructions for dealing with a leak or spill.

Regulations Regarding Hepatitis B Vaccination

Vaccination with hepatitis B vaccine must be made available to all employees who have occupational exposure to bloodborne pathogens and OPIM. The employer must also ensure thorough post-exposure evaluation and follow-up for anyone who may have come into contact with an infectious agent.

There must be complete documentation of the vaccination and follow-up plan. The program must include records of the information and training provided the staff, affidavits of employees who may decline the vaccine (with notification of their right to change their minds), and post-exposure medical treatment. All aspects of the plan, both the vaccination and post-exposure care, must be provided at no cost to the employee.

Communication of Hazard to Employees

OSHA emphasizes the importance of providing information and training about the potential danger, protective measures, and availability of treatment to the persons who may have occupational exposure to blood or OPIM. OSHA requires that communication efforts be focused on two fronts: (1) labels and signs and (2) information and training.

Labels and Signs

Figure 20 – 1 presents the international legend that warns of a biological hazard. This legend is to be posted at the entrance to work areas and on items where bloodborne or OPIM pathogens present a potential hazard. Biohazard warning labels, signs, and containers (bags, boxes, receptacles, etc/) are to be fluorescent orange-red, with lettering or symbols in a contrasting color.

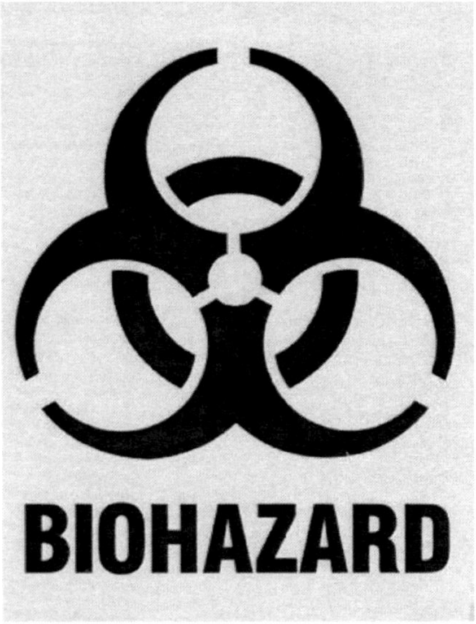

Figure 20 —1. International Biohazard Legend

Information and Training

Employers must ensure that all persons with occupational exposure participate in a training program at no cost to the employee, presented during working hours, completed within 90 days of employment, and repeated at least once a year thereafter, or more frequently if conditions or threats change. The training sessions must be presented by a person knowledgeable in the subject matter and should cover at least the following topics.

- An accessible copy of the regulatory text of the standard and an explanation of its contents.
- A general description of the epidemiology and symptoms of bloodborne diseases and their modes of transmission,
- An explanation of the employer's exposure control plans and the means by which the employee can obtain a copy,
- Instruction on the methods for recognizing activities that may involve exposure and in the use and limitation of methods that prevent or reduce exposure risk,
- Clarification of the types, selection, proper use, location, removal, handling, decontamination, and disposal of personal protective equipment.
- Information on the hepatitis B vaccine, including its efficacy and safety.
- Directions on the appropriate emergency treatment and follow-up action to take if exposed to a bloodborne or OPIM pathogen.
- An explanation of the communication system for biohazards (signs, labels, color code, and so on).
- The opportunity to ask questions of the person conducting the training session.

Employees are expected to demonstrate that they are both knowledgeable in the topics covered in the training sessions and proficient in the use of protective (personal and engineering) equipment.

Record Keeping

OSHA standards require that detailed medical and training records be maintained on all employees who have occupational exposure to bloodborne and OPIM pathogens. Medical records must be available for up to 30 years past the termination of employment. Training records must be held for 3 years after the session. All records are to be confidential and released only to authorized regulatory agencies or with the expressed permission of the employee.

Management of Laboratory Safety

The safety and well-being of its workforce should be one of the highest priorities for any enterprise. Neglect in this area not only brings about a sense of insecurity and concern on the part of the employees but also has a direct negative influence on the productivity and stability of the staff and, in turn, a major impact on the profitability of the company.

To create an environment that is conducive to achievement and worker motivation, safety issues should be an integral part of the management plan. Developing a safety-oriented culture must begin at the very top of management and be imbued in the attitude and leadership at each layer of supervision as well as in every member of the organization. To accomplish this objective, the organization should take two steps: assign direct responsibility for ensuring that safety issues are effectively managed and developed; and implement an active safety management program.

Responsibility for Safety

The chief executive officer must assume total, overall responsibility for the safety of the people working in the organization. Primary responsibility for enforcement of safety rules and procedures lies with the worker's immediate supervisor. However, as discussed in the opening section of this chapter, individuals have the personal obligation for ensuring their own wellbeing by performing their duties in a safe and conscientious manner and promptly reporting any problems to their supervisor.

Because safety affects every aspect of the organization and a wide range of interdisciplinary skills are needed to develop and manage a safety program, the use of safety committees and the appointment of a safety officer to oversee this function have gained wide popularity. This approach has the advantage of using a variety of expertise and resources and assigns the administrative authority to implement, monitor, and enforce the safety plan. In a hospital, for example, an organizational safety committee may be responsible for the coordination of safety policies; the laboratory may have its own specialized team.

Safety Committee

A **safety committee** should consist of representatives from all areas of the organization or department, including administration, pathologists, clinical scientists, managers, supervisors, and line workers. Members must be allowed (i.e., encouraged and solicited) to share their opinions and perspectives with the group and to actively participate in the proceedings of the committee.

The safety committee develops and monitors the safety management program and provides a resource for resolving any special safety problems. The committee members also serve as ambassadors to their coworkers in communicating and disseminating the spirit of the safety program and as mentors to encourage the attitude and leadership so crucial for nurturing a safety-oriented culture.

Safety Officer

The **safety officer** is charged with the implementation and day-to-day management of the safety program. In a small laboratory, the responsibilities of the safety officer may be a part of the duties of a designated tech or supervisor. A hospital or large laboratory usually has a full-time safety officer or includes one as part of a dedicated department such as risk management. The safety officers from each department frequently serve as representatives to the hospital safety committee.

The Safety Management Program

A safety management program, established under the auspices of the safety committee and safety officer, involves specific action plans in at least five areas,

- Policy and procedures
- Communications
- Disaster plan

- Safety audits and inspections
- Accident investigation and accident prevention

Much of the information needed to develop each segment of the safety management program has been covered previously in this chapter and is only highlighted here.

Policies and Procedures

Most accrediting and regulatory agencies strongly recommend that each laboratory have a designated manual dedicated to the specific safety concerns present in that facility, including policies and procedures covering physical, chemical, fire, natural disaster, bloodborne, and OPIM dangers. The safety manual should contain the chemical and exposure control plans dictated by OSHA and the program for identifying and monitoring safety indicators for inclusion in the quality management plan of the laboratory.

Communications

The goal of communications is to ensure that the person who is actually working with a hazardous substance or is in a potentially dangerous situation has the information, training, equipment, resources, and support to perform his or her duties in a safe and secure manner. Communications encompass the management process, education and training programs, and compliance and enforcement monitoring, as well as procedure manuals, signs, and labeling systems.

Disaster Plan

No other situation tests the resources and ability of the laboratory to perform than a major natural or medical disaster. A disaster can arise not only with a massive number of casualties and immense demand for service; but also with the normal resources and capabilities of the laboratory greatly compromised because supplies, equipment, power, or staff are not available to meet urgent patient needs due to circumstances beyond the control of the laboratory.

Situations such as these pose a major threat to the safety of the staff and jeopardize quality of care for the patients, especially if shortcuts and other hasty actions must be taken because the laboratory has not made appropriate plans to handle the emergency. For these reasons disaster plans usually fall under the purview of the safety committee and officer.

In the initial planning process, special demands or threats to service may require special contingency and backup plans. These may be caused either by natural (storms, earthquakes, and so on) or medical emergencies involving large numbers of victims, such as bus, train, airplane, or multi-car collisions. After the types of disasters to which the laboratory may be vulnerable have been defined and identified, contingency plans must be developed for dealing with each kind of emergency. Areas that need special consideration include the following.

- What services must be available and which can be placed on hold until the crisis is over.
- Work flow and plans to handle the expected services demand, such as setting up additional crossmatch stations or starting backup instruments.
- Use of staff from areas not expected to be affected by the disaster.
- Plans for meeting increased demand for blood
- Sources for additional supplies.
- Sleeping and feeding plans for staff who may have to stay in the laboratory for extended periods.
- Sources of additional help and types of staff needed in a particular disaster.

After the disaster plan has been written, the next step is to ensure that the staff is competent to implement the procedures and that the needed resources are available and in good working order. This is normally done through training and regularly scheduled disaster drills.

As a final comment, plans must be department- and section-specific. Not all situations will affect the whole hospital or department equally. For example, a school bus accident might present a major disaster for the radiology department, which must x-ray every patient, but present no particular problem for the laboratory after blood samples have been collected for processing. In the laboratory itself, the same accident may have placed tremendous pressure on the phlebotomy and blood bank staff, but the other areas may experience little, if any, effect. A good plan would be to use the areas not expected to be affected by the disaster to assist other departments or sections, if only to help in processing paperwork or serving as couriers and patient attendants.

Safety Audits and Inspections

An important technique for monitoring and following up on safety rules and procedures is to conduct a safety audit and inspection of the laboratory on a periodic basis. These audits and inspections are not to replace the constant diligence to safety matters required of each member but to provide a mechanism to formalize and document the attention given to this subject.

The safety committee should develop a program that sets the frequency of inspections needed, the members of the inspection team, and the tools (checklists, review forms, and so on) that will be used to carry out the assignment. These factors should be determined by the nature and hazards of the work being done in the laboratory, results of previous audits, and regulatory requirements.

Most accrediting and licensure agencies require that safety audits be completed at least annually and more frequently if circumstances (i.e., inspection results, compliance problems, previous safety records, changes in procedures, or the types of work being performed) warrant more aggressive monitoring.

The safety inspection team should be made up of members with the knowledge and expertise to identify and suggest solutions to problems that may exist in the laboratory: several supervisory and staff laboratorians, representation from the safety committee, the safety officer, and any needed outside experts such as fire or regulatory advisors. The total numbers of members should be small, yet inclusive enough to conduct the review effectively.

Accident Investigation and Prevention

As part of the duties of the safety committee and the annual audit required by regulatory and accrediting agencies, a continual program should be designed for the investigation and prevention of accidents.

Surprisingly, one of the more difficult aspects of this program is to make sure that accidents are reported in the first place. Many employees may be reluctant for a variety of reasons to report what appears to be a relatively minor injury. These reasons may range from simply not wanting to look stupid to their supervisors or coworkers, fear of losing their jobs or receiving negative evaluations, or just not wanting to be bothered with "all that paperwork." However, even the routine investigation of a very minor infraction may uncover clues that will prevent a major accident. To overcome this natural disinclination, the organization must conduct all reviews in a caring, timely, and nonthreatening manner.

A thorough investigation of an accident includes, at a minimum, a review of the following factors.

- Who had the accident?
- When and where it happened?

- What equipment or supplies were being used?
- Any modifications to standard procedures?
- The training of persons involved.
- Use of safety protocols.
- Any unusual circumstances that may have contributed to the accident (power or equipment failures, variation in the work flow, production pressure)?
- Use of necessary precautions.
- Additional steps or actions that could be taken to prevent the recurrence of the incident.

These factors and other information are included in an accident investigation form completed by the workers involved in the accident, their supervisor, and the person conducting the review. The completed form, along with a report of the action taken, is then included in the institution's quality, safety, and risk-management monitoring programs.

Accident investigation and documentation are normally part of the institution's risk management program. Insurance and government worker protection rules all require that the employee and organization report any injuries and accidents to the appropriate authorities within a very short time period, often within 72 hours of their occurrence. Penalties for failure to follow these guidelines are often severe, with fines for the laboratory and possible loss of benefits for the employee. For this reason, and to make sure both the worker and the company are protected, the laboratory must ensure that all accidents are promptly reported, incident forms completed, and follow-up action taken.

The next chapter: Quality Assessment and Performance Improvement

— Case Study —

Chapter Twenty: Laboratory Safety

"Hi, Mark," said John, the second shift tech as he arrived for duty.

"Oh. . . hi," answered Mark, obviously in a hurry.

"Hey, you're not wearing that cover gown, like you're supposed to," remarked John. "You know the microbiology supervisor said at the last meeting that they had to spend a lot of money getting us these gowns, and if anyone is caught not using the proper safety equipment, he would be written up immediately."

"I know. . . but it's too hot in here," quickly responded Mark, trying to finish up his work. "Everybody complains. Engineering said that they checked it last week, and that there was nothing more they could do about it, unless administration wanted to put in a new system. This has gone on now for a year. Anyway those managers don't have to work here, so what do they care?"

"I don't like it either," remarked John, getting ready to take over from Mark. "Last night we were talking about how if an instrument overheats, they all run in with all kinds of fans and everything, but they don't seem to care much about it when we complain about it being so hot."

"Watch out!" John shouted suddenly to Mark, as he knocked over the container of distilled water and it splashed against the centrifuge and spilled onto the floor.

"Oh, my knee," Mark said, rubbing his leg as he picked himself up off from the floor after slipping on the water.

"That was a nasty fall. Maybe you should go over to the ER and let them check it and fill out the forms. Here comes the supervisor now."

"No way. . . don't say a word," answered Mark, gathering up his things and hobbling out the door. "I'm leaving right now for vacation, and I can't waste any more time. If it's still sore after I get back next week, I'll have it checked out then. Maybe you should call engineering and have them check that centrifuge, though. It got pretty wet."

"It'll be all right," answered John, pulling the plug. "I'll clean it up later. We don't use it on our shift, so it'll have plenty of time to dry out before they come in on Monday. Have a nice trip."

Chapter Sections for Review

- The Role of the Individual
- The Role of the Employer
- Electrical Safety and Table 20 – 3 [Water Spills and Electrical Accidents[
- Protective Measures [adequate ventilation]
- Accident Investigation and Prevention

Questions for Discussion

1. What do you think of the attitude and concern about safety of both the employer and employees in this laboratory? Are their concerns genuine or are they only trying to meet regulations? Who is at fault in this situation?
2. If you were the supervisor coming down the hall, and saw the situation, what action would you take? About Mark? About cleaning up the spill?
3. If it turns out that Mark goes away for vacation without reporting the incident and find out that his injury is serious, has he jeopardized his rights for government and insurance benefits? Can the laboratory be in trouble over reporting requirements? Why/why not?

[21]

Quality Assessment and Performance Improvement

— Chapter Twenty–One —

No other subject is as fraught with confusion as that of quality. It is difficult to even decide on the proper term or to settle on a good title for this chapter. One thing has become evident, however, as industry and the health care community continue to grapple with this issue and as new assessment methods are proposed, the old ways continue to increase in value. The analytical tools used in all of the recently acclaimed programs look strikingly similar to the statistical methods that have been used in the laboratory for a long time.

Quality is an extremely broad and all encompassing topic. The specific goal of this chapter is to provide the reader with a conceptual framework for understanding quality assessment and assurance. The following topics are reviewed.

1. A historical perspective of the development and transition of current quality concepts and terminology.
2. Leaders of organizational quality and their theories.
3. Tools of quality monitoring and assessment.
4. Application of these tools to the quality concerns of the laboratory.

Objectives

After completion of this chapter, the reader will be able to demonstrate accomplishment of the following objectives.

1. Define the concept of quality from the perspective of successful management of health care organizations and the provision of services for patient care.
2. Analyze past quality management transitions and philosophies and apply the analysis to future directions.
3. Select the appropriate tools and procedures for monitoring the quality of laboratory services.
4. Design and implement a quality management program for a medical laboratory.

Chapter Highlights and Glossary of Key Terms

I. HISTORICAL PERSPECTIVE: QUALITY CONCEPTS AND TERMINOLOGY TRANSITION

A. Quality control

Quality Control (QC): *Historically, the application of statistical methods to the evaluation of the quality of products and services. In the QA model, quality control refers specifically to the activities directed toward monitoring the individual elements of care (e.g., instrument and test procedures).*

B. Quality assurance

Quality Assurance (QA): *A program in which the overall activities conducted by the institution are directed toward assuring the quality of the products and services provided.*

C. Total quality management and continuous quality improvement (CQI)

Total Quality Management (TQM): *A quality management program that includes each component (customer, producer, and supplier) in the creation process, from the acquisition of supplies to active follow-up after the product or service has been received by a delighted customer.*

D. Quality assessment and improvement and continuous performance improvement

Quality Assessment and Improvement (QA&I): *A quality management program that focuses on the success of the organization in designing and achieving its set goals and objectives.*

E. Six Sigma

Six Sigma *is a quality management collection of practices, intended to focus the business entity on reducing cost and increasing profits by systematically improving the production process by eliminating defects.*

II. MAJOR FIGURES IN QUALITY MANAGEMENT

A. Philip Crosby
B. W. Edwards Deming
C. Joseph Juran
D. James O. Westgard

III. QUALITY MONITORING AND ASSESSMENT TOOLS

A. Basic quality control statistics

1. Accuracy and precision

   Accuracy: *The closeness of a result to the actual value of an analyte when running a test; more commonly called "hitting the bull's-eye."*

   Precision: *How well a procedure reproduces a value.*

2. Data population

   Population: *A term used in statistics to describe and define the items that are being studied at a particular time.*

3. Population sample

   Sample: *A part of a population that is used to analyze the characteristics of that population.*

4. Gaussian distribution

   Gaussian Distribution: *The term that describes the statistical phenomenon whereby members of a population are usually evenly disbursed around the population mean.*

5. Percentage and probability
6. Mean

   Mean ($\bar{X}$): *The arithmetic average for all the data contained in a sample population (or an algebraic set).*

7. Standard deviation

   Standard Deviation (SD): *A measurement of precision, or the tendency of the values in each population to cluster, center, or scatter around the mean.*

8. Coefficient of variance

   Coefficient of Variance *(CV): The standard deviation expressed as a percentage of the mean; considered a measurement of precision and variability.*

B. Graphic and systematic presentations of information

1. Standard data plotting techniques
   a. Basic statistical graphs
   b. Gaussian distribution displays
2. Seven old methods
   a. Flow charts
   b. Control charts

      Control Chart: *A chart used to plot control measurements against standards to identify when a process is in or out of control.*

c. Pareto charts
d. Cause-and-effect diagrams
Cause-and-Effect Diagrams: *Graphical displays with a "fishbone" appearance; used to identify the possible causes of, or contributing factors to, a problem or quality defect.*
e. Run charts
Run Charts: *Line graphs used to display data over a period of time.*
f. Scatter diagrams
g. Story boards
Story Boards: *A story told in sequential pictures displayed on a flip chart or other visual aid.*

3. Specialized laboratory data evaluation methods
a. Levey-Jennings chart
Levey-Jennings Chart: *A control chart used to plot quality control values against previously set limits to determine if a procedure is in or out of control.*
b. Youden plot
Youden Plot: *A technique used to demonstrate and compare the performance of a laboratory on paired samples with other laboratories using common control lots or survey material.*
c. Multi-rule analysis
Multi-rule Analysis: *A set of rules, such as the Westgard rules, that are used for accepting or rejecting a control run.*

4. SBAR
SBAR: (Situation – Background – Assessment – Recommendation) is a format for communicating messages between healthcare professionals.

C. Interpretive strategy
1. Error
Error: *An incorrect accept/reject or problem/no problem decision.*
Random Error: *An error that may occur at any time and place within the production process.*
Systematic Error: *An error that occurs in a predictable direction or pattern.*
2. Manipulation of data
Statistical Bias: *A set of numbers (i.e., sample) that does not truly reflect the characteristics of the whole population.*
3. Examination of control charts
Skewed Curves: *Deviations from the symmetrical bell-shaped appearance of a frequency polygon.*
a. Trends
Trend: *A systematic drift in one direction away from the established mean.*
b. Dispersions
Dispersion: *Control or sample values that are widely scattered in an unusual and unexplained pattern around the control chart.*
c. Shifts
Shift: *A sudden switch of data points to another area of the control chart away from the previous mean.*

D. External quality assessment programs
1. Proficiency surveys
2. Laboratory inspection

E. Indicators of quality performance: Institutional Programs
1. Utilization review and peer review organizations
Utilization Review: *Hospital and physician review of the necessity of care; mainly focused on reducing patient length of stay in the hospital.*
Quality Improvement Organizations (previously: *Peer Review Organization)**:** A federally mandated program that appoints an agency for a state or region to review hospital case* records for quality of care and reimbursement decisions.

2. Critical-care pathways

Critical-Care Pathways: *A hospital-wide quality care management program that places emphasis on the outcomes of treatment received by the patient as the definition of quality.*

IV. MANAGEMENT OF QUALITY
- A. The philosophy of quality
- B. Operational systems
- C. Quality management programs

V. MEDICAL ERRORS
- A. Organizational Focus
- B. Number one Villain to Patient Safety
- C. Non-Punitive Policy
- D. Root-Cause Analysis
  1. Definition
  2. Characteristics of an Acceptable Root Cause Analysis
- E. Failure Mode, Effects, and Criticality Analysis

Historical Perspective: Quality Concepts and Terminology Transition

Defining "quality" has proved to be one of the more frustrating efforts of modern management. Quality is like love: Everyone knows what it is, but no one knows exactly how to describe or measure it.

This search has been equally elusive for the laboratory and the health care community over the past few decades. Although the laboratory has developed excellent tools for determining the precision and accuracy of its procedures; finding indexes that measure efficacy, responsiveness to the needs of the patients and their physicians, and cost effectiveness has been much more difficult. For example, JCAHO has attempted to provide new terminology to nail down a program that both promotes and measures quality in health care institutions.

To develop a plan to assess and ensure the quality of the services delivered by the laboratory, the manager must have a full understanding of both the history and philosophy of quality up to this point as well as knowledge of specific statistical techniques and their application to the laboratory. The following collection of acronyms illustrates this journey:

QC/MBO → QA → TQM/CQI → QA&I/CPI →? QC/MBO?

These initials and monikers illustrate the history of the terminology of quality and the programs that were in vogue in the health care community from the 1970s until today. With the 1995 JCAHO standards, the concepts and principles of quality management have returned to their roots of QC and MBO: that is, to set performance objectives and measure their achievement. This is not to say that we have not learned a lot from our pursuit of a definition of quality and for ways to measure its existence and intensity. We have learned a great deal. Following is a brief review of the ideas and contributions found at each stage of the voyage and the remaining questions that have driven the search for new methods.

Quality Control

Quality control (QC) relies heavily on quantitative statistical methods that focus on the final product, as defined by standards set by the producer. For example, in a manufacturing facility, products are randomly collected from the production run and tested to see if they fall within acceptable QC ranges established for the item. In the laboratory, controls are processed periodically to make sure that the procedure is within control limits. If the controls are within range under the QC model, the techs are secure in the knowledge that they are turning out a high quality result.

The strength of the QC approach to quality management is that precise performance standards can be established and measured with objective analytic tools. The weakness of the QC system lies in its emphasis on the evaluation of the final product; this often makes troubleshooting difficult. Also, QC relies on standards and techniques that measure the quality of the product in isolation from the needs of the customer or patient.

Quality Assurance

Quality assurance (QA) developed out of the limitations of the QC approach and defined quality in health care institutions by the success of the total organization, not just individual components of the system, in achieving the goals of patient care.

When introduced by JCAHO in 1980, *quality assurance* was defined as the overall activities conducted by the institution that is directed toward assuring the quality of the services provided. QA focused on the *recipient,* namely, the patient. Risk management, in-service and continuing education, safety programs, quality control, and peer review were all part of the quality assurance program. In the QA model, the term "quality control" was applied to activities directed toward the monitoring of the individual elements of care — for example, instrument and test procedures — whereas QA focused on the monitoring of *outcomes* or *indicators of care.*

One of the major criticisms of the QA program was the absence of any specific guidelines or reference material for meeting JCAHO QA accreditation standards. In 1985 JCAHO finally published its 1O-step QA monitoring process.

1. Assign responsibility for QA plan.
2. Define scope of patient care.
3. Identify important aspects of care.
4. Construct indicators.
5. Define thresholds for evaluation.
6. Collect and organize data.
7. Evaluate data.
8. Develop corrective action plan.
9. Assess action; document improvement.
10. Communicate relevant information.

The major contribution of QA was to point out that the true indicator of a quality service was patient care, not just the ability of an individual part of the system to do its job well.

Although an improvement over QC, QA overemphasized outcomes; like the QC model, it failed to improve the troubleshooting capabilities of the system or to fully include the patient's viewpoint in the definition or measurement of quality.
JCAHO has now abandoned the term "quality assurance," but it is still being used in the regulatory language of CLIA'88.

Total Quality Management and Continuous Quality Improvement

Total quality management (TQM) and continuous quality improvement (CQI) have previously been discussed in this text within the context of their role as models for the general management of the laboratory (Chapter 1) and in developing performance appraisal instruments (Chapter 10). TQM/CQI quickly replaced the QA model because of its expanded emphasis on satisfying the needs of the customer, especially in its ultimate definition of quality: **"a delighted customer."**

To accomplish this goal, TQM/CQI held that the total enterprise, as well as each unit within the organization (and especially each *employee),* had to successfully perform and meet the obligations of three simultaneous roles: customer, producer, and supplier.

The inclusion of each component in the creation process — from the acquisition of supplies to active follow-up after the product or service has been received by a delighted customer broadens the focus of QC and QA on the end product. This emphasis on the total production process helps to correct a major deficiency of QC and QA by providing tools with which to identify and troubleshoot problems that might occur at each stage of production.

TQM/CQI was initially proclaimed as the elixir for the many ills affecting businesses that were experiencing a steady erosion of market share because of their past emphasis on short–term financial gains. The rush to adopt TQM/CQI was further fueled because it claimed to have been the reason for the dramatic turnaround in the quality of products made by Japanese companies after World War II and their resulting success in the international marketplace.

Many executives incorrectly believed that through the ostentatious adoption of TQM and CQI programs, they could magically wash away past transgressions and convince their customers and employees of their newfound enthusiasm for quality. This wholesale strategy of imposing on the organization TQM/CQI programs designed by outside consultants violated one of the main tenets of TQM/CQI — that of employee participation and major responsibility for decision making and was one of the many reasons for its failure to deliver on its promises.

In addition to the ways it was introduced to employees and the resulting skepticism, TQM/CQI suffered from its reliance on detailed documentation of actions, the avalanche of paperwork generated by this effort, and the tremendous amount of staff time it consumed. Corporate executives, pressed by the urgency of current problems, also realized that they could not wait 10 years until paradigm shifts were completed and promised results materialized. These factors, combined with the demise of several corporations held out as TQM models and the emerging realization that the economic woes of the Japanese economy were actually quite similar to those of the United States, have led managers to look for other means to assess and ensure quality. However, TQM's principles of continuous quality improvement, its focus on the complete *process* (supplies to customers), and its analytical and troubleshooting methodology are contributions that remain an important part of all quality management programs.

Additional information about the origin, concept, and techniques of TQM and CQI is provided in the sections on the leaders and tools of quality management.

Quality Assessment and Improvement and Continuous Performance Improvement

For several reasons, including the reluctance of many hospitals to support the requirement to adopt TQM/CQI and the acknowledged difficulty in defining quality, in 1992 JCAHO introduced a new monitoring standard: **quality assessment and improvement (QA&I)**. In 1996, the standard was renamed —performance improvement (PI). QA&I /PI incorporates the concepts of quality assurance and TQM/CQI, especially the idea that quality is a continuous process of improving the system, not just an end point measurement, and that it requires the direct support and active participation of the leadership of the organization.
Quality assessment and improvement focuses on the success of the organization in designing and meeting set goals and objectives, hence the term "continuous performance improvement (CPI)." With the implementation of the QA&I/CPI in 1994, JCAHO was also able to monitor certain indicators through a computerized reporting and evaluation system as part of their accred-

itation process. "Performance," as the reader has no doubt observed, is a much easier concept to define and measure than the elusive "quality."

Accredited hospital began collecting data on standardized, or “core,” performance measures in 2002. To support JCAHO’s accreditation process they included these measurement requirements (ORYX® report) as part of their quality improvement efforts in 2004.

Certain *Core Performance Measures* are also made available to the public through a JCAHO program called Quality Check® and Quality Reports (National Patient Safety Goals) to allow the consumer to compare hospital facilities.

> Compliance with the Joint Commission’s National Patient Safety Goals, as applicable to the organization, and performance on National Quality Improvement Goals (hospitals only). National Quality Improvement Goals reflect hospital reporting on the key indicators of quality of care in up to five treatment areas: heart attack, heart failure, community acquired pneumonia, pregnancy and related conditions, and surgical infection prevention. As more measures are approved and endorsed by the National Quality Forum, the Joint Commission will explore ways to incorporate that data into Quality Reports
>
> — About Quality Check® and Quality Reports

The College of American Pathologists in their accreditation process also uses the “improvement” model and defines *Quality Improvement* this way:

> Quality improvement in laboratory medicine is the process of assuring that all pathology services involved in the delivery of patient care have been accomplished in a manner appropriate to maintain excellence in medical care.
>
> — Standards for Laboratory Accreditation (2000)

Six Sigma

Six Sigma is a quality management collection of practices, intended to focus the business entity on reducing cost and increasing profits by systematically improving the production process by eliminating defects [i. e., 3.4 or fewer defective parts per million (ppm) – or – 6 Sigma (±6 SD)]. The process was developed at Motorola® by Bill Smith in 1986, and has become part of many Total Quality Management programs.

There are five basic steps in Six Sigma:

Define – Measure – Analyze – Improve – Control.

- Define the goals of the project
- Measure the activities involved in the current process
- Analyze to develop alternatives and possible solutions
- Design solutions
- Control the implement through statistical monitoring

Some modifications to the tools in the steps of the methodology terminology acronyms have been done (e.g., **DMAIC**: Define – Measure – Analyze – Improve – Control; ***DMADV***: Define – Measure – Analysis – Design – Verify)

There are tremendous sources on the web concerning the statistical tool and techniques of Six Sigma which the interested reader may wish to pursue [for example: Six Sigma First (*Sixsigmafirst.com*)]. There is also a training video available on line at *bmgi.com*.

Below is an interesting observation concerning the historical roots of Six Sigma:

> “Bill Smith did not really "invent" Six Sigma in the 1980s; rather, he applied methodologies that had been available since the 1920s developed by luminaries like Shewhart, Deming, Juran, Ishikawa, Ohno, Shingo, Taguchi and Shainin. All tools used in Six Sigma programs are actually a subset of the Quality Engineering discipline and can be con-

sidered a part of the ASQ Certified Quality Engineer body of knowledge. The goal of Six Sigma, then, is to use the old tools in concert, for a greater effect than a sum-of-parts approach."

Answers.com

Like other quality management programs (TQM, Zero-Defects, etc.), Six Sigma is not without major implementation and execution problems which are threaten its adoption by companies. The first is the tremendous commitment of time and resources, both people and facilities, which must be invested to make it work. An example of this is the statement by Larry Johnston (President, Chairman, and CEO) of Albertson's, Inc.: "*We plan to have 300 Black Belts deployed over the next three years managing hundreds of projects across the company*." This is obviously quite a commitment of resources and expectation of results in this cost conscience business environment.

A more direct concern over the effectiveness of Six Sigma is voiced by Mike Micklewright (June 2006):

> I find it interesting that, at least to my knowledge, there has not been a statistical analysis on whether or not the reported millions of dollars companies have saved after having embarked on a Lean/Six Sigma program is statistically significant or not. Were these same companies not enjoying savings, via productivity gains, in the years prior to going Lean Six Sigma?

Major Figures in Quality Management

In any review of quality management, certain names appear over and over, particularly with the current attention on the concepts of total quality management. Armand Feigenbaum coined the term "total quality management." Walter Shewhart (whose work served as a basis for the multirule based Westgard rules) is known as the father of statistical quality control. Several Japanese scholars developed important workplace models for the principles taught by Deming and Juran: Musaaski Imai, Kaori Ishikawa (who designed the cause-and-effect diagram), Shigru Mizuno, and Genichi Taguchi. The most famous "gurus of quality" are Philip Crosby, W. Edwards Deming, and Joseph Juran. These men are discussed in the following section, together with James O. Westgard, who applied concepts and techniques of quality management to the medical laboratory.

Philip Crosby

Frequently referred to as the "evangelist" of quality management, Crosby preached the need for quality practices in the book *Quality Is Free* and through the worldwide consulting network of quality colleges. Crosby propounded that:

- Quality is free. Poor quality is expensive.
- Do things right the first time.
- "Zero defects" is the only legitimate goal of a quality program [root of Six Sigma]

These ideas are also prominent in the writings of Westgard and other laboratorians who were addressing quality issues before TQM gained popularity in the health care community.

W. Edwards Deming

Deming is often credited with providing the Japanese with the information and training that brought them to their position as the world's leader in the production of quality products. Deming, a statistician who worked with Shewhart, introduced the use of statistical tools in decision making, problem solving, and troubleshooting the production process.

Deming is also frequently cited as the source of most of the concepts and methods contained in the TQM model. Among Deming's more prominent contributions to the language of TQM are the "fourteen points" (Table 21 – 1), the "delighted customer" definition of quality, the "seven old tools," and the "seven deadly diseases" (Table 21 – 2).

Joseph Juran

Another person held in high regard by the Japanese is Joseph Juran. Juran established the concept that quality is a *continuous improvement process* that requires managers' active pursuit in reaching and setting goals for improvement.

The *pareto principle,* or 80/20 rule, which states that 80 percent of serious problems arise from only 20 percent of the causes or trouble points, was introduced by Juran. According to the pareto principle, managers should focus their time and efforts on identifying and solving the 20 percent.

Juran was a leader in promoting participatory management styles. He pointed out that it was necessary for all employees to be included in, and committed to, the continual process of designing and producing a quality' product. Quality circles and project teams, which use a wide variety of employee inputs, are two methods that trace their origins to the teaching of Juran.

1. Create constancy of purpose toward service improvement.
2. Adopt the new philosophy.
3. Cease dependence inspection to achieve quality.
4. End the practice of awarding business solely on the price tag.
5. Constantly improve the process of planning production and service.
6. Institute training on the job.
7. Institute leadership for people and systems improvement.
8. Drive out fear in order to encourage employees to work together.
9. Break down barriers between departments and work areas.
10. Eliminate slogans, exhortations, and production targets.
11. Eliminate numerical quotas for management and the workforce.
12. Remove barriers to pride of workmanship.
13. Institute a vigorous program of education and self-improvement for everyone in the organization.
14. Put everyone in the organization to work accomplishing the transformation.

Table 21 — 1. Synopsis of Deming's 14 TQM Points

---

1. Lack of constancy of purpose to improve products and services by providing resources for long-range planning, research, and training.
2. An emphasis on short-term profits and the quarterly dividend.
3. Individual performance evaluations through merit ratings and annual reviews.
4. Managers who are highly mobile, hopping from company to company.
5. Use by management of numbers and figures that are visible and available with no thought of what information may be needed but unknown or hidden.
6. Excessive medical costs.
7. Excessive legal liability costs, swollen by lawyers who work on contingency fees.

Table 21 — 2. Synopsis of Deming's Seven Deadly Diseases

James O. Westgard

James O. Westgard, a professor at the University of Wisconsin Medical School and associate director of Clinical Laboratories-Quality Assurance with the University of Wisconsin Hospital and Clinics in Madison, applied Shewhart's multi-rule system to the evaluation of the quality control data in the medical laboratory, particularly the multi-ranged controls used in clinical chemistry. The six rules for accepting or rejecting a control run are now commonly referred to as the Westgard rules (Table 21 – 3). Additional information on these and other quality management tools are reviewed in the next section.

1_{2S} rule:	The run is accepted when both control results are within 2 SD limits from the mean value.
1_{3S} rule:	The run is considered out of control when one of the control results exceeds the ± 3 SD limits.
2_{2S} rule:	The run is rejected when both controls exceed the mean value +2 SD or the mean –2 SD limits.
R_{4S} rule	The run is rejected when both controls exceed a mean value + 2 SD limits and one exceeds the mean –2 SD limit or when the range of a group of controls exceeds 4 SD.
4_{1S} rule:	The run is rejected when four consecutive control results exceed the mean +1 SD or the Mean –1 SD.
10_{X^*} rule:	The run is rejected when the last 10 consecutive control results fall on the same side of the mean.

SOURCE: From Westgard, JO, and Barry PL: *Cost-Effective Quality Control: Managing the Quality and Productivity of Analytical Processes.* AACC Press, Washington DC, 1986, pp. 93—94. Courtesy of the American Association for Clinical Chemistry, Inc. http://www.westgard.com/mltirule.htm#westgard {other common multi-rules are listed at the site} [connected June 18, 2007]

Table 21 — 3. Westgard Rules

Another word about the contribution of Dr. Westgard to the quality performance of clinical laboratory tests specifically, and major contributions to the application of statistical tools to performance standards in all areas. I would highly recommend a visit to his website, http://www.westgard.com/, to not only avail access to the quality tools offered, but gain insight into the basic philosophy of the pursuit of quality.

Quality Monitoring and Assessment Tools

The precise techniques and mechanisms of quality control are familiar to every technical professional in the laboratory. The objective of this section is to present a short survey of the concepts and terminology frequently found on professional examinations at the supervisory level. These concepts provide a baseline for the discussion of quality management in the medical laboratory. The reader can find more extensive information on each of these methods in the sources cited in the bibliography.

Tools for the measurement of quality and performance in the laboratory can be reviewed in five groups.

1. Statistical techniques that establish performance limits for the analytical accuracy and precision of testing protocols.
2. Graphic and monitoring methods that aid in review, troubleshooting, and decision-making systems.
3. Interpretive strategy for evaluating statistical and monitoring methods.

4. External programs that provide resources for the independent assessment of the technical performance of the laboratory.
5. Methods that are intended to monitor the delivery of the overall services of the laboratory as part of the health care team

Basic Quality Control Statistics

From the multitude of statistical calculations available to the analyst, four measurements constitute the base for most quality assessment efforts. These statistical tools are quite familiar to laboratorians and are particularly applicable to situations in which performance criteria can be quantified. These four measurements are: the mean ($\bar{X}$), or arithmetic average; the standard deviation from the mean (SD); the coefficient of variance (CV); and the most widely used statistical calculation of all, the percentage (%).

These and other statistical terms appear frequently on supervisory examinations. Table 21 – 4 uses these statistical calculations for glucose controls and serves as an illustration of the application of statistical methods to a laboratory example. The reader is encouraged to consult one of the many excellent books listed in the bibliography for additional information about the use of statistical tools.

Quality Control Report: Glucose

		Year to Date	**April**
		Lot 2946, Level I	
$\bar{X}$	=	75.1	74.7
SD	=	2.1	2.2
CV%	=	2.9	3.0
N	=	1,574	
		Lot 2946, Level II	
$\bar{X}$	=	281.9	287.2
SD	=	6.2	6.6
CV%	=	2.2	2.3
N	=	1,574	

Table 20—4. Statistical Calculations

Accuracy and Precision

Accuracy and precision are crucial terms in any analytical process. **Accuracy** refers to the *closeness* of a result to the actual value of an analyte when performing a test, more commonly called "hitting the bull's eye." **Precision,** by contrast, is determined by how well a procedure *reproduces* a value. For example, if you analyze a triglyceride standard with a known value of 200/mg dL five times and obtain values of 169, 167, 170, 168, and 169, you could say you that your methodology is extremely precise. However, its accuracy is way off and the procedure needs to be recalibrated.

Data Population

The term **population** is used in statistics to describe and define the items that are being studied at a particular time. The population may be, for example, all the values obtained on a normal creatinine control for 1 month or the patients who had glucose tolerance tests during the past year. Population is selected and defined by the interest of the person doing the statistical study.

Population Sample

A **sample,** for statistical purposes, is a part of a population that is used to analyze the characteristics of that population. It is a particularly useful technique when evaluating a population with a large number of entities, which makes it impractical to include every member in the study. In general, the larger the sample selected, the more representative of the population; however, as a general rule most statisticians hold that a sample size of at least 30 is satisfactory for most studies (Daniel, p. 110; *Guidelines for Publicizing Hospital National Quality Improvement Goal*) .

To be truly representative, and to avoid bias, samples should be selected at *random* (I,e., *probability sample),* in a manner that ensures that each unit of the population has an equal chance of being included in the study. The letter *N* indicates the number of observations (i.e., individuals, measurements, or values) that make up the sample used for calculating statistical indexes.

For example, the laboratory and the pharmacy may be interested in reviewing the causes for a seemingly high frequency of gentamicin trough levels that exceed acceptable levels. The laboratory may have done several hundred gentamicin trough levels during the period of interest, of which 100 exceeded acceptable dose levels. Instead of an in-depth review of every assay, the study may need to investigate only 30 cases *(N* = 30) to find the cause of the deviations.

Gaussian Distribution

Many terms are associated with the **Gaussian distribution,** including "bell-shaped curve," "normal distribution," "frequency polygon," and "Levey-Jenning charts." All of these terms describe the statistical phenomenon that the members of a population are usually evenly disbursed around the population mean. *(Note:* There are exceptions such as when extreme values are included in the calculations, causing the curve to appear skewed.) This important concept is the foundation upon which the acceptance/rejection criteria of the Westgard rules and the performance limits of Levey-Jennings charts are derived.
Following the rules of a Gaussian distribution, the individual values of a population fall within the following boundaries *(see* Table 20-4):

68.2 percent are within $\pm$ 1 SD of the mean
95.4 percent are within $\pm$ 2 SD of the mean .
99.7 percent are within $\pm$ 3 SD of the mean
[99.99999966 percent are within $\pm$ of 6 SD of the mean (i.e., or Six Sigma {3.4 or fewer defective parts per million})]

With an understanding of these criteria, technologists can make an informed (95 percent certainty factor using the $\pm$2 SD standard) accept/reject decision about the probability of a particular test run being in or out of control.

Percentage and Probability

Two concepts, percentage (%) and probability *(P),* are part of our everyday lives, but the reader may want to note the following points about probability for purposes of review.

Probability is usually expressed in statistical notation as a decimal (0.0 to 1.0) according to the likelihood of an event occurring: the nearer to 0, the less likely it is to occur; the nearer to 1, the more likely the event is to happen.

Probability may also be expressed in the negative; for example, the likelihood of an acceptable control value falling outside the $\pm$3 SD range is only 0.003 (1 – 0.997). In more common language, probability is often expressed as a percentage: "There is a 50 percent chance of rain," or a 0.5 probability of rain.

Mean

The **mean** ($\bar{X}$) is simply the *arithmetic average* for all the data contained in a sample population (or an algebraic set), such as the values obtained by running a normal glucose control for 1 month. The mean is obtained by computing the sum of the values contained in the population and dividing by the number of values included in the calculation.

The mean is easily confused with the *median.* Both mean and median describe the midpoint of a population. However, the mean is a calculated value, whereas the median is obtained by aligning the population from the smallest to the largest unit and selecting the midpoint, the point at which exactly 50 percent of the population falls on both sides.

Standard Deviation

The **standard deviation** (SD) is a measurement of precision, or the tendency of the values in each population to cluster, center, or scatter around the mean. A range of 2 standard deviations ($\pm$2 SD) is generally considered as the minimal limit for an individual control value to be acceptable, because 95 percent of all legitimate values should be within this range. The mean and the standard deviation form the guidelines delineated in the Westgard rules (see Table 21 – 3) and the points plotted on a Levey-Jennings chart. In calculating the SD for a particular control, the difference (or variance) of each value from the mean is used to establish the acceptable range for each control level.

Coefficient of Variance

Calculating the **coefficient of variance** (CV) for each control level and procedure allows a comparison and check on the precision and variability of each method. The CV is expressed as a percent and calculated by dividing the standard deviation by the mean and multiplying the result by 100.

$$CV = (SD \div \bar{X}) \times 100$$

The smaller the CV value, the more precise (actually, the less imprecise) the procedure.

The interpretation of CV numbers must be placed in the context of the methodology of each procedure. Tests that closely follow Beer's law for end-point reactions are expected to have very tight CV percentages, whereas the rate reactions used to measure enzyme activity usually experience a much larger range.

Many other statistical tools are useful in studying both qualitative and quantitative problems. The preceding list covers only the basic techniques used in the laboratory.

The next section reviews some popular quality management methods that organize and present data in graphical and other monitoring formats to expedite analyses.

Graphic and Systematic Presentations of Information

One of the more difficult, yet important tasks of any quality management program is turning the data collected from the monitoring process into information that can be used to troubleshoot and improve the production process. Data alone have no particular interpretive value. If placed within the context of other data points or material, however, they can become extremely useful in the decision-making process. This section outlines the most popular techniques in quality management for organizing, grouping, and sorting data into formats that assist the manager in evaluating the situation and in taking the necessary action to bring about improvement.

With the advent of computer technology and desktop publishing, the boundaries for the graphical display of information have exploded. Bar and circle graphs are now being drawn in three-dimensional, multicolored, topographical schematic figures that can incorporate and demonstrate the relationships between numerous factors on a single graph. The future of the graphical presentation of data is limited only by the imagination of the analyst.

Standard Data Plotting Techniques

The first task of any evaluation plan is to arrange and present the data in a manner that facilitates further analysis. This procedure is referred to as the "orderly array of data " — from lowest to highest value, chronologically by run or date, in groups by sex and age, and so on. This step is usually part of the data collection plan; with continuous monitoring systems such as for a laboratory instrument, it is accomplished by plotting the QC data on a chart or graph as the test is performed.

Once the data have been arrayed in an orderly manner, the results can be presented in an informative format as a chart, graph, or other pictorial display intended to demonstrate problems and potential solutions.

Most of the methods are familiar to the reader both in the laboratory and from everyday life because they frequently appear in news broadcasts, advertisements, classroom training material, and anywhere people may desire to make a certain point or pitch a product. Examples include bar and pie charts and graphs, as well as the control charts used to plot QC data.

Among the list of standard data plotting techniques reviewed next are Deming's "seven old methods," which have been around a long time and form the base of most quality assessment and management programs.

Basic Statistical Graphs

The three most basic methods of presenting information — circle, bar, and line graphs — are used to illustrate the comparative size of different components or factors. Most other graphical display techniques are modifications of these three methods.

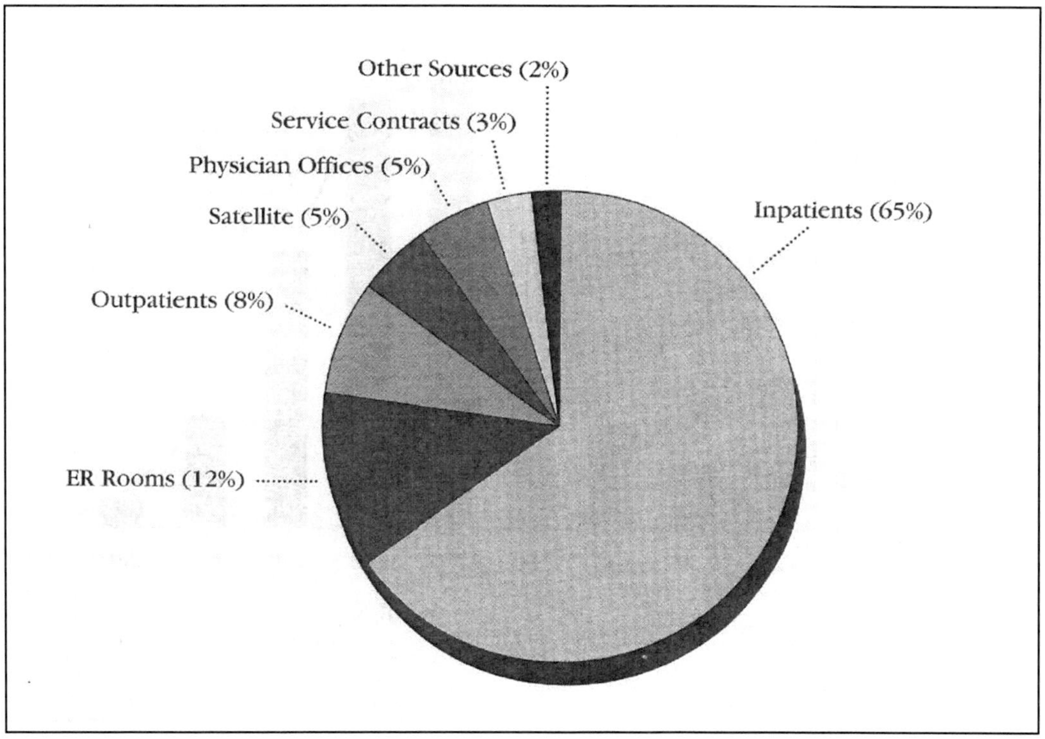

Circle, or pie, charts are circular figures with areas marked off, shaded, or sketched according to the percentage of each component, compared to the whole. In Figure 21 – 1, a pie chart shows the types of clients who make up a laboratory's patient mix.

Bar graphs may be helpful in presenting comparative inter-population and intra- population factors. These may range from showing the makeup of a population to comparing different populations with a key indicator or measurement. The bars on the graph may extend vertically or horizontally according to the preference of the preparer. The point is to present the information in the manner that best demonstrates and clarifies the information being detailed and that assists the users in their evaluation. The bar graph in Figure 21 — 2 displays the same information as is shown in Figure 20—1.

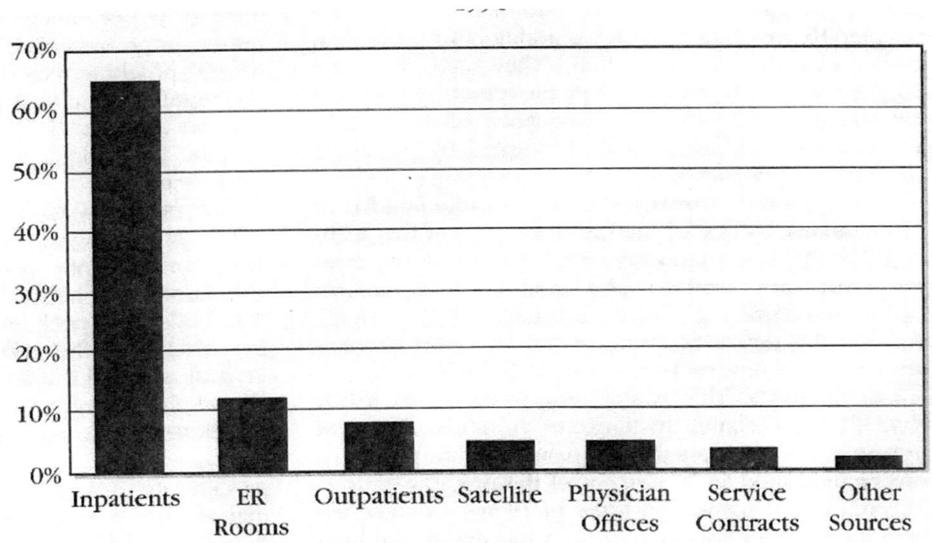

Patient Base of LabTest Medical Laboratory: 2007

Figure 21 — 2. Bar graph

Gaussian Distribution Displays

There are two popular methods of displaying the frequency distribution characteristics of a population: histograms and frequency polygons. Both illustrate the features of the bell-shaped Gaussian distribution curve.

A *histogram* uses a bar graph format to show the relative size or frequency of each "class interval." A class interval is the statistical term for each part of the population. For example, one bar may represent the age group 20 to 30 in a patient population.

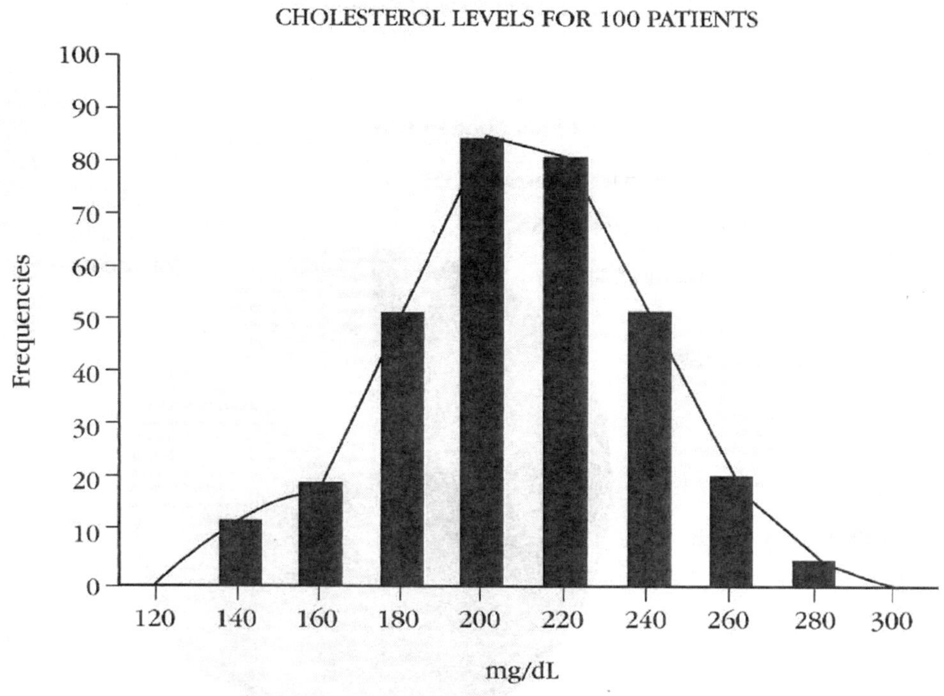

Figure 21 — 3. Histogram with frequency polygon superimposed

Frequency polygons are the very familiar line graphs that give the frequency distribution its descriptive name, "bell curve." In both a histogram and a frequency polygon, a relative frequency scale represents the vertical axis of the graph; the values of the variable being studied are located on the horizontal axis. The values for each class interval are then plotted on the graph using the heights of the bars on the histogram to show the relative size and dots connected by a line for a frequency polygon. If the distribution of the population follows a normal pattern, the classic bell shape appears. Figure 20-3 provides examples of both methods in combination, used to show the reference values for a cholesterol test.

Seven Old Methods

Many other methods may be used to organize and summarize information in quality management studies. Each has its own distinct advantage and analytical purpose. Deming has suggested seven techniques with which the quality manager should be familiar, one of which is the histogram already reviewed. The remaining six, along with the story board technique, which has gained popularity in TQM programs, are briefly described now.

Flow Charts

Quality management borrows the techniques and symbols of logic flow charts used by management information systems specialists to chart and analyze the specific process of information flow. (See Chapter 17 and Figure 17 – 4 for additional information and an example of a flow chart.) They serve the same purpose in quality management programs by identifying and describing the exact sequence of work tasks and checking out ways for improvement by modeling alternative work routes.

Control Charts

Control charts are quite familiar to laboratorians, as one of the best examples of this technique is the Levey-Jennings chart. By definition, control charts are used to plot control measurements against standards (i.e., upper and lower limits, usually equal to the numerical value of $\pm$ 2 SD) used to identify whether a process is in or out of control.

Pareto Charts

This is the term assigned to a bar chart that is designed to illustrate the classical pareto principle, which states that 80 percent of all problems can be attributed to 20 percent of the possible causes. According to this concept, if the problems are matched with their causes and plotted on a bar graph, the area in which managers should devote the majority of their attention and energy become readily apparent.

Cause-and-Effect Diagrams

Cause-and-effect diagrams have several other names, including "Ishikawa diagrams," after Kaoru Ishikawa, who introduced this tool, and "fishbone diagrams," because of their appearance. This method, as the name implies, is used to identify the possible causes or contributing factors of problems or quality defects. The problem is placed at the "head" of the diagram, with possible causes branching out of the backbone, in the work flow direction.

Run Charts

A **run chart** is a line graph used to display data over a period of time. Run charts are also called *trend charts,* as they are designed to show patterns of performance. These may be used in the laboratory in a variety of ways, for example, tracking missed phlebotomies or redraws, data entry errors, or the number of tests that have to be rerun. The charts can be as general (shift, section, department) or as specific (individual, instrument, AM collection) as the study warrants.

Scatter-Diagrams

This method is used to show the relationship between one variable and another. A study may, for example, review the level of an antibiotic maintained in a patient compared to the time a sample was collected (peak and trough studies). A graph is prepared with the concentration of the drug on the vertical axis and the time of collection after administration as the horizontal base. The results of each sample are plotted at the appropriate site on the graph and the pattern analyzed to check dosage and collection timing procedures. A big advantage of a scatter diagram is that all data points, not just the summary statistical indexes, are plotted on the graph.

Story Boards

Story boards refer to the technique of using a pictorial sequence on a flip chart or other visual aid to "tell the story" of a quality management project. The presentation may be very elaborate, containing many of the previously discussed methods to illustrate how the investigators conducted the study, or may be a simple outline of each stage of the project.

Specialized Laboratory Data Evaluation Methods

From the basic methods of organizing, presenting, and analyzing statistical information, three techniques have been developed that have proved to be especially useful in the medical laboratory: Levey-Jennings charts, Youden plots, and multi-rule analysis.

Levy-Jennings Chart

Levey-Jennings (L-J) charts are control charts used to plot quality control values against previously set limits to determine if a procedure is in or out of control. As may be noted in Figure 21 – 7, L-J charts can be described as Gaussian distribution curves turned on the side with lines extended from the mean (X) and each SD ($\pm$ 1, 2, or 3 SD) level.

Youden Plot

Youden plots are used to demonstrate and compare the performance of a laboratory on paired samples with other laboratories using common control lots or survey material. Youden plots use the mean and SDs from all participants to prepare a chart on which each laboratory's results can be marked to show its performance in relationship to the whole group. Youden plots are divided into four areas with a 45-degree line drawn from the X–Y intercept separating the graph into two halves. Depending on the location of a laboratory's results on the Youden plot, the degree of accuracy, precision, and type of error may be inferred.

Youden plots are now frequently being discontinued or replaced with other graphical or numeric displays because of the voluminous amount of computer paper it takes to print out a plot for each analyte and the expense associated with mailing this bulky material. The *Instrument Performance Matrix* used by Coulter® Hematology Reports for its interlaboratory quality assurance program is an example of a technique that has replaced Youden Plots.

Multi-Rule Analysis

Multi-rule analysis, commonly referred to in the laboratory as the "Westgard rules," has formalized the application of multi-rule techniques to the medical laboratory. The six rules proposed by Westgard and Barry for accepting or rejecting a control run are based on the expected Gaussian distribution of sample values. Implementing a multi-rule program involves management choices about the degree of error that the laboratory finds acceptable when making decisions about the possibility of correctly accepting or rejecting a control run. The Westgard rules and a *logic diagram* are given in Table 21 — $3_{(above)}$ and Figures 21 — 4 and 21 — 5. Each rule is designed to detect or warn of an impending error or malfunction that may either halt the reporting of results until the problem is corrected or signal the need for preventive maintenance.

SBAR (Situation – Background – Assessment – Recommendation)

SBAR is a format tool developed by the U. S. Navy and adapted to healthcare situations, intended primarily to aid nurses to communicate patient care needs to physicians [INI.org, Safer Healthcare, Ang]. This technique was designed by Dr. M. Leonard, along with colleagues from Kaiser Permanente of Colorado (Kaiser Permanente of Colorado, 2006). Because of its success in the nurse–physician role; attempts have been made to utilize it in other healthcare settings.

SBAR adoption has not been without problems. John Whittington (Healthcare Risk Management) point out the culture of healthcare has been a problem: "*While SBAR (Situation, Background, Assessment, and Recommendation) technique is a fairly straightforward concept, implementing the methodology can be more difficult than you might expect.*"

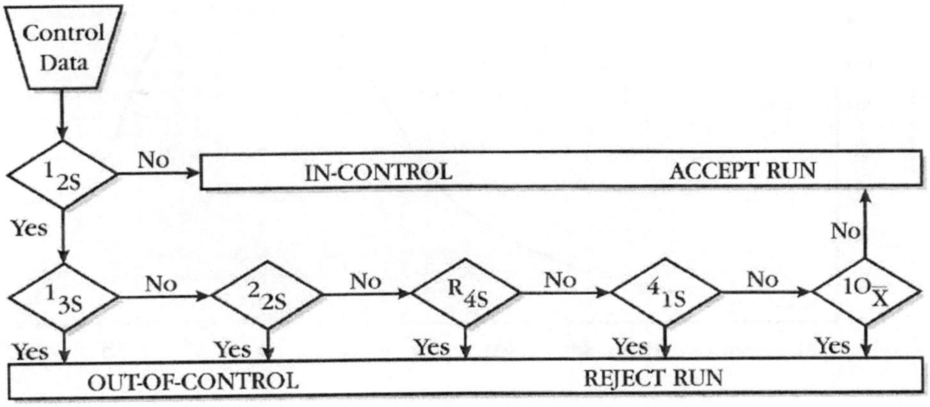

Figure 21 — 4. Westgard logic diagram 1

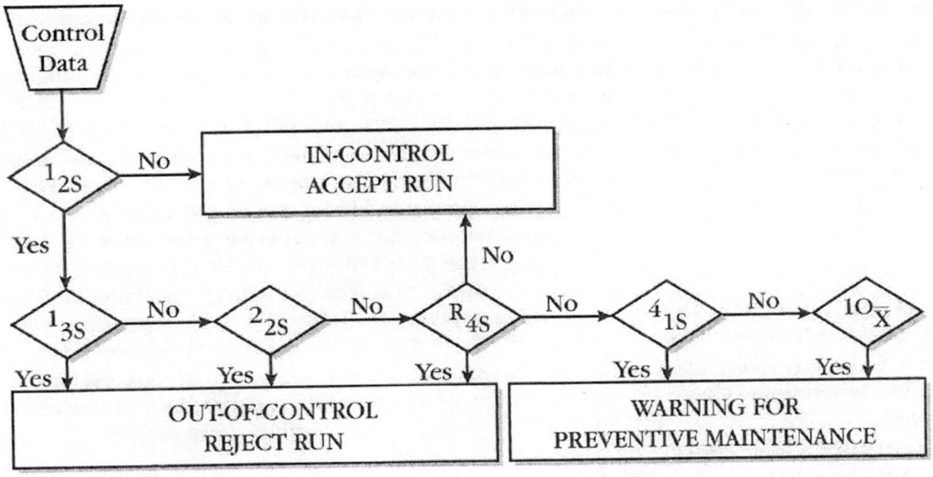

Figure 21 — 5. Westgard logic diagram 2

SOURCE: Reprinted from Westgard, JO, and Barry PL: *Cost-Effective Quality Control: Managing the Quality and Productivity of Analytical Processes*. AACC Press, Washington DC, 1986, pp. 95, 114. Courtesy of the American Association for Clinical Chemistry, Inc.

In the laboratory, for example, efforts have been made to use the SBAR format in instrument troubleshooting and communication logs between personnel. This has meet with limited success, and have resulted in extensive attempts to explain and even change the terminology; particularly since most communiqués do not need to include all the steps. For example, a note "*reran QC material, results are within* $\pm$*2SD*," is enough with the other information simply being implied.

Basically the SBAR model follows the pattern:

- **S** – Situation – what is happening at the present time?
- **B** – Background – what are the circumstances leading up to this?
- **A** – Assessment – what do I think the problem is?
- **R** – Recommendation – what should we do to correct the problem?

> For an example of a SBAR report to physician about a critical situation which resulted because of a failure to properly report a PT IRN; and a table describing Mechanisms to Spread Use of Situation, Background, Assessment, and Recommendation (SBAR) see: http://w3.ouhsc.edu/pcep/documents/SBARWorksheet.pdf
> [connected July 18, 2007

Interpretive Strategy

The detection and correction of errors, both technical and administrative, are a major mission of quality management programs. All of the preceding methods are useless if the technologist or manager is not aware of the types of problems, errors, or malfunctions that can occur in a process and of the clues that may trigger their recognition and resolution. The old microbiology adage, "We tend to find what we are looking for," applies here as well. Following is a list of some statistical terms and clues that may tip the analysts to possible problems.

Error

The concept of **error** is related to accept/reject and problem/no problem decisions. An error can be made in either direction. A decision can be made to accept a run incorrectly with the laboratory reporting out incorrect values, or a legitimate test result may be rejected, resulting in a loss of time and reagent expense. Control limits must be set with both potentials in mind.

Errors may be classified into two types: **random errors**, which may occur at any time and place within the testing or service process, and systematic errors, which occur in a consistent direction or pattern. Random errors are indicative of imprecision in an analytical process; problems of inaccuracy show up as **systematic errors**.

Identifying the type of error is crucial to determining the extent, nature, and timing of action necessary. For example, a random error may need only to be closely monitored for possible recurrence; a systematic error may need immediate remedial action. Control charts (following) and multi-rule analysis may both give clues to the type of error. Violations of Westgard rules 1_{3S} and R_{4S} may reflect random errors; 2_{2S}, 4_{1S}, or 10_{X^*} rule failures may indicate that the error is systematic (Westgard and Barry, p. 99).

Manipulation of Data

Decisions about what to include in a population or sample are often criticized by those who question the validity of statistical figures. Having a set of numbers that do not truly reflect the characteristics of the whole population is referred to as **statistical bias,** which may be either circumstantial or intentional. The exclusion of a number that does not appear to belong in a group of data, an "outlier," is an example of the purposeful manipulation of data.

Manipulation of data is not an uncommon occurrence in the laboratory. If a control was run 30 times and all the values were between 19 and 31 except for one, which was 54, the exclusion of the "outlier" from statistical calculations is an example of an intentional bias. This may also be called "cleaning up the data," a term particularly attractive to the person doing the refinement.

Examination of Control Charts

Clues about data problems are often revealed in the shape of the Gaussian distribution curve. Deviations from the symmetrical bell-shaped appearance of a frequency polygon are called **skewed curves** (Fig. 21 – 6) and serve as a signal that the data do not accurately reflect the parameters of the population. Distribution curves can become skewed in either direction (i.e., to the right or left of the mean) because of a nonrepresentatively small sample size or by the inclusion of data that are flawed because of sampling or process (technical, administrative) errors. Problems that are not rectified may translate into misleading inferences or incorrect range limits on L-J control charts. This, as every tech knows, may trigger unnecessary out-of-control flags, causing much frustration and wasted troubleshooting time.

Three problem related patterns may be detected by studying how data appear when plotted on a control chart: *trends, dispersions,* and *shifts.* These patterns have also been matched with probable causes for their occurrence. The analyst must also be aware that these patterns may all occur at the same time and be constantly alert to the clues provided by each type of change in data configuration.

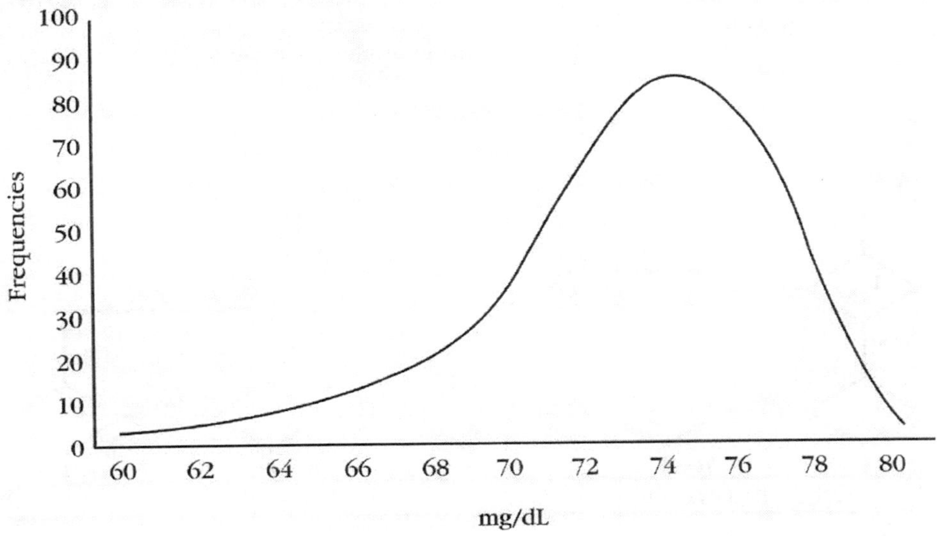

Figure 21 – 6. Example of skewed curve

<u>Trends</u>

Trends (Fig. 21 – 7, pattern 1) are marked by a systematic drift in one direction away from the established mean. Trends may also be detected by 4_{1S} or 10_{X^*} Westgard rule failures. Trends signal the gradual deterioration of procedure components such as reagents, standards, or instrumentation (e.g., light bulbs, electrical elements, filters, and so on).

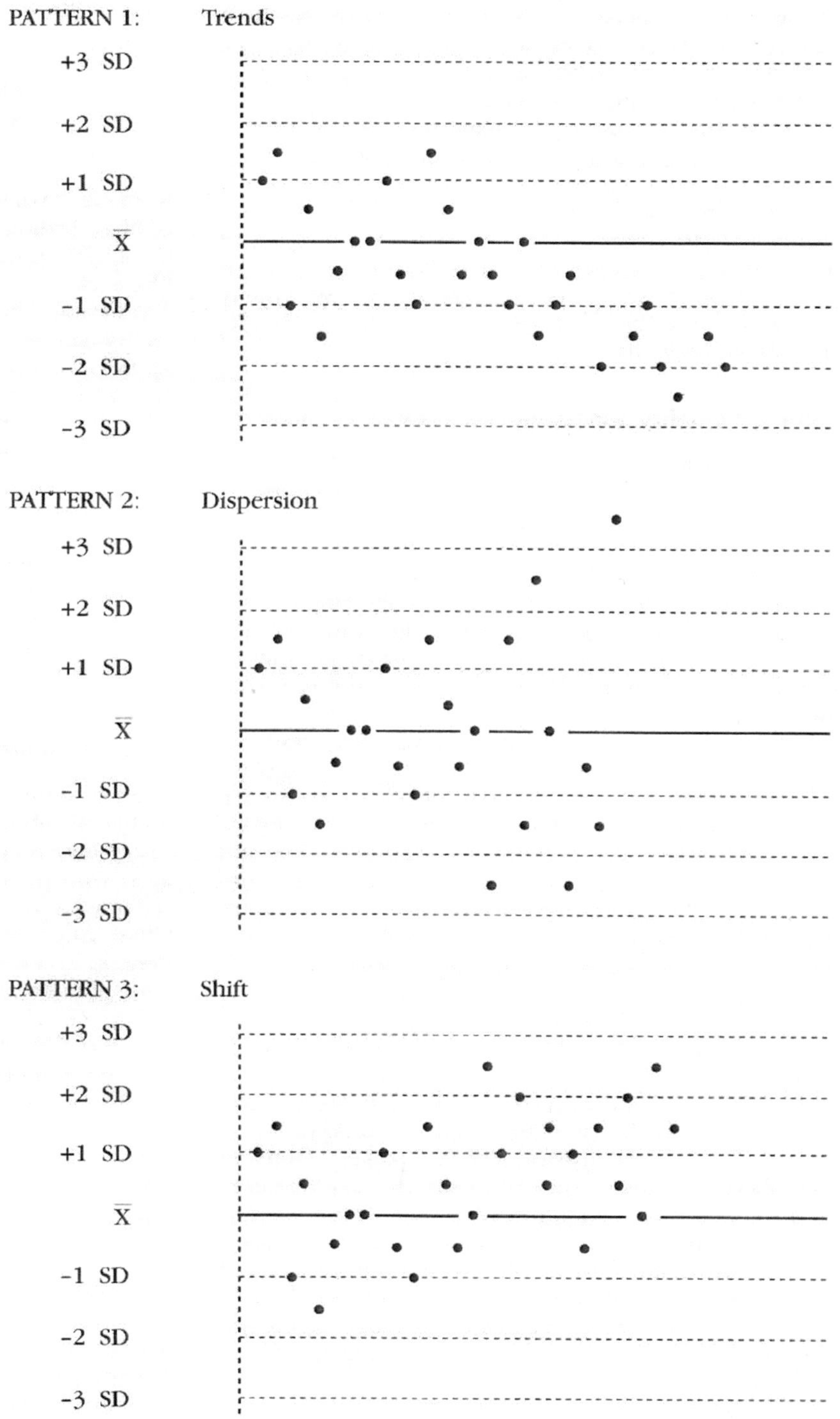

Figure 21 — 7. Interpretation of Levey-Jennings control charts

<u>Dispersion</u>

Dispersion (Fig. 21 – 7, pattern 2) occurs when control values are widely scattered in an unusual and unexplained pattern around the control chart; particularly, with increasing out-of-control (i.e., exceeding $\pm$2 SD and $\pm$3 SD) results and Westgard rule violations 2_{2S} and R_{4S}. Dispersion is a sign of loss of precision and may be caused by inconsistency in such areas as a malfunctioning automatic dispenser or variations in technique by testing personnel.

Shifts

Shifts (Fig. 21 – 7, pattern 3) are a sudden switch of data points to another area of the control chart away from the previous mean. They are usually associated with a change or replacement of some component of the analytical system, such as a new lot of reagents, repair or installation of an instrument part, or

recalibration of the method. These are not necessarily bad and may reflect only some action taken to correct a problem previously noted.

External Quality Assessment Programs

The laboratory may participate on a voluntary or mandatory basis in external programs initiated through the laboratory community, such as proficiency testing, accreditation, and licensure activities in hospital programs such as PRO, risk management, JCAHO, Medicare, and facility licensing. This section focuses on laboratory-based programs, and the next section reviews the other plans as part of the indicators for the overall quality performance of the institution.

External quality assessment programs may be roughly divided into two types for review purposes: (1) proficiency surveys, in which blind specimens are sent by an external agency for analysis and comparison with other laboratories, and (2) licensure and accreditation programs, which involve on-site inspections. The line between these two groups is often blurred because they are so closely intertwined, but the division provides a means for review. Accreditation and licensure plans, for example, may frequently produce their own proficiency surveys or use participation in these plans as a major evaluation criterion.

Possible conflicts of interest arise from the requirement that only the proficiency survey products of a specific inspection agency are acceptable. Frequent complaints are also expressed over the interpretation and enforcement of arbitrarily set "successful" performance levels by some government licensure agencies, despite disclaimers issued by almost all proficiency plans that the results should not be used as a sole indicator or assessor of performance because of the intended design and unreliability of the material for this purpose.

Proficiency Surveys

Proficiency surveys are programs that allow a laboratory to compare its performance on a common sample with a group of peers based on size (number of beds, specimen volume) and methodology (instrument, reagents). The most widely known programs are those issued by the American Association of Bioanalysts (AAB) and the College of American Pathologists (CAP). Some state health departments may produce specialty proficiency material for monitoring syphilis or infant thyroid testing facilities. Most suppliers of commercial quality control samples also include, as part of their report, interlaboratory comparison statistics.

These organizations offer a variety of surveys, which can be tailored to the specific requirements and needs of each laboratory based on the sophistication and extent of services offered. Survey material may range from basic packages for physician office laboratories or satellite testing stations to comprehensive options for the highly specialized procedures performed in areas like toxicology and microbiology.

Although the selection and enrollment in a proficiency survey service may be theoretically voluntary, participation is normally required for accreditation and licensure. Failure to meet designated performance criteria or to demonstrate appropriate corrective action may lead to sanctions including loss of accreditation or license.

In addition to providing an objective means to assess the effectiveness of internal quality control procedures, the studies provide the laboratory community with information about the performance of different methods and instruments. This allows managers and manufacturers to make more informed selection and marketing decisions.

Laboratory Inspection

The laboratory may justifiably feel bombarded with the multitude of entities seeking to inspect its facilities. These may range from those seeking voluntary compliance with professional standards to the local code inspector looking to enforce fire and safety regulations. Often rules and missions may appear redundant or even in conflict, a complaint shared by the laboratory with all business organizations.

The American Association of Blood Banks (AABB) and the College of American Pathologists (CAP) are two professional laboratory organizations that have been leaders in offering inspection and accreditation programs. Both provide extensive educational and resource material about their review processes, including accreditation standards and inspection guidelines. This information has proved useful for developing and monitoring quality management plans for the laboratory as well as preparing for site inspection.

JCAHO, as part of its accreditation programs, maintains standards for the laboratory and also includes a designated member of their site visit team to review the laboratory. In addition to these professional activities, the laboratory has also attracted increasing regulatory interest at both federal and state levels, most notably for CLIA'88 and Medicare certification.

Driven by the criticisms and complaints about redundancy and costs, many of the government and private inspection agencies are working on reciprocal, equivalency, and deemed-status agreements or attempting to coordinate site visits to avoid frequent repetitious inspections of the same services. However, because of territorial issues (not an uncommon characteristic of most organizations), progress in this area has been slow, especially among competing laboratory organizations.

Indicators of Quality Performance: Institutional Programs

The discussion of quality management has, up to this point, reviewed programs with which the laboratory evaluates itself. The laboratory has also begun to play an increasing role, starting with the advent of quality assurance and the indicators of care, in the assessment of the overall care that patients receive in the hospital. This has happened because of the type of information the laboratory provides and its relative ease of quantification and monitoring potential. This role has coincided with the renewed realization that the laboratory's success can be measured only within the context of the total care received by the patient.

The laboratory's increasing participation in these institutional programs is reflected in the JCAHO's quality assessment and improvement (QA&I) and continuous performance improvement (CPI) programs, previously covered, and in the issues associated with caring for, and receiving reimbursement for patients covered by Medicare, Medicaid, and so on. The major hospital based quality activities and their historical transition are reviewed now.

Utilization Review and Quality Improvement Organizations

The federal government, aligned with the states, has devised programs that are designed to assess the quality of care delivered and provide some means of cost containment for the patients enrolled in their plans. These efforts and their terminology have followed a route similar to that of quality management.

Beginning as a **utilization review** plan in 1966, local physician committees were required to review the medical necessity of care, with the main focus on reducing the patient's length of stay in the hospital. In 1972, noting the failure of utilization review to curtail rising health care costs, Congress made major changes and passed a law providing for *professional standards review organizations* (PSRO). This act emphasized cost containment and strengthened the role of individual physician's participation in developing local norms, criteria, and standards of care in a peer review process.

Many of the methods for assessing the total quality of care received by patients and identifying indicators of the quality of performance by the institution were developed under the PSRO program. This was particularly true of techniques for identifying records for *chart audits* and guidelines for utilization review committees.

Ten years later, as part of the Tax Equity and Fiscal Responsibility Act (TEFRA, 1982), the same act that ushered in DRGs, PSRO was replaced by **peer review organizations** (PRO) now renamed as **Quality Improvement Organizations** (QIOs). Under TEFRA this program moved from a local orientation to a single contracted QIO association responsible for an entire state or region. The current program is based on the QIO review of a nationwide beneficiary-specific sample representing about 10 percent of the patients enrolled in federally sponsored plans.

This action does not relieve the local hospital of conducting utilization review studies. On the contrary, this activity and its methods are still a major part of the overall quality management program of hospitals required to meet JCAHO and state standards and to defend or challenge reimbursement decisions made by the PRO.

The federally mandated PRO for each region is charged with reviewing hospital case records for quality of care and reimbursement decisions in the following areas.

1. Validity of diagnosis and suitability of services provided.
2. Completeness, adequacy, and quality of care received by the patient.
3. Necessity of admission and appropriateness of discharge.
4. Congruous care given to "outlier cases," exceptional cases because either cost-of-care or length-of-stay criteria are exceeded.
5. Appropriateness of transfer of patients between facilities.

Critical-Care Pathways

A major hospital-wide quality care management program has developed that places emphasis on the outcomes of treatment received by the patient as the definition of quality. This program, called **critical-care pathways,** or simple *care paths,* was driven by the total-care concept lessons of QA, TQM/CQI, PRO, and the specific performance improvement indicators of QA&I/CPI. This plan incorporates all the resources of the health care system into the delivery of an exact series of interventions or treatments that are to be received by the patient in a designated time period in response to a specific set of symptoms.

Under the critical-care pathways, the patient is expected to respond and progress along a specific care plan. This includes the coordination of both patient-initiated activities (eating, breathing, exercise, and so on) and treatment plans (laboratory tests, medications, x rays, physician care, and so on), usually related to a DRG classification. For example, in a patient manifesting the symptoms of pneumonia (Southwick) a chest x ray is performed within 1 hour of arrival and sputum collected for culture and evaluation within 2 hours.

Management of Quality

Many entities offer advice and programs for the management of quality in an organization. These include the promise-all, prepackaged programs designed by expensive consultants and the theory-based concepts of MBO, QA, TQM/CQI, and CPI/PI. No matter which approach the manager takes, three areas, or ingredients, must be properly aligned if the institution is to achieve its quality performance goals: (1) the philosophy or attitude of its people, (2) the operational system of the enterprise, and (3) the actual quality assessment and monitoring program in place.

The Philosophy of Quality

The attitude of the people toward their work, themselves, the organization, and their customers is reflected in how they treat each other, view their shared interest in achieving common goals, and view their professionalism in the delivery of their product or service.

The philosophy of caring and commitment to the delivery of a high-quality service starts at the very top and permeates every crevice of the institution. It is directly tied to the priorities placed on quality by the organization's leadership and is demonstrated in how managers spend their time, what attracts and consumes their attention, and to whom they issue rewards. If the proper philosophy is not present, efforts expended on the remaining two ingredients — operational and quality management systems — are wasted. Tokenism and symbolism are not character traits of quality.

Operational Systems

Quality management begins with how well managers incorporate quality practices into their management functions. Operational systems represent the actual practices taking place in an organization — not good intentions, wishes, or future plans.

Several authors, most notably the two authors Lundberg (GD) and Bozzo (P), point out that the laboratory's testing cycle begins with the doctor's request for laboratory services and continues when the information is received by the physician and new requests are issued. The laboratory must have operational systems in place that ensure that every step flows smoothly and continually toward the final delivery of a high quality service. The following model illustrates the steps in the testing cycle that are part of the operational systems and quality practices of the laboratory.

From Patient Needs to Patient Needs

Service assessment →
Physician utilization →
Service requisition →
Specimen collection →
Specimen process →
Analytical process →
Results assessment →
Information report →
Service assessment →

Quality Management Programs

Quality management programs differ from operational systems. The former address specific issues and goals and are plans for ensuring compliance or bringing about change; the latter represent the final results of all efforts and are the actual practices taking place. The wide variety of high-quality management programs available to managers includes MBO, quality circles, and, of course, the elements of —

QC/MBO → QA → TQM/CQI → QA&I/CPI/PI →? QC/MBO?

Quality management programs also include the specialized functions that are part of the technical operations of the laboratory and so crucial to the delivery of a high quality service. Ongoing activities that can be defined directly as part of quality management programs include:

- Preventive maintenance (PM)
- Policy and procedure manual writing and review
- Quality control functions
- Staff orientation, continuing education, and development
- Participation in proficiency testing
- Problem solving and troubleshooting
- Laboratory inspection, accreditation, and licensure process

Philosophy, operational systems, and quality management programs combine to create the integrity of the quality management plan. Each is crucial to the success of the laboratory in achieving its goal of delivering high quality services to its patients.

Medical Errors

The laboratory is familiar with medical errors: the origins of the "Panic, or Critical," values; INR; blood transfusion, and PAP smears are just examples. Medical Errors have become major journalistic headlines, and a primary interest to JCAHO and other healthcare accrediting agencies.

Organizational Focus

> **26 Aug 2005** — *World Health Organization officials on Tuesday announced that the Joint Commission on Accreditation of Healthcare Organizations, which inspects the safety of hospitals, and its affiliate, the Joint Commission International, will head an international effort to reduce medical errors.*
> http://www.medicalnewstoday.com/articles/29660.php
> [connected August 7, 2007]
>
> ... the all-day special topic symposium on patient safety and error reduction, entitled "Error in Pathology and Laboratory Medicine: Practical Lessons for the Pathologist," which was held at the College of American Pathologists annual meeting in Scottsdale, Ariz, on September 20, 2004.
> http://arpa.allenpress.com/arpaonline/?request=get-document&doi=10.1043%2F1543-2165(2005)129%5B1226:COAPST%5D2.0.CO%3B2
> [connected August 7, 2007]

Think this is not serous?

> **23 Jun 2007 —** Medical errors are the fifth-leading cause of deaths in the US, with up to 98,000 deaths annually.
> http://www.medicalnewstoday.com/articles/75042.php
> [connected August 7, 2007]

Number one Villain to Patient Safety

This has been an identified problem, way back into the 1980s. Why have things not progress or improved?

> Because: **The number one villain to patient safety is fear, both for themselves (healthcare workers) and for their co-workers.**

There are two exclusive Oxymorons in patient care —

That the healthcare worker will:

- DO something to harm a patient
- DO something to harm themselves or their co-workers

For these reasons two basic solutions have been proposed, but have experienced great difficulty in being implemented:

1) a "**non-punitive**" policy focusing on improvement, elimination, and prevention of errors, RATHER than the assignment of blame and punishment; and because of this failure to focus on solutions rather than blame –
2) **root-cause analysis** has been greatly hindered.

Non-Punitive Policy

Once you find out that someone has made a mistake, especially one which has endangered the health of a patient, *what do you do*? This is the dilemma faced by managers.

Even a verbal reprimand will be seen as threatening by the employee; and dismissal will surely trigger and reinforce an attitude of "not me" and cover-up by the staff; rather than encouraging an open problem solving investigation, intended to find and correct the factors which caused the incident. By taken no action toward the employee the manager will face the push from the organization and public demanding to know "*what has been done.*"

Knowing that it is unthinkable that a healthcare worker would intentional harm a patient, a solution for this dilemma is to fully investigate exactly what contributed to, or "set-up" the person to make this error. This is the tools of Root-Cause analysis. Most certainly after a through investigation there will be found problems with both the ability of the person and design factors within the institutional procedures or product which lead to the error.

Root-Cause Analysis

All of the techniques included in the chapters *on Decision Making and Problem Solving* and *Quality Assessment and Performance Improvement* are directly applicable in investigating and resolving the causes of a medical error. Emphasizing those techniques and specifically highlighting Root-Cause analysis are the focus of this section. Since the goal of this discussion is to direct the reader's attention to the availability of these resources; the definitions of error identification and characteristics of an acceptable Root-Cause analysis comprise the subject.

Definitions

Patient Safety: freedom from accidental injury

Accident: An event that involves damage to a defined system that disrupts the ongoing or future output of the system.

Adverse Event: an injury resulting from a medical intervention, or in other words, it is not due to the underlying condition of the patient.

Sentinel Event (JCAHO): an unexpected occurrence involving death or serious physical or psychological injury, or the risk thereof.

AHRQ Error: the failure of a planned action to be completed as intended or the use of a wrong plan to achieve an aim. (Agency for Healthcare Research and Quality [US department of Health and Human Services])

Quality Interagency Coordination Task Force (QuIC) Error: the failure of a planned action to be completed as intended or the use of a wrong plan to achieve an aim. Errors can be in practice, products, services, procedures, and systems.

Deviation: A one-time, random, human error.

Effectual Problem: The symptom or surface sign that may hide the real cause of a problem.

Casual Problem: The root cause of the problem

Two key concepts are extremely important in the final resolution; that is that all error possesses almost certainly have two types of failures, contributable to **both** the person **and** the institution.

- **Active Failures**: Errors made by the operators performing the processes.
- **Latent Failures** (closest thing to the Root Cause): Errors attributed to the people who influence the system but who are not active participants.

Characteristics of an Acceptable Root Cause Analysis

The characteristics of an acceptable root cause analysis (JCAHO as of Fall 1998) are provided in a checklist prepared by Jerod M. Loeb.

It must be **thorough**

- Proximate factors
- Analysis of systems and processes
- Identifies possible underlying "systemic" factors (enablers)
- Potential improvements
- Action plan
- Measurement strategy

Must be **Credible**

- Participation by leaders and those closest to the process
- Internally consistent
- Considers relevant literature

and,

- Applicable to multiple "events"
- Same "root causes" derive from different events

Failure Mode, Effects, and Criticality Analysis

One other tool mentioned often and associated with Medical Errors and Root-Cause analysis is Failure Mode, Effects, and Criticality Analysis (FMECA) [or simply (FMEA)] which declares that "Variation is Present in *ALL* Processes."

FMEA points out that there are two sources: common cause variation and special cause variation.

- Improvement strategies are determined by sources of variation.
- Process improvement comes from **elimination** of **special** cause variation and **reduction** of variation in a process. The **less** variation, the **more predictable** the result.
- Inappropriate reaction to variation leads to many negative outcomes.

In summary do not focus on finding out who made the error; but on making sure the system itself is error free

---

Medical errors conclude the discussion of *Quality Assessment and Performance Improvement*. Next: *Work Flow and Laboratory Design*.

— Case Study —

Chapter Twenty-One: Quality Assessment and Performance Improvement

"Here . . . please check these numbers before I post the QC data for the new lot numbers," said the chemistry tech, handing the supervisor the data sheets in the laboratory break room.

"Let's see. . . seems OK . . . good job," answered the supervisor, looking over the calculations. "Wait . . . it looks like there are fewer values for the BUN controls."

"Remember, we had to use the back-up procedure for the BUN at the beginning of the month, because of problems with the reagent module. We are only missing four values, I thought it would be all right."

"You need at least. . . ," said the supervisor, pausing at the laughter of another tech in the room. "What's so funny?"

"I don't know," answered the laughing tech. "It just seems that the latest quality programs quickly fade, and we always go back to basic QC."

"What do you mean?" asked the supervisor.

"You know. . . QA, TQM, Peer Review.. . now QA & I. . . I don't see why they just don't stick with what we have been doing for years. Good old SD and CV."

"Well, they're not the same . . . " the supervisor stopped as the evening shift tech came rushing into the room.

"Look at this!" complained a frustrated evening tech. "This computer rejected my control, even though I got the same number as first shift. It's not fair! The repeat was also flagged. I haven't calibrated this procedure in a long time so you'll have to stay and help me, if it must be recalibrated. Anyway, we're getting a new lot of reagents on Monday, and it has to be recalibrated then."

"Let me see," sighed the supervisor, looking at the other techs making a hasty retreat to start their weekend. "Oh, no," she thought to herself, "not this test. When will they deliver that automated method from the manufacturer?" she asked herself, as she grabbed the papers and headed toward chemistry to see what had to be done.

Chapter Sections for Review

- Historical Perspective: Quality Concepts and Terminology Transition
    - Quality Control
    - Quality Assurance
    - Total Quality Management and Continuous Quality Improvement
    - Quality Assessment and Improvement and Continuous Performance Improvement
- Utilization Review and Peer Review Organizations

- Population Sample
- Specialized Laboratory Data Evaluation Methods
    - Multi-rule Analysis, also Table 21 — 3, Westgard Rules: Figures 21 — 4 and 21 — 5, Westgard logic diagrams

Questions for Discussion

1. As a general rule, what sample size should the supervisor and tech be looking for to approve the QC data?
2. What are the main differences in each of the quality management programs mentioned by the tech? Do you agree with the comments?
3. Below are the results obtained on the last 10 runs of the controls. Which Westgard rule(s) is violated? What should the supervisor do in this case?

DATA:	Control Level I	Control Level II
MEAN:	100	200 units
SD:	3.0	5.1
Last 10 Values		
	101	203
	97	206
	103	198
	102	209
	101	200
	98	196
	96	197
	94	198
	95	204
	95 flag	201
	96 repeat flag	

Solutions

Question 1. 30

Question 3. 4_{1S}. See Figures 21 — 4 and 21 — 5 for recommended action

[22]

Work Flow and Laboratory Design

— Chapter Twenty–Two —

Work flow and laboratory design is a significant fulfillment of the planning and organizing management functions. Where the laboratory is located, how it receives and processes its specimens, the spatial relationship of each section, and the physical layout and arrangement of work areas and instruments are all factors that directly affect the operations of a laboratory. This topic is closely aligned to the subjects of work flow, work process, and the analysis of work itself reviewed in Chapter 9.

This chapter addresses the *physical,* or structural, relationships of work and the workplace and falls into the branch of management called "industrial engineering," which deals with job analysis.

Physical and structural work flow and design have two components that are recapped in this chapter: (1) the interface with customers, patients, and other users; and (2) the internal processes, or how the work is done within the laboratory itself. The concepts and topics presented in this chapter are equally applicable to all laboratory settings, including large university and reference laboratories, as well as the small workplace of a physician's office laboratory

Objectives

After completion of this chapter, the reader will be able to demonstrate accomplishment of the following objectives.

1. Evaluate and propose solutions for first directional (specimen and requisition procurement) problems in relationship to the customer interface needs of a laboratory.
2. Describe the work flow and spatial design factors that must be incorporated into the physical layout plan of the laboratory.
3. Use the tools of work flow and design in preparing a functional narrative document for a laboratory building or remodeling project.
4. Work with architectural, engineering, and construction firms in overseeing the completion of a building or remodeling project.

Chapter Highlights and Glossary of Key Terms

I. INTERFACE WITH CUSTOMERS, PATIENTS, AND OTHER USERS

Work Flow and Laboratory Design: *The planning and design of the physical and structural relationships of work and the workplace.*

A. First directional (specimen procurement) problems
B. The case for centralized laboratories

II. INTERNAL WORK PROCESSES OF THE LABORATORY

A. Flexibility and modulation
B. Functional and spatial design
C. Lean Management

III. ORGANIZING AND BUDGETING A PROJECT

A. Project design team

Project Design Team: *A group of laboratorians responsible for overseeing a workflow and laboratory design venture.*

B. Project budgeting

IV. PROJECT DESIGN AND CONSTRUCTION

A. Functional Narrative Document

Functional Narrative Document (FND): *A document prepared by the project design team to describe the purpose, functions, relationships, and activities that will be conducted in an area, with the specific goal of providing architects and engineers with the information needed to prepare the formal plans and construction agreements.*

1. FND content
2. FND preparation

Spatial Relationships: *The distance and physical structures (walls, halls, and* so *on) between two or more areas that must closely interact for the work to be completed.*

Bubble Drawings: *A series of circles (or bubbles) that represent a function or area and depict the flow of information and work tasks by using lines and arrows to show direction and connections in the relationships.*

Block and Schematic Drawings: *Variations of floor plans and sketches that are to be used as the preliminary edition of the schematic design drawing*

Department Relationship Matrix: *A matrix technique for illustrating and defining how each section or function interacts with other areas.*

Building Models: *Lifelike, built-to-scale replicas or color-coded blocks that represent people, counters, furniture, and instruments; that can be moved around on a floor graph to display a variety of configurations and design options.*

B. Architectural and engineering documents

1. Graphical depiction documents

a. Schematic drawings

Schematic Drawings: *The descriptive title given to the first attempt and draft of how the architects have interpreted the information provided them in the FND.*

b. Design development drawings

Design Development Drawings: *A preliminary floor plan or blueprint draft that includes construction details and layout patterns.*

2. Working drawings and project manual

Working Drawings: *The final blueprints that will be used for construction of the project.*

Project Manual: *A document that contains the working drawings and detailed information on the types of building material and construction techniques to be used, informally called the "spec book. "*

Construction Guidelines Proposal: *An edition of the project manual supplied to vendors to prepare construction and material bids on the project.*

Bibliography: Work Flow and Laboratory Design

Interface with Customers, Patients, and Other Users

The laboratory must interact in two directions with patients, clients, and other users of its services: (1) the intake or requisition of specimens and requests for services; and (2) the return of information and results. The resolution of these directional problems usually determines the geographical service base of a laboratory.

The second of these directions, the return of information and results, has for all practical purposes been resolved. What this means is that with worldwide instant telecommunications, computer linkage, and a fax machine, the physical proximity of the laboratory is of no relevance when it comes to releases results. The other direction [specimen (*first*) intake] is, of course, another story.

First Directional (Specimen Procurement) Problems

The laboratory is a relatively unusual entity in health care — it does not need direct contact with the patient. Specimens can be collected and transported to the lab either by laboratory personnel or by intermediaries. This feature has made the laboratory the center of efforts to consolidate health care services. Up to this point, the time involved in delivering the specimen to the testing site has made in-house laboratories the most viable option for inpatient testing. However, this is changing because of improvements in delivery systems and collection routes.

- Technological advances will bring about changes in both satellite and centralized laboratories. Ease of use and modularity make it possible to perform tests at the patient's bedside and in near-care areas such as operating and emergency rooms, intensive care units, and physicians' offices. Then again, the improved cost-benefit economics of procedures and profiling instruments continue to support centralized centers.
- Drawing stations placed at strategic locations in the hospital (outpatient departments, oncology, admissions) and in satellite facilities (physicians' offices, shopping centers, walk-in clinics) permit the laboratory to control the collection and delivery of specimens.
- Overnight or same-day delivery services eliminate the need for physical proximity of the laboratory. As a result, the local lab is feeling increased competitive pressures from regional and national laboratories seeking to attract additional clients.

We can also expect increased application of robotics in the laboratory. Writing in *MT today,* Denise Leathers (**1993**) describes just one situation in which robotics is being explored in the laboratory and may serve to presage the future:

> At the University of Virginia . . . laboratorians are experimenting with a robotics center in the ICU. A nurse draws a blood sample, then hands it over to the robotics unit, which actually performs the tests. Results are transferred back to the central lab via computer link. Medical technologists review the results to ensure proper quality control. They approve the results and release them to the unit. (p. 13)

Bringing us up-to-date on robotic automation Ron Berman (**2006**) points out that: "*By the end of 2005, about 25 percent of large hospitals in the United States had purchased some form of automation for their laboratories*." Add the introduction of Autoverification, even the delay created from the tech's review of results before release, is being eliminated.

The Case for Centralized laboratories

Although the benefits of near-care testing are tremendous, especially in remedying space and logistical problems, it does not offer a panacea. Accessibility and cost-of-care concerns will continue to have a major impact on the delivery of health care services. For this reason the manager must carefully weigh the advantages and disadvantages in each service option.

The centralized laboratory with enhanced specimen intake strategies will remain a viable delivery mechanism. Once immediate STAT and triage concerns are satisfied, specimen procurement becomes mainly a transportation problem.

The case for a centralized laboratory is strong. Economies of scale are possible in a centralized lab, which can handle a large volume of tests and afford the highly efficient, though costly, profiling instruments and the well-trained staff necessary to run such equipment.

Managers must pay attention to the marketing of laboratory services (i.e., convenience, public visibility, ability to attract clients) as well as the timely receipt and delivery of specimens at the testing site.

Internal Work Processes of the Laboratory

The laboratory, as part of the health care community, will continue to undergo an explosion of change. A whole array of work flow and design factors must be incorporated into the physical layout of the laboratory, including planning for known and anticipated needs as well as possible use for an entirely different purpose in the future. Laboratory areas may need to be adapted during the life of the building to totally unrelated functions because of changes in technology or service needs. Sound planning reinforces the value and justification of a building or remodeling project.

Flexibility and Modulation

The literature on work flow and laboratory design centers around two closely related concepts: flexibility and modulation. Flexibility in design and physical layout allows the laboratory to readily adapt to changing space needs. Modulation in the structural components enables the laboratory to achieve flexibility.

These two principles, flexibility and modulation, should imbue each stage of the design and planning process, including decisions about floor space and room size, cabinetry, electricity, plumbing, ventilation, and even the movability of the walls. Plumbing (sinks, drains, pipes, and so on) used to severely limit the rearrangement of an area; however, with new grid installation methodology similar to the electrical ceiling matrices now available, even plumbing designs can contribute to the flexibility of a space.

Functional and Spatial Design

The goal of planning the physical and structural aspects of work flow and laboratory design is optimal productivity. The space should enhance the work being performed and adapt to the needs of the people rather than being an impediment that must be adapted to.

With this goal in mind, work flow and laboratory design deals with the spatial relationships between people, equipment, supplies, and the traffic generated by laboratory activities.

For optimum functioning, laboratory design must take into account the following factors.

- *Space allocation* (in square feet) for the tasks to be performed, with sufficient room for personnel, equipment, supplies, patients, and the traffic generated by the activities involved.
- *Ergonomic planning* of cabinetry and workstations for enhanced productivity
- Placement of *utilities* — plumbing, ventilation, lighting, electrical outlets for computers and other equipment.
- *Traffic flow* of personnel, equipment, and patients.
- Sufficiency and convenience of *storage areas.*
- *Safety equipment and design,* including ventilation, showers, egress, containment and disposal of hazardous waste, and a changing area for removal of contaminated clothing and protective equipment.
- *Staff facilities* such as lavatories, locker rooms, and eating areas.

These factors must be considered in light of the guidelines and regulations of accreditation and licensure agencies.

Lean Management

A discipline which attempts to bring tools to work flow and space design is **lean management**. Lean management traces its principles from Toyota® and Ford® (Taichi Ohno) and many of its actual techniques from the time-motion studies of industrial Engineering (Chapter 1). It is based on eliminating "waste:" waste in time (work flow), motion, effort/energy, space, and costs (Ohno's 7Ws).

- **Defect** – do it right the first time.
- **Over-Production** – doing tests not necessary or clinically indicated (Diffs, Urine Microscopy, repeat testing).
- **Waiting** – e.g., Tech's waiting for samples to be collected/received; samples setting in racks waiting on one test to be done, before carry it to another station (UA, before Culture or Drug Screen).
- **Transporting** – unnecessary movement, sample having to be carried a long way (down several halls, different stations) to be processed.
- **Movement** – Supplies not handy; extra/unnecessary steps in the testing process; production stops required to do routine calibrations of test before processing (e.g., calibrations expiring during evening/night shifts or morning run).
- **Inappropriate processing** – do only what is necessary
- **Inventory** – eliminate back orders, forgotten orders; "just-in-time" material management (chapter 15).

(Note: Suggestions for the work flow concerns of the actual, live, ongoing processing of the work in the laboratory [*micromanagement of work*], may be reviewed under the General Comments on Staffing and Scheduling section of Chapter 19: Staffing and Scheduling – *p. 325*).

Organizing and Budgeting a Project

Work flow and laboratory design involves four stages: organization, which includes the management planning process; written narrative description; budgeting; and graphical displays. These four stages can be further divided into two phases: the internal aspects of planning and budgeting for a project and the process of working with architectural, engineering, and construction firms to bring the project to fruition. Although parts of these phases are going on simultaneously, the laboratory should have a good idea of its needs, preferences, and financial resources before approaching outside agencies.

Skills necessary for a manager to guide a project from inception to completion have been presented throughout this book. Principles of leadership (Chapter 7), management of work groups (Chapter 8), communications (Chapter 3), and decision-making and problem-solving skills (Chapter 4) are key elements in organizing the project design team and developing a budget.

> **Bibliography: Work Flow and Laboratory Design**
> Because of the many building regulations and rules, both governmental and professional construction standards, several references pertaining to specific guidelines for laboratories are included at the end of the chapter for the reader's consultation as needed.

Project Design Team

A **project design team** should include both laboratorians and construction specialists. The team should solicit input from pathologists, technical and administrative managers, clinical scientists, supervisors, and especially the bench-level staff who will work in the area. It is also important to obtain suggestions and advice from those who will be actively interfacing with the users; namely, phlebotomists, clerical staff, and supply stock personnel. Once the design team is in place and information has been gathered and prepared, it is time to meet with the architects and engineers who will be working on the project.

Project Budgeting

The budgeting process is detailed in Part 3 of the text. Chapter 16 reviews the preparation of the capital budget and contains specific tools and techniques for justifying and preparing a budget for expensive and long-term projects such as building or remodeling a laboratory. Capital budget topics that are pertinent for building and renovation plans are the narrative and quantitative tools of analysis and justification for a capital expenditure.

Although the internal project planning process is quite similar to other management functions, a manager may be somewhat intimidated by the language and techniques used to put the plans on paper and deal with the formal documents of the building profession. For this purpose, the next section offers a description of the types of documents, graphical displays, terminology, and steps that are common in most professionally designed construction projects.

Project Design and Construction

Like all professions, the building trade has a wide variety of documents and visual aids that can be used for planning, contracting, and constructing a project. Computer simulation programs have reached the point in which real life pictures and scale models can easily be produced to demonstrate how different options and decisions affect the final structure.

From conception to production of the final construction models and contracts, several steps or phases are common to most project plans (Table 22 – 1). Much of this work may be overseen in cooperation with the engineering department for hospital-based laboratories. In a large multi-hospital system, the corporation may have a separate architectural and construction division assume responsibility for the project.

Development and Review Process	
Phase 1:	Laboratory responsibility • Functional narrative document • Initial schematic drawings
Phase 2:	Architectural and engineering responsibility • Design development drawings • Final working drawings • Project manual
Phase 3:	Construction

Table 22 — 1. Work Flow and Laboratory Design Project

The manager should be familiar with the functional narrative document, graphical depictions, and the contract documents produced in cooperation with the architect.

Functional Narrative Document

The **functional narrative document (FND)** describes the purpose, functions, relationships, and activities of the area under consideration. It is prepared by the project design team for the engineers so that they can prepare formal plans and construction agreements.

This is a crucial planning stage. The temptation to skip or shortchange is strong in the excitement of drawing floor plans and getting on with describing the new desirable features. However, careful planning at this point avoids mistakes and costly corrections later in the process.

This phase is also strikingly similar to the process of planning and designing a laboratory information system (LIS; see Chapter 17). Many of the steps, techniques, and process analysis methods are the same. In each process, attention to detail at the earliest planning stage is a key factor in the success of the project.

FND Content

Specific detailed information must be provided in the functional narrative document about space, spatial relationships, utilities, lighting, ventilation, and so on. These factors can be organized by discipline (hematology, chemistry) or function (clerical, specimen processing, supply storage, waste disposal, personnel lounges), but each component must be addressed. The following list contains a sample of the topics that should be reviewed in the FND:

- Types of tasks and movements, especially in terms of space and coordinated efforts.
- Volume of activities including the amount of traffic generated by the number of tests performed, supply restocking, specimen processing, telephone and other communication transactions, and the movement of people.
- The nature and structural needs (power, utilities, counter space, protective equipment such as hoods and safety showers, waste disposal, and so on) of the tests and procedures to be performed in the area.
- The kinds of instruments and equipment that will be present and their space specification.
- Communication links both inside and outside the laboratory, including telephone, intercom, fax machines, and all parts of the LIS.
- The number of personnel and the staffing patterns (24-hour coverage, number of persons on each shift, and so on) and their support needs. This includes space for activities such as break areas, work-stations, lavatories, changing areas for protective clothing, and the possible need for sleeping or resting facilities in case extended coverage is required. (For example, the spatial needs of a couple of techs running the lab on the night shift are usually quite different from those of the day staff).
- Supply requirements in consideration of requisitioning, storage, and dispensing.
- Detailed description of the plans for the computer system (LIS) including wiring, location of the central processing unit and terminals, as well as outside linkage.

Much of the information needed in preparing the FND will come from members of the project team and through interviews with the architects and engineers involved in the project.

FND Preparation

Information about most of the items in the FND is readily available in the laboratory or easily obtained from an architect. Sources for the information are historical workload data, charts showing minimum square footage allocation and structural requirements for people and equipment, manufacturer installation specification manuals, and code enforcement regulations. However, spatial relationships must be evaluated for each situation.

Spatial relationships are the distance and physical structures (walls, halls, and so on) between two or more areas that must closely interact for the work to be completed. For example, spatial relationships may hinder or expedite the flow of specimens within the laboratory. If a sample must travel down two halls or pass through several other sections before being delivered, these spatial relationships must be planned into the work flow and design of the laboratory. This factor is even more pronounced in the case of pediatric specimens or tests that are dependent on the completion of other procedures.

Koenig (AS) offers several ways to incorporate spatial relationships into the functional narrative document, including bubble, block, and schematic drawings and the department relationship matrix. These techniques demonstrate the extent of interaction between each section or laboratory function.

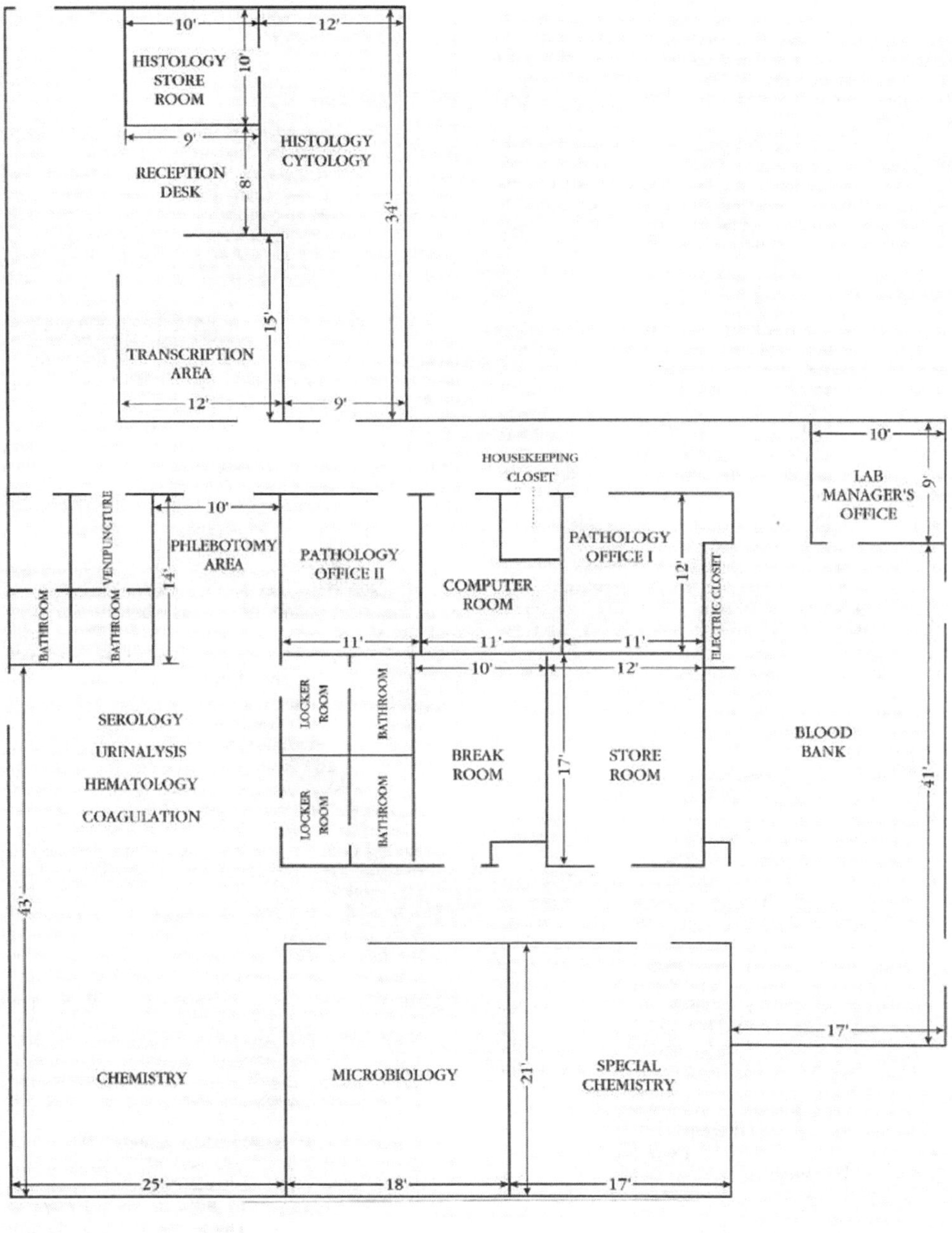

Figure 22 – 1. Initial schematic drawing (floor-plan sketch)

Bubble drawings are a series of circles, or bubbles, that represent a function or area (e.g., specimen processing, hematology) and depict the flow of information and work tasks using lines and arrows to show the direction and connections in the relationships. They are similar to the flow charts described in Chapter 17, but much less formal, allowing both the laboratorian and the architect to describe and experiment with work flow and design options.

Block and schematic drawings are preliminary floor plans or sketches (Fig. 22 – 1), representing the first efforts of the architect to put the functional narrative document on paper. Like the bubble drawings, they are intended to be used to explore alternate layouts without regard to traditional boundaries and space limitations. They start out as very rough sketches, gradually increasing in refinement to include scale and structural details as the model progresses and layout decisions are made.

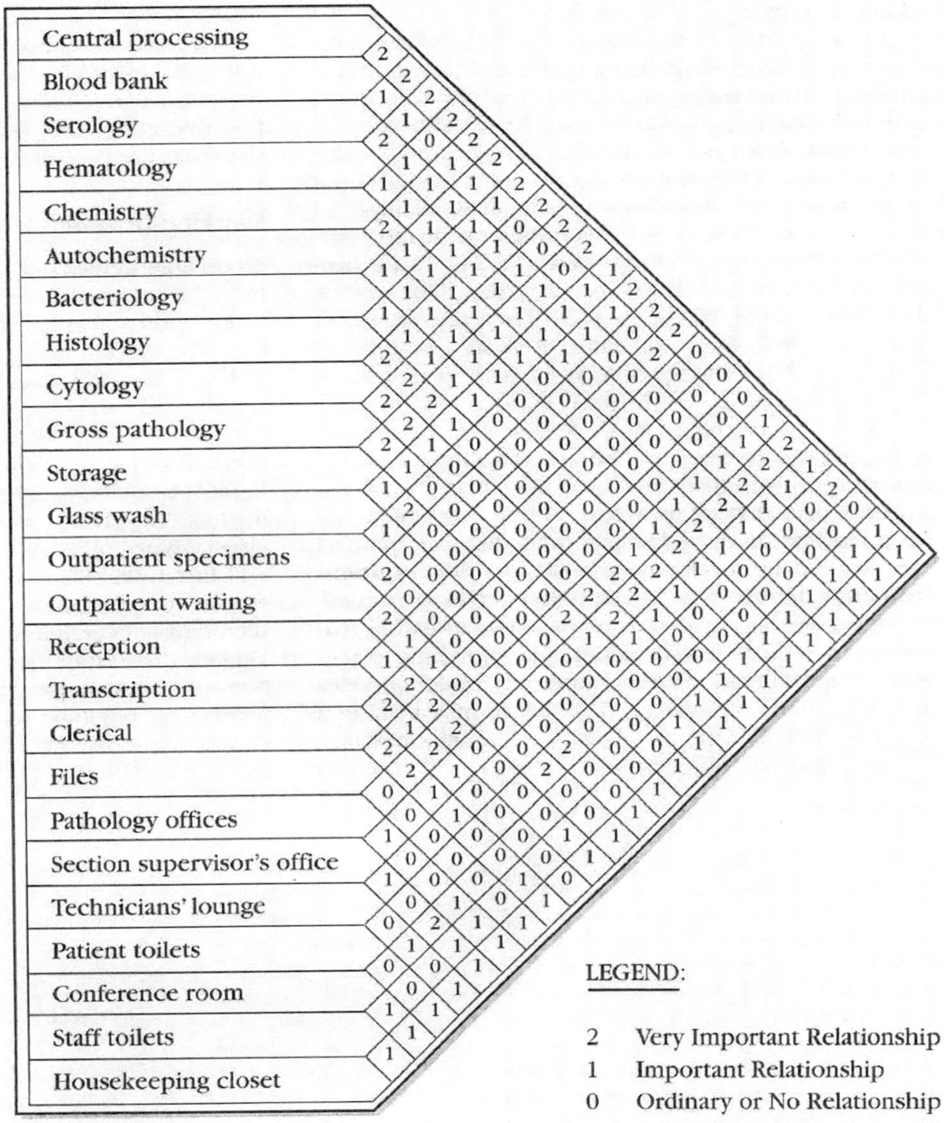

Figure 22 – 2. Department relationship matrix

(From the Laboratory Function and Design Committee, Koenig, AS [Chairman]; Medical Laboratory Planning and Design, Skokie, IL. College of American Pathologists, 1985, p. 41, with permission.)
see also DiBerardinis et. al., p. 15

The **department relationship matrix** (Fig. 22 – 2) shows areas that interact and also quantifies the degree of coordination involved in the interaction. This allows the design team to set priorities in space and location arrangement and in determining the spatial and structural characteristics of the facility.

In addition to line drawings, miniature building block modules can be used to try out various structural arrangements and layouts. The **building models** may be lifelike, built-to-scale replicas or color-coded blocks that represent people, counters, furniture, and instruments. Components can be moved around on a floor graph to display a variety of configurations and design options.

The functional narrative document is an extensive, detailed package covering all aspects of the work flow and project design. It is intended to give the architects a comprehensive overview of the purposes, functions, and needs of the user and provide the information needed to prepare the initial schematic design drawings of the facility. These drawings also go through several revisions before being given to the construction company.

The review and revision process (See Table 22 – 1_{above}) may be summarized in three graphic phases critiqued in the next section from the point at which the architect receives the FND until agreement is reached on the final blueprints and construction documents.

Architectural and Engineering Documents

Upon receipt of the functional narrative document, the architects and engineers assume direct responsibility for preparation of the formal construction plans.
The laboratory — and frequently regulatory agencies — is asked to review, approve, and sign off on each phase of the design process as it progresses through the graphical depiction documents to the final approval and issuance of a project manual.

Graphical Depiction Documents

Graphical design documents commonly go through three editions or phases before completion: the initial schematic drawings of the facility developed from the functional narrative document; design development drawings, from which building codes and material specifications can be prepared; and the final working drawings, or blueprints, that will be used for construction.

Schematic Drawings

Although the functional narrative document frequently contains sketches of floor plans, **schematic drawings** are the first attempts of the architects to interpret the information in the FND.

Schematic design drawings (see Fig. 22 – 1_{above}) are usually straightforward, single-line drawings that outline the various areas of the project. They are drawn to scale with preliminary estimates of square footage allotments and key elements such as instruments, sinks, and workstations outlined. These drawings are used by the laboratory and architect to review how the project is shaping up, correct any misunderstandings, and correct any problems that have been identified.

Design Development Drawings

When agreement has been reached on the schematic drawings, the architect can proceed to developing the **design development drawings.** In this stage, construction details are added, including specific space layout patterns, structural features and requirements, utilities and plumbing placement, ventilation and airflow plans, and building codes and regulations compliance. This phase may include a full-scale model of the project as well as line drawings.

From this point on, it becomes increasingly costly to make changes because of the professional time and research already invested in the project. For this reason, it is crucial that all aspects of the project be extensively reviewed and double-checked for agreement by both the laboratory and architect before the final working drawings are prepared.

Working Drawings and Project Manual

Once final agreement has been obtained from all parties, the architects complete the **working drawings,** or blueprints, that are used for construction of the project. The design process culminates in a **project manual or construction guidelines proposal,** which contains the working drawings and detailed information on the types of building materials and construction techniques to be used. Informally called the "spec book," it includes specific, itemized information and instructions about *everything:* construction schedule targets; types of wiring, light fixtures, carpet, cabinetry, and furniture; ceiling heights; wallpaper patterns; decorative details; door knobs; cement reinforcement; plumbing — everything, down to and including the kitchen sink. From these final documents the construction project can be completed, and because of the meticulous planning that has taken place, the laboratory workers will be able to enjoy their new facilities and achieve their goal of better patient care.

The documents and steps which are used in professionally designed construction projects concluded this chapter. The next chapter examines the *Regulatory and Professional Oversight* of the medical laboratory.

Bibliography: Work Flow and Laboratory Design

Because of the many building regulations and rules, both governmental and professional construction standards, several references pertaining to specific guidelines for laboratories are included here for the reader's consultation as needed.

Committee on Design, Construction, and Renovation of Laboratory Facilities; Laboratory Design, Construction, and Renovation; National Academy Press, Washington, D.C.; 2000

DiBerardinis, Louis and Janet S. Baum, Melvin W. First, Gari T. Gatwood, and Anand K. Seth; Guidelines for Laboratory Design 3rd edition; A. John Wiley & Sons, New York, 2001

Griffin, Brain; Laboratory Design Guide 3rd edition; Elsvier (Architectural Press), Boston; 2005

— Case Study —

Chapter Twenty-Two: Work Flow and Laboratory Design

"I wonder who designed this lab," expressed a frustrated tech, trying to find room to store the shipment of supplies that had just arrived. "Must have been someone who never worked in a lab, or it was built in the stone age!"

"I know what you mean," added another tech, attempting to locate a place to put up the new Performance Improvement charts, suggested by the hospital's quality leader.

"Just the people I'm looking for!" The two techs turned in surprise toward the sudden voice speaking behind them, and saw the smiling laboratory manager.
"We just got approval to remodel this part of the laboratory, and I need some volunteers to be on the project design team. We're meeting in my office at eleven o'clock. I'd appreciate it if you would join us then. See you?"

Chapter Sections for Review

- Internal Work Process of the Laboratory
- Project Design Team
- Functional Narrative Document
    - FND Content
    - FND

Questions for Discussion

1. Can the students think of similar situations with which they may be familiar and reasons for the problems present (i.e., functional spatial design problems: e.g., space, traffic flow, safety).
2. Prepare an outline of an FND for a laboratory or section in which the students may be interested, including a draft of the initial schematic design drawing (i.e., floor plan), covering the issues listed in the FND content description.

[23]

Regulatory and Professional Oversight

— Chapter Twenty–Three —

Encounters with regulatory and professional agencies begin with our very first introductions to the medical laboratory and continue throughout our professional careers. Checking into career options and professional qualifications introduces the potential student to the agglomeration of agencies and acronyms that affect the laboratory profession. CAP, ASCP, NCA, CLIA'88, HCFA, AABB, JCAHO, CDC, and CLSI are only some national groups; in addition are a number of state agencies.

Laboratorians gain familiarity with the credentialing, licensing, and accreditation process early in their career and gain expertise in compliance during the performance of their technical duties. This chapter presents a broad overview of the regulatory, inspection, accreditation, and credentialing process from a management perspective.

It provides a survey of general legal issues common to all health care providers, regulation and licensure of medical laboratories by governmental agencies, professional personnel certification, and laboratory inspection and accreditation programs.

Objectives

After completion of this chapter, the reader will be able to demonstrate accomplishment of the following objectives.

1. Explain the workplace environment and social forces directing the legal and professional surveillance of medical laboratories.
2. Recognize past efforts, present requirements, and future directions in the regulation and licensure of medical laboratories by governmental agencies.
3. Identify key elements of CLIA'88 as they apply to the reader's laboratory situation.
4. Describe current professional personnel certification and laboratory accreditation programs.

Chapter Highlights and Glossary of Key Terms

I. WORKPLACE LEGAL ISSUES
- A. Records and documentation
- B. Professional standards
  Peer and Community Review Standards: *Level of service expectations and standards of care applied in the legal system to establish or disprove malpractice in specific geographical and practice situations.*
- C. Properly qualified and trained personnel
- D. Malpractice

__Malpractice:__ Incorrect performance or improper conduct on the part of a purveyor, especially professionals, either through negligence or by a violation of ethical standards for the business or profession.

__Tort:__ A willful and harmful act (e.g., malpractice), not involving a contract, which can result in a civil law suit.

E. Professional liability insurance for laboratorians

II. REGULATION AND LICENSURE OF MEDICAL LABORATORIES

__Regulation:__ A rule or requirement imposed by a government agency.

__Licensure:__ Government permission to operate or engage in a business practice or occupation, usually requiring some type of formal training and/or testing to demonstrate competency.

A. Federal regulation of medical laboratories

B. CLIA'88

__Clinical Laboratory Improvement Amendments of__ **1988** *__(CLIA'88):__ Federal law governing the conduct and practice of medical laboratories as of 1988.*

1. Complexity classification of laboratories
2. Classification criteria
3. Practice standards for moderate-complexity and high-complexity laboratories
   a. Certificate of waiver or registration
   b. Quality control and quality assurance
   c. Patient test management
   d. Inspection
4. Personnel qualifications for moderate-complexity and high-complexity laboratories

C. State regulation of the medical laboratory

III. PROFESSIONAL PERSONNEL CERTIFICATION AND LABORATORY INSPECTION AND ACCREDITATION PROGRAMS

A. Laboratory inspection and accreditation programs

__Accreditation:__ Certification, usually by a professional organization, that designated standards have been achieved.

1. Joint Commission on the Accreditation of Healthcare Organizations
2. College of American Pathologists
3. American Association of Blood Banks

B. Professional certification of laboratory personnel

__Credentialing:__ The process of establishing qualifications to perform a duty or job, usually through the formal recognition of professional or technical competence to an institution or person as having met certain requirements or standards.

__Certification:__ The process of establishing and declaring that a person has met the standards established by a professional organization or commercial service.

Workplace Legal Issues

The "litigious society" refers to this society's propensity for resolving disagreements and conflicts through the court system rather than through traditional routes of family, church, and social discourse. This trend is particularly pronounced in business relations and is rapidly infecting the health care community. Legal actions involving business and customers, employer and employee, professional and client, physician or health care provider and patient, and now even attorney and client are flooding the already jammed court docket.

The laboratory itself is not immune to litigation. Actually, the laboratory's involvement in legal cases is growing because of the value placed on test results in resolving conflicts over the quality of care patients may have received from their physician. For this reason laboratorians are being subpoenaed as witnesses for both sides of a case.

Even though legal issues may be handled by a risk management department or the counsel retained for this purpose; managers should be aware of certain things in order to protect themselves, their staffs, and the laboratory from legal problems. As well as the sound management and professional strategies described throughout this book, managers should pay particular attention to records and documentation, the qualifications and training of personnel, malpractice, developments in the tort and legal system, and personal liability insurance.

Records and Documentation

An almost audible groan can be heard as the reader contemplates this first topic — an indication of the general recognition of the importance of this point. Good records are a major element of sound management and good legal defense. An old inspection adage, familiar to all laboratorians, states: "If it is not written down, it is not done." The same is true in legal matters.

Professional Standards

The courts have long held the concept of professional standards as the measure against which performance, customer expectations, service complaints, and damage assessment can be measured. This principle is reflected in **peer and community review standards** common to a broad range of situations, including product performance, claim satisfaction, and the quality of care received by a patient as compared with the level of service offered by the business' peers.

A major way the laboratory can demonstrate compliance with peer and community review standards is through participation in accreditation programs such as those offered by CAP, ASCP, and JCAHO, as well as by meeting the criteria for licensure.

Properly Qualified and Trained Personnel

Closely aligned with professional standards are the selection and training of the laboratory staff. It is one thing to have documentation of how work is to be done. But if the personnel do not follow these guidelines or are not prepared to meet the standards detailed in the procedure manual, the laboratory is especially vulnerable to charges of malpractice.

There are two sides to the personnel issue: how the employees actually perform their duties; and how they interact with and treat clients. Numerous studies have shown that the number of litigation claims filed against an individual or organization is directly tied to customer or client treatment. If the relationship is courteous, friendly, and satisfaction-oriented, the probability of a claim being filed is greatly reduced. Training employees in customer relations appears to be one of the better ways to decrease lawsuits.

Malpractice

Malpractice is defined as incorrect performance or improper conduct on the part of a purveyor, especially a professional, either through negligence or by violating ethical and professional standards. Malpractice can be difficult to determine, fraught with controversy, and open to disputed interpretations. For this reason, the courts apply professional peer and community review standards to the particulars of the situation to determine if the patient or client has been a victim of malpractice. Closely align with malpractice is the "tort system'" A **Tort** is a willful and harmful act (e.g., malpractice), not involving a contract, which can result in a civil law suit

As the litigious society continues to expand, the probability grows that laboratorians will be called on either to defend their performance or to testify in another type of case. Having a sense of control and comfort with the legal system is a big advantage, either as a defendant or as a witness. The key to achieving this familiarity is to work closely with the attorney representing the case, making sure that each stage of the process is fully explained and understood, and to know what to expect. Obtaining counsel and practicing for testimony are especially crucial in preparing to be a witness or giving a disposition.

Professional Liability Insurance for Laboratorians

Do laboratorians need professional liability insurance? Some say that it is not necessary because the employee is most likely already covered under the policy of the organization, and there is very little probability of the employee's being named as a defendant because the jury may base an award on the financial worth of the worker rather than on that of the corporation.

But attorneys are actually paid by and represent the *company,* leaving the employee vulnerable and basically without legal representation in situations in which the potential financial liability can be staggering. The cost is almost negligible compared with the potential risks [$193 annual premium quoted on June 26, 2007 through ASCP (Lockton Companies) for a Medical Lab Technician: $1 Million per incident/$3 Million annual aggregate].

Regulation and Licensure of Medical Laboratories

Government rules and regulations include labor relations, OSHA, and rules affecting the general conduct of business. Many of these laws and regulations were covered in previous sections (see chapters on Human Resource Management and Laboratory Safety). This section focuses on direct governmental monitoring of the laboratory's professional practice.

Federal and state government **regulations** and **licensure** include rules that regulate the laboratory facility itself and rules that establish the professional credentials of the technical staff.

Federal Regulation of Medical Laboratories

The federal government generally exercises its authority to regulate medical facilities through the financial reimbursement process for medical services. The catch 22 of this approach is that, although a laboratory may not be "required" to meet the rules promulgated by federal agencies, if it wishes to deliver and be paid for services to patients in federal programs, it must meet their criteria.

The federal process of validation is usually referred to as registration and certification of laboratories, although there are instances in which federal licenses are issued. The terminology of actual *licensure* of laboratories (i.e., permission to engage in a business activity) and personnel (i.e., permission to practice an occupation) is generally considered a function of local and state entities. Federal oversight of laboratories is encompassed in CLIA'88.

The first efforts by the federal government to regulate medical laboratories can be traced to the enactment of Medicare legislation in 1965 as an amendment to the Social Security Act and the provisions to monitor the quality of care received by its beneficiaries in hospitals and other health care facilities.

Shortly thereafter, in 1967, the first edition of the Clinical Laboratory Improvement Act (CLIA'67) became law. Although administration of Medicare was carried out through regional and local peer review programs such as PSRO and PRO (see Chapter 21), CLIA'67 was at first centralized under the control of the Centers for Disease Control (CDC) in Atlanta and applied to laboratories that processed more than 100 specimens per year in interstate commerce (i.e., specimens that crossed state lines). For this reason, CLIA'67 usually affected only large, independent laboratories because most hospitals and physicians' offices performed tests only on their own patients or for clients in a relatively restricted geographical area.

In 1988, CLIA was revised and became the Clinical Laboratory Improvement Amendments of 1988 (CLIA'88). These amendments were enacted to revise and expand the authority of both CLIA'67 and Medicare and Medicaid provisions. Further revisions were made as part of the FDA Modernization Act of 1997.

An updated CLIA was needed because of growing evidence of fraud and errors in test procedures and results. There was considerable confusion and overlap in the rules and regulations of various agencies, so CLIA'88 was also a major consolidation of regulations.

CLIA'88

CLIA'88 classifies and regulates laboratories based on the complexity of procedures being performed rather than on location, as under previous rules, and establishes personnel qualifications. CLIA'88 rules were also expanded to apply to all testing sites; however, they do allow generous waivers for many procedures and levels of testing complexity. Table 23 — 1 highlights the main provisions of CLIA'88; the complexity categories and personnel qualification guidelines are outlined in the following sections. The reader is also referred to the bibliography for more extensive coverage. Especially recommended are the 11 articles written by Richard B. Passey and published in *Medical Laboratory Observer* from August 1992 through July 1993.

1. Classifies laboratories based on the complexity of procedures performed
   - Low-complexity (waved) testing
   - Moderate-complexity testing
   - High-complexity testing
   - Provider-performed microscopy procedures (PPMP)
2. Sets personnel qualifications for six groups
   - Director
   - Technical consultant
   - Technical supervisor
   - Clinical consultant
   - General supervisor
   - Testing personnel
3. Rules apply to all testing sites
4. Baccalaureate laboratorians at four levels
   - Director (moderate-complexity testing
   - Technical consultant
   - General/technical supervisor
   - Testing personnel

Table 23 — 1. Highlights of CLIA'88

The latest update on CLIA'88 issued by CDC may be found on the following website, which includes particulars of the law itself as well as access to chronological, demographics and regulations.

> CDC: Current CLIA Regulations
> (including all changes through 01/24/2004)
> http://wwwn.cdc.gov/clia/regs/toc.aspx
> "page last reviewed: 7/7/2004" [connected July 26, 2007]

Complexity Classification of Laboratories

The regulations implementing CLIA'88 separate laboratories according to complexity, as follows:

- Category 1: waived tests, considered to have a low-complexity testing methodology
- Category 2: moderate-complexity testing methodology
- Category 3: high-complexity testing methodology
- Category 4: provider-performed microscopy procedures (PPMP)

Each level has specific rules governing the types of tests that can be performed, level of proficiency testing and quality management monitoring required, and designated personnel standards. The procedures that can be performed by each category of laboratory are limited to those specifically listed by the Department of Health and Human Services (DHHS).

Tests in the waived categories consist mainly of procedures like dipstick or tablet urinalysis, occult blood, non-automated Sed Rates, pregnancy test kits based on color comparison methodology, and blood glucose analyzers for home use. In conjunction with the tests listed in the waived category, a group of procedures may be performed personally by a physician or other health care practitioner, such as a midwife, nurse practitioner, or physician assistant. Provider-performed microscopy procedures (PPMP) include wet mounts, KOH (potassium hydroxide) preps, pinworm examinations, and urine microscopes.

Classification Criteria

DHHS uses seven criteria to differentiate tests that may be performed by moderate-complexity laboratories and high-complexity laboratories. Each test or procedure is scored on a scale of 1 to 3, with 3 the highest level of complexity. These seven criteria are:

1. The level of knowledge needed
2. Training and experience required
3. Complexity of the preparation of reagents and materials
4. Operational steps required in the procedure
5. Characteristics and availability of calibration, quality control, and proficiency testing material
6. Extent of troubleshooting and maintenance required
7. Degree of interpretation and judgment necessary in the testing process

Two *very* frequent qualifiers found in the moderate complexity category are (1) "automated procedures that do not require operator intervention during the analytic process" and (2) "manual procedures with limited steps and with limited sample or reagent preparation." This differentiation allows a moderate-complexity laboratory to perform a manual white cell differential without identification of atypical cells and assigns more definitive procedures, such as microbial identification and susceptibility and blood bank compatibility testing, to high-complexity laboratories.

Practice Standards for Moderate-Complexity and High-Complexity Laboratories

CLIA'88 rules set minimum standards and requirements for laboratory practice in seven areas for moderate complexity and high-complexity laboratories. Facilities performing only waived or PPMP tests are generally exempt from these rules; however, they must maintain records of the types and volume of tests performed. Specific requirements must be met in the following areas: certification, proficiency testing, quality control, quality assurance, patient test management, inspection, and personnel.

Certificate of Waiver or Registration

All laboratories are initially required to obtain either a certificate of waiver or a registration certificate from the Health Care Financing Administration (HCFA). They must also participate successfully in proficiency testing (PT) programs for each specialty and subspecialty in which they perform tests. As part of any PT program, documentation of remedial action is expected whenever acceptable performance (usually 80 percent) is not achieved.

Quality Control and Quality Assurance

Quality control and quality assurance standards are similar to those established by the practice parameters of the professional laboratorian, as reviewed in the chapter on Quality Assessment and Performance Improvement. Close adherence to the manufacturers' instructions when using prepackaged test kits, reagents, and instruments and detailed documentation of procedures when modifying or using in-house methods are CLIA'88 guidelines recommended by all laboratory associations.

QC and QA requirements also include the preparation of a procedure manual, calibration of procedures at least twice a year, a minimum of two levels of controls each day of use, and the establishment of a comprehensive QA program for monitoring the overall quality of the testing process. Following manufacturers' instructions on such products as FDA-approved test kits and instruments meets most of the general QC requirements of CLIA'88.

Patient Test Management

Patient test management covers the system designed to protect the integrity of specimens and the reporting of accurate results. It provides regulations regarding the following aspects of practice: processing and receiving service requisitions; specimen integrity in submission, handling, and referring; and the issuance and maintenance of results and records.

Inspection

CLIA'88 requires that both records and facilities of certified laboratories be available for unannounced inspection to check for compliance with its rules and regulations. These inspections are to be conducted on a biannual basis, either by DHHS or by a designated representative such as a state agency or approved accreditation program.

Details of specific CLIA'88 rules and compliance guidelines in each of the seven areas are available from regulations published by DHHS in the *Federal Register* and by the proliferation of articles, booklets, and other publications issued by laboratory journals and associations to assist in complying with these requirements.

Personnel Qualifications for Moderate-Complexity and High-Complexity Laboratories

CLIA'88 sets personnel qualifications in four groups for moderate-complexity laboratories: (1) laboratory directors, accountable for the overall operation of the laboratory; (2) technical consultants, who are responsible for the technical and scientific aspects of the services; (3) clinical consultants, who are expected to be available for results reporting and interpretation; and (4) testing personnel, who actually perform the tests. Additional provisions for a general or technical supervisor, who must be responsible for day-to-day supervision, are stipulated for laboratories doing high-complexity testing. Qualifications for each position are summarized as follows.

- **Director.** Directors for moderate-complexity laboratories are required either to be physicians or to hold a bachelor's degree or higher in a science discipline with corresponding experience. For high-complexity level facilities the director must be a doctoral-level scientist with an appropriate laboratory specialty or a physician with training or experience in laboratory medicine. In some situations (e.g., oral pathology and special clinics), directors may also be other doctoral-level health care professionals such as dentists. There are also liberal exemption clauses for persons who could have qualified under previous federal or state rules as directors.
- **Technical consultant.** In a moderate-complexity laboratory, the same general director qualifications apply for technical consultants.
- **Technical supervisor.** In high-complexity laboratories, the same general qualifications apply as for the technical consultant.
- **Clinical consultant.** A physician or a doctoral level clinical scientist may provide the services of a clinical consultant.
- **General supervisor.** A laboratorian with an associate's degree or higher in medical laboratory technology and two years of training and experience in a high-complexity laboratory may perform the duties of a general supervisor. There are also exceptions for individuals who could have qualified under previous regulations.
- **Testing personnel.** As of September 1, 1997, all persons performing tests in a high-complexity laboratory must have at least an associate's degree. Until this date, the minimum qualification for both moderate- and high-complexity laboratory personnel who are processing specimens and performing tests is a high school diploma with appropriate experience.

In addition to these regulations, several laboratory and related disciplines have special exceptions. Individuals performing and supervising blood gas analysis, histopathology, dermatopathology, ophthalmic pathology, and cytology must have designated training and experience in their discipline, usually at the same level as for the clinical laboratory.

There are many special-interest groups, both within the laboratory community and in other health care areas, who are not happy with all aspects of DHHS's propagation of the CLIA'88 rules. Physicians and hospital associations, especially, want changes ranging from the total repeal of the act, to expansion of the PPMP category to allow "midlevel" practitioners (nurse practitioners, physician assistants, and so on) to perform these tests, to the total exemption of physicians' laboratories. All of these requests and suggestions are under consideration for possible change. This is indeed an uncertain and exciting time to be part of the laboratory community as our practice parameters continue to unfold.

State Regulation of the Medical Laboratory

At the state level, regulations encompass a broad variety of laws. Some states, such as California and Florida, have comprehensive regulations governing both facilities and personnel. Except for possible public health screening tests like cholesterol or HIV, 10 states have no laboratory facility regulations: Iowa, Missouri, North Carolina, North Dakota, Ohio, Oklahoma, South Carolina, Texas, Vermont, and, Virginia (Martin).

As of the last check (July 26, 2007), 12 states and the territory of Puerto Rico have licensure programs for medical laboratory personnel: California, Florida, Hawaii, Louisiana, Montana, Nevada, North Dakota, Georgia, Rhode Island, Tennessee, New York, and West Virginia (ASCLS, Med-

Hunters). Licensure of medical laboratory personnel is an issue actively pursued by many laboratory organizations and has resulted in legislation pending in several states.

The qualifications and levels of personnel licensure vary by state. Florida, for example, licenses laboratorians at four levels, each requiring specific qualifications and the passing of an examination: director, supervisor, technologist, and technician. Each level of licensure is offered separately in nine areas (microbiology, blood gas analysis, hematology, and so on) with a generalist examination for technicians.

Professional Personnel Certification and Laboratory Inspection and Accreditation Programs

A wide range of professional organizations offer educational, accreditation, and certification services. Because laboratorians become familiar with these groups early in their educational and professional careers, this section presents only a brief overview of the organizations that offer programs for accreditation of facilities and the certification of laboratory professionals.

Laboratory Inspection and Accreditation Programs

Three organizations are active in the inspection and **accreditation** (I&A) of medical laboratories: the Joint Commission on the Accreditation of Healthcare Organizations (JCAHO); the College of American Pathologists (CAP), which sponsors I&A for hospital and independent laboratories; and the American Association of Blood Banks (AABB). A separate organization, the Commission on Office Laboratory Accreditation (COLA), offers programs for physicians' office laboratories. Highlights of the JCAHO, CAP, and AABB programs are provided next.

Joint Commission on the Accreditation of Healthcare Organizations

JCAHO includes the inspection of laboratories as part of its overall review of medical facilities and issues standards and scoring guidelines in a publication entitled *Accreditation Manual for Pathology and Clinical Laboratory Services.* Even though promoted as a volunteer peer system, successful participation is essential to the professional reputation of the facility. It is also vital for reimbursement and regulatory compliance because most federal and state programs (Medicare, Medicaid, and so on) recognize JCAHO accreditation as equivalent to, or as having, *deemed status* in meeting their criteria.

The JCAHO accreditation manual details standards in the following six areas of laboratory practice that meet the CLIA'88 requirement for moderate- and high-complexity testing facilities.

- Availability of appropriate services to meet the needs of the hospital
- Sufficiency of space, equipment, and supplies to perform the workload
- Communication requirements
- Maintenance of records and reports
- Management of quality
- Enforcement of specific testing requirements

College of American Pathologists

The College of American Pathologists sponsors a laboratory accreditation program (LAP) for hospitals and independent laboratories. Like the JCAHO surveys, CAP provides standards and criteria for monitoring specific testing parameters and operational factors such as facility suitability, staffing, quality management, and safety. In addition to JCAHO, many federal and state programs also recognize accreditation by CAP as acceptable in meeting their requirements.

A frequent recommendation of laboratory managers is to include the use of CAP's inspection checklists and site visits as part of the overall management plan of the laboratory because of their detailed and specific guidelines for each area of laboratory practice.

American Association of Blood Banks

The American Association of Blood Banks (AABB) was the first laboratory organization to develop an I&A program. Their *Standards, Accreditation Requirements Manual,* and *Technical Manual* have served as the principal guidelines of blood transfusion services for over 30 years. Standards have been established for blood and organ donations, component processing and preparation, and transfusion and transplantation practices.

Many laboratories, particularly those that are hospital-based, have traditionally participated in both CAP and AABB programs, in addition to meeting the blood process and products regulation of the FDA. Even though these organizations have sometimes issued conflicting opinions, they have generally been complementary in their efforts to standardize and improve the quality of the blood supply.

Professional Certification of Laboratory Personnel

Compared to the few agencies that offer I&A programs for laboratories, a whole array of organizations seek to provide professional credentials for laboratorians. This is a unique situation; most other health care professions have only a single **credentialing** organization. This feature has resulted in much confusion on the part of laboratorians, other health care practitioners, and the public about the nature and qualifications of the persons working in laboratories.

Organizations providing **certification** programs for laboratory personnel can be grouped into two broad groups: (1) those that offer a traditional generalist certification, and possibly additional specialty categories (e.g., hematology, blood bank), at several levels such as for specialists, supervisors, or technologists; (2) those that certify doctoral-level scientists in areas like clinical chemistry (American Association of Clinical Chemistry) and microbiology (American Society for Microbiology).

The oldest of all certifying agencies is the Board of Registry, sponsored by the American Society of Clinical Pathologists (ASCP). The board provides certification programs in a variety of specialties as well as for generalists. Offering similar programs are the National Certification Agency for Medical Laboratory Personnel and the American Medical Technologists. Two other organizations with smaller memberships, the International Society for Clinical Laboratory Technology and the American Association of Bioanalysts, also have programs that certify several levels of laboratorians.

There are also commercial companies which have specific credentialing and educational programs. **PriorityEd** (*PriorityEd.com*), for example, which is owned by the author offers continuing education programs for medical laboratory professionals. We also provide a **management and supervision competency certification and credentialing program for medical laboratory professions** as a three day seminar, design to prepare the experienced as well as aspiring laboratorians with the knowledge necessary to run the modern medical laboratory. The program meets the Florida State continuing education criteria for a supervisor license.

Despite a consensus in the laboratory community that professional laboratorians (technologists and clinical laboratory scientists) should have a bachelor's degree, there is considerable disagreement about the acceptability of alternative routes to practice and recognition of nonacademic training and experience. This range of opinions about qualifications also holds true for the other categories of laboratory professionals.

The review of professional personnel and laboratory accreditation and credentialing programs conclude this chapter.

The next chapter will cover marketing strategies for medical laboratories.

— Case Study —

Chapter Twenty-Three: Regulatory and Professional Oversight

"Tom is making a killing working as a consultant to doctor's offices in helping them meet CLIA'88 requirement," stated John to a couple of his fellow techs during coffee break.

"I don't know about a 'killing,' but he does seem to be doing pretty well," remarked Bill.

"My friend, Betty, who also works as a lab consultant, told me that she was doing real well and likes the opportunity very much," added Ann, finishing up her coffee.

"You know what?" said a thoughtful John, "I know we all have families and don't want to take the risk of leaving our jobs, but if we got together, maybe we could do some labs together and still keep our jobs here."

"I like that." agreed Ann. "We could stop by the offices after work and on our days off. We all work in different sections, so that should make things easier."

"I already have one lead," Bill said, nodding his head in agreement. Dr. Smith asked me about the new regulations when she stopped by yesterday to check some results."

Chapter Sections for Review

- Workplace Legal Issues
- CLIA'88
  - Complexity Classification of Laboratories
  - Personnel Qualifications for Moderate-Complexity and High-Complexity Laboratories

Questions for Discussion

1. Does this seem like a potentially successful plan on the part of John, Ann, and Bill? What are the career and personnel obstacles that they may face? Is success guaranteed? How might their employer look at their plans? Is such a plan ethical (e.g., should they get the approval of the laboratory before the do start their business)? What do you think about these issues?

2. What kind of qualifications must these techs have to offer these services? Assuming that all three techs have a bachelor's degree in science, have completed a formal medical technology program, have over 7 years of laboratory experience, and are certified as medical technologists or clinical laboratory scientists by a national laboratory organization, which positions are the techs qualified to perform, under CLIA' 88 provisions?

<u>Solutions</u>

Question 2: These techs are qualified to fill all the positions except Clinical Consultant and Director in high-complexity laboratories. (Note: They are qualified as directors in moderate-complexity laboratories).

[24]

Marketing Laboratory Services

— Chapter Twenty–Four —

In 1987, I made the following statement:

> Never before has the laboratory manager been called upon to respond to such a rapid change in environment. The laboratory has come to accept rapid technological advances as commonplace and has learned to develop strategies for assimilating this new knowledge. We must now develop similar strategies to deal with the challenges of new reimbursement mechanisms and the restructuring of the laboratory delivery system. (Varnadoe, 1987, p. 397)

This statement is even more applicable today, in 2007, as the laboratory faces new health care delivery alliances, organizational re-engineering, managed care, changes in reimbursement practices, and increasing competition from all sides. A quick look on the internet for medical laboratory testing or the business section of the phone book, will demonstrate just how important marketing laboratory services has become.

The concepts, topics, and strategies covered in this chapter apply to all types of laboratories. However, because of marketing changes in the hospital-based laboratory and the resulting impact on the whole testing community, it is used for the baseline examples for our discussion.

One note about terminology: "customers;" "client;" and "market share" describe users of laboratory services — that is, patients, physicians, nurses, and third-party payers such as insurance companies and government agencies. This terminology may offend the sensibilities of some laboratorians, as we are all taught that our first priority is to the "patient." However, if there are no customers for our services, there is no need for our particular laboratory. This is the purpose of a marketing plan — to ensure the economic survival of the laboratory so that the patient can receive the highest quality care possible. The ability to respond to a rapidly changing market environment is a skill especially crucial to the manager of today's laboratory.

Objectives

After completion of this chapter, the reader will be able to demonstrate accomplishment of the following objectives.

1. Identify the customers and products of the laboratory.
2. Determine the market potential (clients, geographical area) for the services provided by a laboratory.
3. Analyze the four market variables as they relate to laboratory services.
4. Develop a marketing plan to enable the laboratory to achieve its outreach goals.

Chapter Highlights and Glossary of Key Terms

I. LABORATORY-CUSTOMER RELATIONSHIPS

II. THE MARKETING PHILOSOPHY

Marketing: The *strategic process of attracting and maintaining a customer base.*

Public Relations: *A communications tool designed to influence attitudes toward the organization.*

III. THE MARKET ENVIRONMENT FOR MEDICAL LABORATORY SERVICES

Market Environment: *Such factors as patient population, purchasing habits, and competition, which determine the opportunities and limitations of a potential customer base.*

IV. THE LABORATORY CUSTOMER

A. Marketing target: the customer

Customer: The *discretionary buyer who selects where a laboratory test is performed.*

1. Captive market

Captive Market: *Customers whose tests must be performed by a specific laboratory (e.g., hospital in-patients).*

2. Discretionary buyers

Discretionary Buyer: The *entity that decides which laboratory will perform the test.*

B. Customer expectations

Customer Expectation: *The dimension of value (i.e., hest products, best total solution, or hest total costs) the customer is seeking to satisfy.*

V. THE FOUR P'S OF MARKETING

A. The laboratory product

Marketing Variables: *Factors such as price, packaging, product, and. convenience that can be manipulated to attract customers.*

Product Differentiation: *Factors such as convenience, turnaround time, and price that make a product or service attractive to a customer.*

B. Price

C. Place

D. Promotion

Advertisement: *Commercial presentations paid for by the organization to promote its products and services.*

Sales Promotion: *Short-term purchase incentives such as discounts and gift programs.*

Personal Selling: *Selling through personal contact; using sales representatives to explain and sell a product or service.*

Publicity: *Noncommercial educational materials, news releases, and seminars designed to influence purchasers' decisions or improve the organization's image.*

VI. THE MARKETING PLAN

Marketing Proposal: *A formal strategy for maintaining, identifying, and attracting customers.*

A. Market research

B. The market proposal

Laboratory–Customer Relationships

Theoretically, all laboratories are competing for the same market. In actual practice, the current competitive environment is driven by changes in directly affecting the role of the hospital laboratory.

Until fairly recently, the typical institutional laboratory served a captive in-house market. Although lip service was given to attracting outpatient work, it was generally understood that a hospital laboratory could not compete with an independent laboratory for the outpatient market because of the expense involved in providing a 24-hour, on-demand service. With rare exceptions (high degree of specialization or unique geographical advantages), this was true for one reason: Medicare patients had to be charged the lowest price offered to any client. Hospitals tried all types of legal, organizational, and marketing maneuvers to circumvent this rule — all to no avail. A multi-tiered pricing structure was out of the question. Then came DRGs.

Today, the hospital is released to explore selective pricing and develop multi-tiered charges for different categories of customer or service, including discounts for payment in cash, price breaks on courier routes, and price menus based on different categories of patients. Under DRGs the laboratory is no longer classified as a revenue profit center; rather, it is now an accounting cost center, similar in the ledger status to Housekeeping. Hospital administrators eye the laboratory with the hope that it can provide a possible entry into new areas of health care marketing. It has been identified as an "asset" that can be sold off, or "merged," with other laboratories to provide a major reduction in hospital expenses and deliver a guaranteed profit per test regardless of occupancy.

Whereas previously laboratory managers were concerned primarily with operations, today they need to generate business in addition to maintaining the current clientele. The laboratory must defend itself from assaults on its client base and increase its contributions to the financial well-being of the organization.

The Marketing Philosophy

Why an organization exists, its plans for the future, and how it attracts and services its users are all part of the marketing philosophy of every organization. This applies especially to how the organization views its customers and internalizes their needs into the core of its operations.

Marketing, as a specific function of management, may be defined as the strategic process of attracting and maintaining a customer base. Without success in this area, the very survival of the organization may be placed in jeopardy. Marketing has to do with how *your* laboratory deals with the new reimbursement mechanisms and the restructuring of the laboratory delivery system.

Public relations often confused with marketing, serves a different but complementary function. It is a communications tool, designed to influence public *attitudes* toward the organization. It has to do with the organization's public image. Marketing, by contrast, tries to influence specific consumer *behavior* in making purchasing decisions.

Marketing philosophy and strategy have to do with how the laboratory interfaces with the marketplace. A wide range of entities call themselves "medical laboratories." Each type, from the small labs in physicians' offices to the huge corporate structures, has its strengths and vulnerabilities; they have all survived and flourished up to this point by identifying and serving special niches in the testing market.

But times have changed. The laboratory, like all businesses, must also change how it views, attracts, and deals with its customers. The new market philosophy must be one of exploration, openness, risk taking, and savvy — of being able to identify and pursue market opportunities.

The Market Environment for Medical Laboratory Services

Many forces influence the delivery of laboratory services. Many of these are outside the control of the manager, but all must be understood and factored into the marketing strategy. The **market environment** is a vibrant, interactive ecosystem where conditions are constantly changing. The manager must be alert to its evolving character and develop strategies that turn these events to the laboratory's advantage.

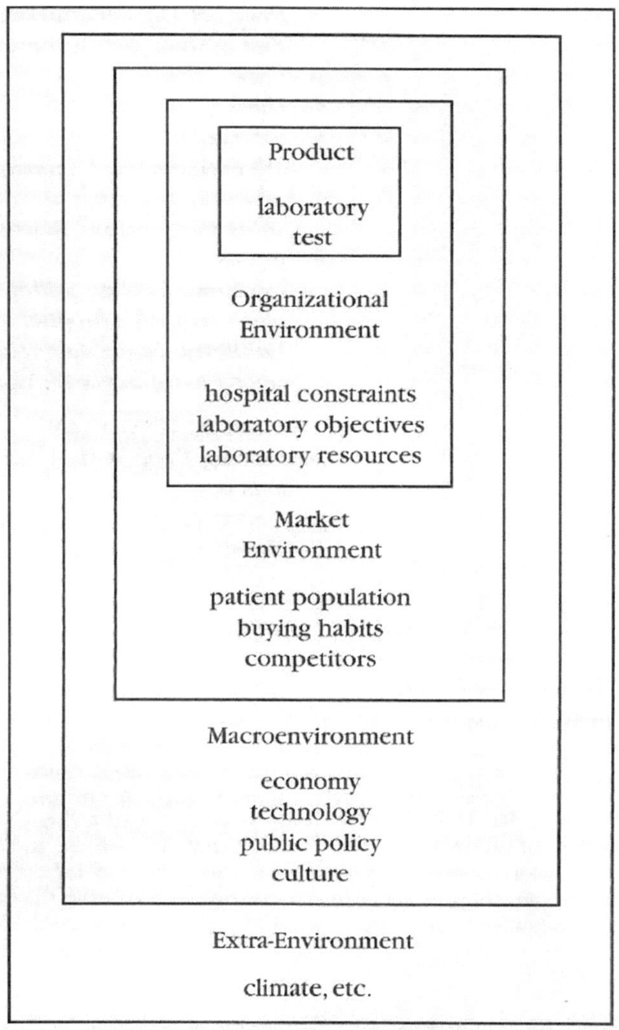

Figure 24 — 1. Laboratory marketing environment (from Varnadoe, LA; Marketing the hospital laboratory. Laboratory Medicine 18:397 — 401. © 1987 by the American Society of Clinical Pathologists. Reprinted with permission.)

Macrofactors (events outside the organization) such as the total patient population, their purchasing habits, and competition determine opportunities and limitations of the potential customer base (Figure 24 –1).

The market environment is beyond the control of either the manager or the organization. However, these macrofactors set the possibilities and limitations common to all providers of laboratory services. Extraenvironmental forces include such things as the characteristics of the population, climate, and geographical features of the service area. The radical changes in Medicare reimbursement and the introduction of DRGs are striking examples of the impact macroenvironmental factors can have on the way laboratories do business.

With these factors in perspective, managers can focus on the parts of the market environment that may be responsive to the actions taken by a specific laboratory or its competitors. These include the objectives, resources, organizational flexibility, and commitment of the laboratory to meeting the needs of its customers.

The Laboratory Customer

Determining exactly who the customer is and what the customer wants is a crucial aspect of any market plan.

Marketing Target: The Customer

There is no question that the person toward whom the laboratory directs its professional concerns is the patient. However, the laboratory must also identify the **customer** — the entity (patient, physician, parent, employer, insurance company, government agency) that sends the patient to the laboratory. The laboratory manager must further understand why a patient comes to this particular laboratory and the factors that influence this decision.

Within the laboratory community, many places can perform a test (Figure 24 — 2), each with its own traditional patient base. Influencing and changing the purchasing decisions (Figure 24 — 3) of the entity that selects where the test is performed is the goal of the marketing strategy. This is an important concept in any marketing plan, but it is especially crucial that the hospital based laboratory understand this concept, given its traditional in-house orientation.

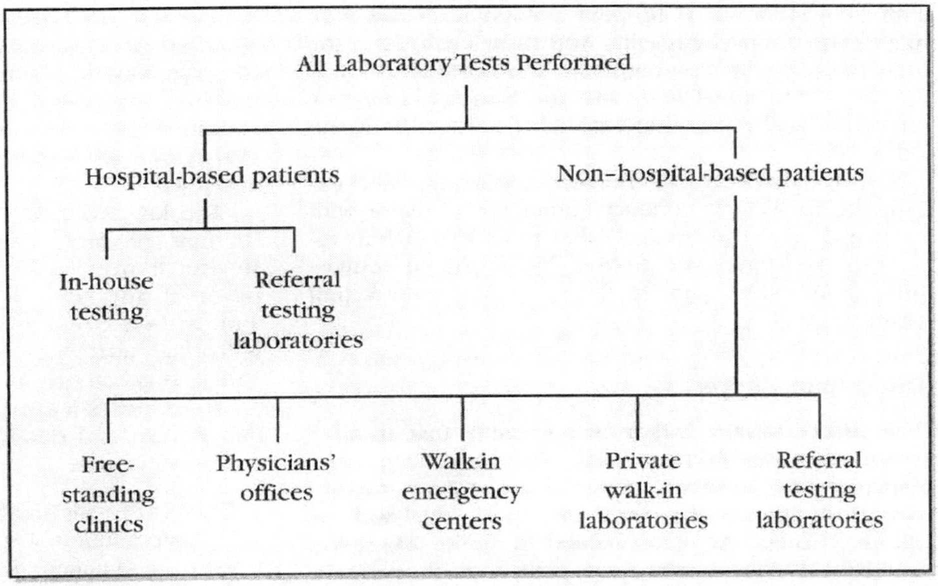

Figure 24 — 2. Where laboratory tests are performed (from Varnadoe, LA; Marketing the hospital laboratory. Laboratory Medicine 18:397 — 401. © 1987 by the American Society of Clinical Pathologists. Reprinted with permission.)

For marketing purposes, the purchasing decision makers can be divided two basic groups: (1) captive users (those who are committed to a specific laboratory); and (2) discretionary buyers (those who can choose among several laboratories).

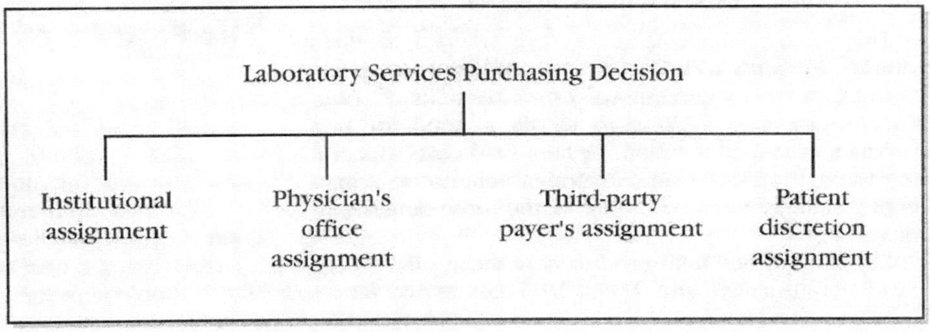

Figure 24 — 3. The buyer's decision from Varnadoe, LA; Marketing the hospital laboratory. Laboratory Medicine 18:397 — 401. © 1987 by the American Society of Clinical Pathologists. Reprinted with permission.)

Captive Market

Having a captive patient population for its testing services has been a distinct advantage of hospital-based laboratories in the past. However, this advantage is rapidly changing as more patients receive their care at outpatient surgery centers and walk-in medical clinics and even show up at hospital admission centers with their own laboratory results. Add these changes to the new medical alliances, corporate and hospital mergers, HMOs, PPOs, and DRGs, and the hospital laboratory may find itself competing with what used to be its referral lab.

Captive markets for laboratory services are also expanding to include contract commitments made with managed-care alliances and other providers such as insurance and employer groups. These patient sources are an important part of the laboratory's marketing plan.

Discretionary Buyers

The **discretionary buyer** is the entity that decides where a service is performed. This may be a large managed-care alliance capable of delivering a captive base of thousands of patients or an individual walk-in self-pay patient. As demonstrated in Figure 24 – $3_{(above)}$, the discretionary buyer may be a patient, a physician, a third-party payer, or even another institution.

Market research shows that the mother is usually the one who decides where the family receives medical care. For this reason much of health care's promotional focus is on the mother and on women in general and associated family issues. This is similar to the marketing tactics of fast-food restaurants, which focus their advertising on children for the same purpose.

Customer Expectations

Which customers to target are determined to a large extent by the laboratory's ability to satisfy certain **customer expectations.** Treacy and Wiersema point out that this problem is faced by all organizations, not just those involved in health care. Talking about "leaders" as organizations rather than as persons, they list three important truths that market leaders believe characterize the new world of competition.

- Different customers buy different kinds of value. You can't hope to be the best in all dimensions, so you choose your customers and narrow your value focus.
- As value standards rise, so do customer expectations; you can stay ahead only by moving ahead.
- Producing an unmatched level of a particular value requires a superior operating model — a "machine" dedicated to just that kind of value.

Treacy and Wiersema group customers into three *market segments* with specific but different needs according to their expectations, or *dimensions of value.* Each segment is looking to satisfy a need for best product, best total solution, or best total costs. According to these authors, laboratories can choose as a marketing strategy to excel in one of the three dimensions of value.

Excelling in *best total product* may mean offering the most sophisticated and specialized laboratory procedures or highly attentive service (e.g., elaborate personal attention and facilities). *Best total solution* may mean providing a complete package (test menu, phlebotomy, turnaround time) of services designed for a specific type of customer (single or group practice). *Best total costs* may involve concentrating on volume and price.

The key word in this model is *total.* It may mean (in best products) individualized, highly customized service; it may mean (in best solution) relieving the buyer of any paperwork or lab-associated problems; and (in best costs) it may mean not only the price of individual tests but all associated expenses such as billing, phlebotomy, and specimen transportation.

Treacy and Wiersema also list four new rules that govern and describe market leaders' actions and market strategies:

Rule 1: Provide the best offering in the marketplace by excelling in a specific dimension of value.
Rule 2: Maintain threshold standards on other dimensions of values.
Rule 3: Dominate your market by improving value year after year.
Rule 4: Build a well-tuned operating model dedicated to delivering unmatched value.

For example, a hospital laboratory may attract business by linking physicians' offices to its computer systems to provide a common carrier for all its patient needs (best total solution). A small independent laboratory may set up a lab or phlebotomy center in the physicians' office complex with hand delivery and charting of results (best product). A national laboratory may offer to perform tests for a managed-care system at a big discount (best total costs). The point is, basic standards must be met in all three areas, but a laboratory can achieve success only by *excelling* in one of the dimensions of customer value.

To become a market leader, organizations must have in place the *operating models,* or process, to deliver this customer value: "business structure, management systems, and culture, all of which are synchronized to create a certain superior value" (Treacy & Wiersema, p. 30). What this means is that the customer, like quality, must be an integral part of each management function: planning, organizing, directing, and controlling (see Chapter 1).

The Four P's of Marketing

According to Kotler and Clarke, there are "four major instruments — product, price, place, and promotion — that constitute the organization's strategic and tactical means for attracting and retaining customers". These four **marketing variables,** used in the context of dimensions of value, provide the framework for developing a marketing strategy and identifying the way to implement the plan.

The Laboratory Product

What is the laboratory's product? The answer to this question may seem so obvious as to appear ridiculous: *performing tests and giving results.* But a quick glance outside the walls of the standard lab reveals that many other entities perform tests. A better answer might be the sophistication, expertise, and technological ability to perform a large number of tests or carry out complex procedures.

The difficulty in reaching a professional definition of product is evident in the ongoing debate within the laboratory community about these and similar concerns. This issue is further complicated by the pressure on all economic concerns to refine their products and services in response to changing market realities.

The laboratory must deal with this reality. Only a definition of product that allows the laboratory to see its market potential from a broad *service* perspective gives it the capability of responding to a new competitive market characterized by managed care and other health care alliances. Focusing on doing only traditional testing outside the context of the total health care system ensures the erosion of the patient base. Direct-access pathology, whereby patients can come directly to the laboratory and request a test without referral from a physician, is an example of the changes taking place in the way the laboratory has traditionally approached its market.

The *product* of the clinical laboratory is *information* (Varnadoe, 1978) Daniel F. Cowan underscores this point: "*The business product of the laboratory, aside for the exception of blood and blood products is information.*" (p. 3).

Providing support and *information* to the medical community through its analytic resources and talents, the laboratory is able to research, identify, and respond to a dimension of value demanded by this changing market environment. Information (*its delivery speed and format*) is what distinguishes one product from another, why a consumer selects one detergent over another or one laboratory's glucose from another. In market language, this is called **product differentiation.**

Differentiation comes from service-related items such as turnaround time, price, convenience, test mix, payment options, and reputation for quality. These are part of the arsenal of the marketing manager and are service variables that directly influence the buying decision.

Price

The inability of the laboratory to develop and administer a multi-tiered pricing structure based on competitive factors and cost-revenue considerations was the single most crippling liability in marketing laboratory services. Medicare patients had to be charged the lowest price offered to any patient. However, in many ways this factor also protected the hospital laboratory's traditional patient base from assault from other institutions. Both situations have now changed.

Price has become a major competitive factor, and those laboratories that have been able to control expenses and offer attractive prices to discretionary buyers now enjoy a distinct advantage in this crucial service component. This ability to compete based on price is especially important in bidding for the laboratory portion of managed care and prepaid capitative programs (HMOs and PPOs).

Laboratories that have not yet realized the new market sensitivity to price, even from individual self-paying patients, need only to see the headlines appearing in their local newspaper. Both the consumer and the press are now "shopping" and comparing medical care costs.

A story that appeared in the Fort Pierce, Florida, *Tribune* (1995) described the dilemma of a Tampa hospital when a patient complained of what appeared to be excessive charges for laboratory work. The newspaper then surveyed other laboratories in the area and found that several would have charged only $22, compared with $278 at the hospital where the tests were performed. This story was then picked up by other news services, illustrating the national interest in this issue and the importance of price in the marketing plan of a laboratory.

Place

"The location of a health care organization is often such a dominant factor that it dictates what the rest of the marketing mix looks like," say Kotler and Clarke *(1987). Place* affects service distribution and entails three decisions: (1) physical access, which covers channels of care (physician's office, emergency room, clinic, and so on), location, and facilities design; (2) time access, including travel and waiting time; and (3) information and promotional access, involving obtaining referrals and getting the consumer to the provider.

Place is a factor in designing how convenient the laboratory service is to its clients. Remote drawing stations, frequency of pickups, and hours of operation are examples of practical variables that have to be considered.

Promotion

Products and services are constantly promoted through commercials and **advertisements** in newspapers, on car windshields, TVs, radios, in our mailboxes, and even on computer networks. In the laboratory community the ongoing campaign to increase our visibility as professionals includes promotional activities such as *Lab Week* and publications designed to inform the public of our contribution to its health (Mooney; Robinson).

We are all familiar with customer service representatives who visit the laboratory every day. However, the direct selling of medical services, particularly professional diagnostic and treatment procedures such as laboratory tests and physician services is a very recent phenomenon. However, to catch a glimpse at how common advertisement has become in healthcare; scan your morning newspaper, and notice the billboards along the roads.

Kotler and Clarke divide promotional tools into four groups:

- **Advertising:** any type of nonpersonal presenta tions such as displays and ads in newspapers and journals, as well as brochures and flyers
- **Sales promotion:** short-term discounts, product incentives, and so on
- **Personal selling:** selling through personal service representatives
- **Publicity:** noncommercial informational presentations issued through the news media and other public forums such as social clubs and educational institutions (print, radio, and TV news releases, public information sessions)

Large commercial laboratories have always had to use all of these techniques to reach their hospital and physician market. Now other laboratories must follow this model in developing promotional strategies for their marketing plan.

The Marketing Plan

The marketing plan is a formal strategy for maintaining, identifying, and attracting customers by incorporating all of the concepts and ideas discussed in this chapter. Like all plans, it goes through the basic steps of needs awareness, research, analysis, alternative solutions identification, selection, action plan, and implementation.

A laboratory marketing model includes the following steps (Varnadoe, 1987):

- Evaluation of the laboratory service area
- Determination of test demand
- Development of the appropriate test mix
- Development of the market through concerted efforts
- Systematic evaluation of all tests and services

Figure 24 – 4 suggests a **marketing proposal** format for laboratory services in five parts:

1. Purpose of proposal
2. Market overview SWAT analysis (strengths, weaknesses, analysis, and tactics)
3. Opportunities with recommendation and implementation suggestions
4. Approval request for implementation of the plan

Important to the design of any plan is the extent and accuracy of the information upon which it is based. This information is obtained through a continual process of market research.

Marketing Proposal for Laboratory Services
(Outline)

Plan objective

I. Market overview
  A. Market segments available
    1. Outpatients
    2. Physicians' offices
    3. Institutions
    4. Other
  B. Competition
    1. Present consideration
      a. Institutions
      b. Private (small) laboratories
      c. Independent (including national) laboratories
      d. Clinics
      e. Other
    2. Anticipated developments

II. SWAT (Strengths, weaknesses, analysis, and tactics) analysis
  A. Strengths and weaknesses of competition
    1. Lab A
      a. Strengths
      b. Weaknesses
    2. Lab B
      a. Strengths
      b. Weaknesses
  B. Strengths and weaknesses of your laboratory
    1. Strengths
    2. Weaknesses

III. Opportunities
  A. Outpatients
    1. Recommendation(s)
    2. Implementation
  B. Physicians' offices
    1. Recommendation(s)
    2. Implementation
  C. Institutions
    1. Recommendation(s)
    2. Implementation
  D. Others (clinics, satellite drawing stations, etc.)
    1. Recommendation(s)
    2. Implementation

IV Approval requested

(Here, clearly and specifically, state what steps need to be approved by administration and what resources are necessary, if any, to initiate the plan immediately

---

Figure 24 — 4. Marketing proposal outline for laboratory services. (from Varnadoe, LA; Marketing the hospital laboratory. Laboratory Medicine 18:397 — 401. © 1987 by the American Society of Clinical Pathologists. Reprinted with permission.)

Market Research

To provide the information necessary to effectively market the services of a health care organization, Kotler and Clarke suggest that four marketing research systems be in place:

- *Internal record system,* in which medical, financial, and operational parameters are monitored for marketing information
- *Marketing intelligence system,* to obtain everyday information about developments in the marketplace
- *Marketing research system,* organized to systematically collect, study, and report findings about specific marketing opportunities
- *Analytical marketing system,* using statistical and marketing model techniques to evaluate the data obtained from these systems

The emphasis of market research is on the continuous systematic monitoring of the laboratory's market environment, not simply on occasional questionnaires or surveys to provide decision-making information.

The Market Proposal

Although marketing is an ongoing process and part of the management function, putting a specific plan to capture a targeted customer into action is the purpose of the market proposal. The plan details the research conducted, opportunities identified, and suggested implementation strategies. Figure 24 – $4_{(above)}$ outlines a format for the proposal, and Figure 24 – $5_{(end\ of\ chapter)}$ presents a marketing proposal for a hospital based laboratory that has decided to go after the local testing market by seeking to offer the best total solution dimension of value for these customers.

The proposal outline divides the presentation into four parts, after clearly stating the objectives or purpose of the plan.

Market overview: In this first section, market segments, competitors, and anticipated changes in the marketplace are identified and reviewed.

SWAT analysis: The relative strengths, weaknesses, and market tactics of each competitor, along with those of your laboratory, are analyzed to place the proposal into the perspective of the market overview.

Opportunities: In this area the specific dimension of value and operational modes needed to take advantage of the market opportunities are identified. They may be listed by each customer, or market segment, giving first the recommendations and followed with the steps needed to implement the plan.

Approval: In the final section of the proposal, request permission to pursue the plan and state exactly what action is needed from the organization, including approval of staffing and budgeting requests.

Paul Howie, administrator at the International Medical Laboratory in Sarasota, Florida, provides a concluding perspective on the realities of the new competitive marketplace for laboratory services: "*Even though it's a medical procedure, it's still a retail business*" (*Tribune,* p B2).

Marketing Laboratory Service concludes the book. <u>Medical Laboratory Management</u> and <u>Supervision</u>.

Figure 24 — 5. Marketing proposal for laboratory services (from Varnadoe, LA; Marketing the hospital laboratory. Laboratory Medicine 18:397 — 401. © 1987 by the American Society of Clinical Pathologists. Reprinted with permission.)

Metropolitan Medical Center
— Marketing Proposal for Laboratory Services —

Purpose: The purpose of this study is to identify and expand the user base for the laboratory services of the Metropolitan Medical Center.

This program is based on the premise of a multi-tiered pricing structure.

Market Overview

Market Segmentation:
Three potential market segments have been identified as offering major opportunities for expanding our services:

Outpatients: This term is defined specifically to apply to the patients who make the decision as to where their laboratory work will be performed.

Physician offices: This term is used to describe laboratory work that is drawn in a physician's office and sent to an outside laboratory for completion.

Institutions: This segment refers to institutions that have a concentration of persons who may need laboratory work. This category includes not only nursing homes, but can include apartment complexes and other areas that can be processed as a single entity.

Competition:

Present Considerations:

River County is now served by two local hospitals-one small independent laboratories that accept only walk-in clients and three major national laboratories that cover the county using courier services.

In addition to Metropolitan, City Hospital and Clinical Medical Laboratory offer laboratory services to the outpatient clients. The three national laboratories that compete for the physician's office business are LabCorp, ChemLab, and PathService.

Future Consideration:

By the end of the year, four additional laboratories will begin operations in the immediate area of City Hospital, covering the southern part of the county:

- City Hospital will open a separate outpatient facility.
- General Hospital, from a neighboring county, will open an emergency walk-in center.
- A private pathologist will open a medical office complex laboratory.
- A health care corporation will open an "emergicare" facility that will accept outpatient work.

These five organizations will be competing with each other for the outpatient business in the southern part of the county. They will, of course, make some attempts for the physician office business also.

SWAT Analysis

Strengths and Weaknesses of Competition:

This analysis is confined to the geographical area of the middle and northern parts of River County because of the market saturation around City Hospital.

Clinical Medical Laboratory

Clinical laboratories is the only independent lab in the county at present. Located in the downtown area, Clinical has benefited from the price structure at Metropolitan, which has caused us to forfeit a major portion of the outpatient work.

Strengths:

- 25-year reputation in the county
    - Price differential advantage
    - Known by medical staff and patient population
- Can compete on turnaround time
- Can choose type of patient to serve (no charity, Medicaid)
- Can choose test mix on profit factors alone

Weaknesses:

- Patient base has a high sensitivity to price.
- No price constraints, except to be lower than Metropolitan.
- Probably has limited financial resources with which to offer services that have low profit margins. This could make them vulnerable to competition when turnaround times are important.

National Laboratories

Strengths:

- Extremely low price
- Mechanism for physician or patient billing
- Courier pick-up service
- Well-trained sales staff to call on clients

Weaknesses:

- No local technical support
- Quality of services can be difficult to ascertain because of remote locations
- Slow turnaround time
- No professional or personal interface by physicians with pathologists, which creates impediments to building strong relationships

Metropolitan Medical Center

Strengths:

- High reputation for quality and delivery of service
- Local technical and professional support for the medical staff
- Instrumentation available to support an increase in test volume, without additional capital outlays

- A captive patient base, so that services can be priced selectively, without fear of market erosion

Weaknesses:

- High prices
- Reputation for high prices-would be a liability even if charges were lowered

Opportunities

Given the previously detailed analysis, the following programs would be recommended:

1. Approach nursing homes in the area about doing their laboratory work. Offer the following:
    - Fast turnaround time for results
    - 24-hour services
    - Phlebotomy and pick-up services
    - Special discount prices, which may be retailed to their patients (wholesale to retail)

    Implementation:
    - Letter of introduction, listing programs and announcing that services are available
    - Personal visit to the facility to sell services and negotiate a contract
2. Physician Offices:
    Because most of the tests available from this source are not STAT, price plus turnaround time will be the competitive factors.
    - High, known quality of services available
    - Technical and professional staff available locally for problem solving
    - Specimen picked up and results delivered to office several times a day
    - Personalized billing programs to fit the needs of individual practices
    - Technical support could be offered for in-office testing

    Implementation:
    - Letter introducing the availability of services to the physician's office and the new discounted prices
    - Establish a pick-up and delivery schedule
    - Set up a personal meeting to sell and establish contracts
3. Outpatients:
    - While this market segment may appear the easiest to tap, it will prove the most difficult because:
    - Patients perceive prices are high at Metropolitan.
    - Established habits of obtaining laboratory tests.
    - Patient chooses the laboratory, so advertisements and solicitations are made difficult, because you are dealing with many individual choices rather than a single entity.

    Suggestions and implementation:
    - Establish a separate location, or name, that can be used to recruit patients. This could be as simple as setting up a remote drawing station.
    - Explore setting up joint ventures with independent laboratories to attract business. This would reduce any
    - costs involved in setting up satellite stations and would take advantage of their sales staff.
    - Develop a price schedule that undercuts Clinical lab.

4. Management services:
   There are numerous physician offices that perform laboratory work for their patients but are unable to accept work from other physicians because of licensing limitations. A relationship could be developed with these physicians so work could be accepted. This may be a mechanism to open a laboratory in areas where there are large concentrations of physicians' offices.

Approval Requested:

1. Authorize the preparation of a letter announcing our new services.
2. Request that the hospital public relations department prepare a questionnaire to explore what types of services are needed by the physicians.
3. Authorize a survey of charges of competing facilities with which to develop a multi-tiered price schedule

End of Figure 24 — 5. Marketing proposal for laboratory services

— Case Study —

Chapter Twenty-Four: Marketing Laboratory Services

CASE A

"Hello Bill . . . Ann," John greeted the two, as he set down his tray for lunch. "Giving our plan any more *thought?" [See previous (Regulatory and Professional Oversight) case study(Chapter 23)]*

"Yes, we have," answered Ann. "We both like it. However, Bill thinks we should look at our options and not just head out without planning first."

"See here," Bill said, holding up a book for John to see. "Maybe we should develop a marketing plan first. That way we'll know what we're facing and have a plan for dealing with it."

"I see," answered John, taking the copy of *Medical Laboratory Management and Supervision,* as he sat down. "Sounds like a pretty good idea to me. What do we do first?"

CASE B

"Yes, Betty, come in," the administrator greeted the laboratory manager, pointing her toward a seat. "Thanks for coming by so soon."

"Look here," continued the administrator, handing Betty some papers. "We have the opportunity to join with several doctors in a managed care arrangement to provide health care services for the employees of Standard Corporation. This would include both their local plant and the two over in the next town."

"As you can see, we have a lot of competition from the other hospitals and doctors in the area for this contract, but I think we can win. We have to win! If we don't, it could mean at least 20% of our patients might go to another hospital for their care," emphasized the administrator.

"I understand," Betty nodded in agreement.

"The laboratory will be a big part in this contract, because of the type of work they do. These patients will to be monitored regularly, in addition to their other health care needs. Here's a list of some important tests I want you to pay special attention to. The controller will work-up an overall proposal of price breaks, but I want you to see if we can do these tests at a special price. You might have to get with our reference lab and have them work up a proposal also."

"I'll get right on it," promised Betty, as she prepared to leave the office.

"Look for any way we can cut costs," concluded the administrator. "Our very future depends on how well we handle this proposal. Check with the controller if you need any help."

Betty nodded in agreement and hurried back to the lab to make her report.

Chapter Sections for Review

- The Market Environment for Medical Laboratory Services (Figure 24 – 1)

- Marketing Target: The Customer
    - Discretionary Buyer
- Customer Expectations [dimension of value] . The Laboratory Product
    - Product Differentiation
    - Price
- The Marketing Plan
    - Market Research
    - The Market Proposal

See also:

- Chapter 13: Revenue and Cost Accounting for Medical Laboratories
    - Break-Even Analysis
    - Break-Even Point in Test Volume
    - Break-Even Point in Revenue
    - Break-Even Point and Profit Requirements
    - Gross Profit or Gross Margin

Questions for Discussion

CASE A

1. Is taking time to study the market a good idea for the techs? Why?

2. At which "dimension of value" do you think the techs can best excel (i.e., best total product, best total solution, or best total cost)?

3. Using the dimension of value selected in Question 2 and the marketing proposal model presented in Figures 24 – 4 and 24 – 5, prepare a marking plan or strategy for the techs' consulting business. Specifically include a survey of market segments available (i.e., physician offices with laboratories) and SWAT analysis of other laboratory consultants that may be already offering this services. Sources of information include personal knowledge of physician office labs, laboratory and other health care colleagues working in doctor's offices, and phone book listings by practice types of physicians who use a lot of laboratory tests.

CASE B

1. Using the local market environment in your community (see Figure 24 – 1): patient population, buying habits, and competitors) prepare a market proposal (examples Figures 24 – 4 and 24 –5) based on a "dimension of value" advantage. This could be, for example, a plan to offer microbiology or special services to other laboratories, a plan to open a remote outpatient or drawing center, or a plan to customize laboratory services for the elders. Use your imagination. Look at your laboratory situation and develop a plan for its survival.

2. Based on the information provided by administration, Betty has estimated that at least 25% of the laboratory's business would come from the managed care contract. She has also found from this information that each patient would need the following tests at each check-up, and bas decided to use these data as the basis for her calculations. Use the information below to help Betty determine the break-e\en point for revenue and test volume to prepare for her meeting with the controller. What recommendation would you make to administration?

    - Current mark-up policy: 500%.

- Total fixed costs of the laboratory: $1 million
- Average revenue generated per test: $27.50
- Variable [fixed] costs per test performed: $3.90
- (Each employee will need this panel of tests at each check-up).

Test	Current Charge	Direct Cost
CBC	$50	$4.50
UA	$43	$3.10
BUN	$20	$0.90
Cholinesterase	$53	$10.50 (ref. lab charge)

Solutions

CASE B

Question 2:

Test	Direct Cost	Direct + Fixed Cost
CBC	$4.50 (+$3.90)	$ 8.40
UA	$3.10	$7.00
BUN	$0.90	$4.80
Cholinesterase	$10.50	$14.40

Revenue per panel: $34.60
No. of tests in panel: + 4
Average revenue/test $ 8.65

Proposed average revenue generated per test = $8.65
Proposed variable cost per test performed = $3.90
(remains the same unless cost-cuts imposed)

Using the Break-Even Point in Test Volume and Revenue equations we can determine the following values:

Fixed costs *(F)* for this part of the laboratory patient base could be estimated on its share of the fixed costs [$1 million **x** .25 = $250,000]

$$R = \frac{F}{CM} = \frac{\$250{,}000}{.549} = \$455{,}373 \text{ in revenue is needed}$$

$$CM = \frac{A - V}{A} = \frac{\$8.65 - \$3.90}{\$8.65} = .549$$

$$T = \frac{F}{A - V} = \frac{\$250{,}000}{\$8.65 - \$3.90} = \frac{\$250{,}000}{\$4.75} = 52{,}632$$

So ... 52,632 tests a year are needed from this source to break even.

The recommendation may be to go with these prices plus an additional profit requirement determined by administration in their overall consideration of the situation. (see break-even point and profit requirements formulas).

PART 4: BIBLIOGRAPHY

This book is presented as a 2nd edition, revision, update, additional text content, and sequential of: Varnadoe, Lionel A; Medical Laboratory Management and Supervision: *Operations, Review, and Study Guide*; F. A. Davis Company, Philadelphia; 1996. Following is the initial bibliography (p. 305,306) plus additional current citations.

Accreditation Manual for Hospitals: Quality assessment and improvement Joint Commission for Accreditation for Healthcare Organizations, Chicago, 1993

Accreditations Manual for Pathology and Clinical Laboratory Services: Joint Commission for Accreditation for Healthcare Organizations, Chicago. 1993.

ASCLS
http://www.ascls.org/jobs/grads/personnel_licensure.asp
This site also provides a list of the states with laboratory personnel licensure and contact information:
[July 26, 2007]

Baer. OM: Designing a lab that meets evolving needs. Medical Laboratory Observer, 27:22-25, 1995.

Barker, JH: Designing a Laboratory. American Public Health Association, Washington, DC, 1989.

Barnes, PW: Forging partnerships that work: A strategy for near-patient testing. Clinical Laboratory Management Review, 8:106, 1994.

Berkowitz, Eric N.; Essentials of Health Care Markething, 2nd ed.; Jones and Bartlett Publisher, Sundbury, MA; 2006.,m

Black, HS, Gart, RC, and Peterson, OM: Laboratory Management Principle and Practice. Van Nostrand Reinhold, New York, 1988.

Bozzo, P: Implementing Quality Assurance. ASCP Press, Chicago, 1991.

Brocka, B, and Brocka, M: Quality Management: Implementing the Best Ideas of the Masters. Irwin Professional Publishing, Burr Ridge, IL, 1992.

Brzezicki, LA: Target marketing. Advance for Administrators of the Laboratory, 4:37, 1995.

Chapman, B: Getting lab safety practices to stick. CAP Today, 6:1, 1992.

Check, WA: Should consumers order lab tests? CAP Today, 5:1, 1991.

CLIA Q&A. Clinical Laboratory Management Association, Malvern, PA, and American Association for Clinical Chemistry, Washington, DC, 1993.

College of American Pathologists: Inspection Checklist-Laboratory General. Northfield, IL, 1994.

Cowan, Daniel F., editor; *Informatics for the Clinical Laboratory A Practical Guide*; Springer-Verlag, New York; 2003

Crosby, PB: Quality is Free. McGraw-Hill, New York, 1979.

Daniel, WW: Biostatistics: A Foundation for Analysis in the Health Sciences, 5th ed. Wiley, New York, 1991.

[Dissemination] Institute for Health Improvement - Program on SBAR - Communication between care providers
http://lists.von.ca/pipermail/dissemination/2006-June/000057.html
[connect July 18, 2007]

Fairburn, C: Different strokes for different folks-the modified work week as a management tool. Advance, 6:5, 1994.

Feichter, M: Microscope on Washington: Keys to understanding state licensure. Laboratory Medicine, 26:238-239, 1995.

Fort Pierce, Florida, Tribune: Medical lab fees cause sticker shock; January 23, 1995, P B2.

Gile, TJ: Ergonomics for the laboratory. Clinical Laboratory Management Review, 8:5, 1994.

Gore, MJ: Personnel licensure: Making slow inroads. Medical Laboratory Observer, 27:24-29, 1995.

Hillestad, Steven G. and Eric N. Berkowitz; Health Care Market Strategy;Jones and Bartlett Publishers, Sudbury, MA; 2004

IHI.org

http://www.ihi.org/IHI/Topics/PerinatalCare/PerinatalCareGeneral/EmergingContent/SBARTechniqueforCommunication.htm
[connect July 18, 2007]

http://www.ihi.org/IHI/Topics/PerinatalCare/PerinatalCareGeneral/EmergingContent/PerinatalSBARTools.htm
[connect July 18, 2007]

Joint Commission for Accreditation for Healthcare Organizations: Improving Organizational Performance. Chicago, 1993.

Koenig, AS: Medical Laboratory Planning and Design. College of American Pathologists, Skokie, IL, 1985.

Kotler, P: Marketing Management, ed 8. Prentice-Hall, Englewood Cliffs, NJ, 1994.
Kotler, Philip; Marketing Management 11th ed.; Prentice-Hall, Upper Saddle River, NJ; 2003

Kotler, P, and Clarke, R: Marketing for Healthcare Organizations. Prentice-Hall, Englewood Cliffs, NJ, 1987.

Lang, HK: Licensure legislation update: '93-94 victories/disappointments. Advance, 6:7, 1994.

Lang, HK: Professional organizations agree: 4-year degree benchmark for MT/CLS. Advance, 6:7, 1994.

Leathers, D: Inside out, upside down. MT Today, 3:12, 1993.

Lehmann, C, Leiken, A, and Branchflower, R: Workflow analysis, a tool for laboratorians-case study: A drug-testing laboratory. American Clinical Laboratory, 13:12, 1994.

Loeb, Jerod M.; "Sentinel Events and Root-Cause Analysis; A Workshop by the Joint Commission;" in Scheffler, Adam and Zipper, Linda, editors; *Enhancing Patient Safety and Reducing Errors in Health Care;* National Patient Safety Foundation, 1999

Lundberg, GD: Managing the Patient-Focused Laboratory. Medical Economics Book Division, Westwood, NJ, 1976.

MacDonald, J, and Piggott, J: Global Quality: The New Management Culture. Pfeiffer, Amsterdam, 1993.

Martin, BG, ed: The CLMA Guide to Managing a Clinical Laboratory. Clinical Laboratory Management Association, Malvern, PA, 1991.

McLendon, WW, and Barnes, CC: Organization and management on the clinical laboratory. In Henry, JB (ed), Clinical Diagnosis and Management by Laboratory Methods, ed 17. WE Saunders, Philadelphia, 1984.

MedHunters.com Article published on Aug 23 04 12:59AM.
http://www.medhunters.com/articles/licensingMedLabTechUsa.html
[July 26, 2007]

Mooney, B: One laboratory's video-other labs' promotional tool. Advance, 7:17, 1995.

Murand, JL, and Litle, LM: Guide to safety in the workplace, Part III: Ergonomics: The study of work. Clinical Laboratory Science, 6:215-216, 1993.

Nace, L: Ready to renovate your laboratory? Advance, 5:8, 1993

Nace, L: Blood bank redesign: An effective business strategy. Advance, 7:6, 1995.

National Committee for Clinical Laboratory Standards (NCCLS [now CLSI]), Villanova, PA.

Clinical Laboratory Procedure Manuals, Vol 4, No. 2.

Clinical Laboratory Hazardous Waste (proposed guidelines), Vol 6.

Protection of Laboratory Workers from Instrument Biohazards (proposed guidelines), 11: 1991.

Protection of Laboratory Workers from Infectious Disease Transmitted by Blood, Body Fluids, and Tissue (tentative guidelines), 11: 1991.

Clinical Laboratory Technical Procedure Manuals, ed 2, 12: 1992.

OSHA: Bloodborne facts. OSHA Publications, U.S. Department of Labor, Washington, DC, 1993.

OSHA: "Occupational Exposure to Bloodborne Pathogens; Final Rule;" Federal Register: 29 CRF Part 1910. 1030; Friday, December 6,1991; Washington, DC.

Passey, RB: *Medical Laboratory Observer,* August 1992- July 1993.
How to obtain a CLIA certificate.
How to meet the new personnel requirements.
How to read the Federal Register.
A master plan for implementing CLIA.
How to prepare for a proficiency testing event.
How to follow the rules for patient test management.
Walking the straight and narrow on quality control.
How to prepare for and survive a CLIA inspection.
CLIA's quality assurance: A study in total devotion.
CLIA'88 penalties and how to avoid them.
Proving performance.

Robinson, AT: "PR" good lab practice-all year long! Advance, 7:16, 1995.

St. John, N, and Reed, RG: Point-of-care testing: Meeting regulatory guidelines with nonlaboratory personnel. American Clinical Laboratory, 14:11, 1995.

Sazama, K: Licensure of laboratory personnel. Laboratory Management, 24:216, 1994.

SBAR: A Communications Framework And Technique
Romilda Ang, May 1st, 2006
Journal SCI Nursing
http://www.unitedspinal.org/publications/nursing/2006/05/01/sbar-a-communications-framework-and-technique/
[connect July 18, 2007]

Seems simple, but culture change can be difficult.(d)
Source: Healthcare Risk Management
Publication Date: 09/01/2006
http://www.accessmylibrary.com/coms2/summary_0286-17511517_ITM
[connected July 18, 2007]

Seckinger, DL: Competing amidst consolidation. CAP Today, 9:5, 1995.

Safer Healthcare
http://www.saferhealthcare.com/sbarinfo.html
[connect July 18, 2007]

Southwick, K: Labs step in to help map care. CAP Today, 8:1, 1994.

Stern, A, et al: Fire safety in the laboratory. Laboratory Medicine, 24:275, 1993.

Stewart, CE, and Koepke, JA: Basic Quality Assurance Practices for Clinical Laboratories. Lippincott, Philadelphia, 1987.

Swayne, Linda E., W. Jack Duncan, and Peter M. Ginter; Strategic Management of Health Care Organizations; Blackwell Publishing, Malden, MA; 2006.

Treacy, M, and Wiersema, F: The Discipline of Market Leaders. Addison-Wesley, Reading, MA, 1995.

U.S. Department of Health and Human Services: CLIA'88. Federal Register: Rules and Regulations. Part 1910 (amended), No. 235. Washington, DC. 56:64175, 1991. Also No. 40. 57:7001-7288, 1992.

Varnadoe, LA: Designing a mission-oriented laboratory. American Journal of Medical Technology, 44:1145, 1978.

Varnadoe, LA: Designing a mission-oriented laboratory. American Journal of Medical Technology, 44:1145, 1978.

Varnadoe, LA: Requesting help: Laboratory work group staffing. Generalist Series, ASCP Tech Sample, October, 1995.

Westgard, JO, and Barry, PL: Cost-Effective Quality Control: Managing the Quality and Productivity of Analytical Processes. American Association for Clinical Chemistry, Washington, DC, 1986.

Weiss, RL, Ahlin, PA, Hawker, CD, et al: Transition in quality: From quality assurance to strategic quality management. Clinical Laboratory Management Review, 9:27,1995.

Weissman, D: Legislative and regulatory update. Paper delivered at CLMA 1994 Annual Conference, Orlando, August 29,1994.

Wrobel, S: Space wars. CAP Today, 7:42, 1993.

— Content Outlines —
Professional Examinations for Medical Laboratory Supervisors, Managers, and Directors

---

Diplomate in Laboratory Management

American Society for Clinical Pathology
ASCP Board of Registry
33 W. Monroe Street – Suite 1600
Chicago, Il 60603-5617
(312) 541-4999
(800) 267-2727
bor@ascp.org
Contact information: http://www.ascp.org/certification/Contacts/
[connect July 30, 2007]

CONTENT OUTLINE

http://www.ascp.org/Certification/CertifyingExaminations/cert_procedures/eligibility/dlm.aspx
http://www.ascp.org/Certification/CertifyingExaminations/cert_procedures/content/dlm.pdf
[connect July 30, 2007]

DIPLOMATE IN LABORATORY MANAGEMENT
"Refer to the DLM Competency Statements for the competencies tested in each subtest. The percentages indicate the percent of items that will appear on the examination in each subtest. Included within each subtest are items on planning, organizing, directing, controlling, coordinating and integrating."

I. Financial Management (33%)
   A. Budgets
   B. Capital Equipment Acquisition
   C. Cost Analysis
   D. Materials Management: Purchasing
   E. Financial Accounting
   F. Reimbursement Issues
   G. Materials Management: Inventory Control
   H. Contract Negotiations
   I. Cash Flow Analysis
   J. Billing and Collection

II. Operations Management (29%)
   A. Performance Improvement
   B. Licensure/Accreditation
   C. Safety
   D. Intra/Interdepartmental Relations,(e.g. Physician Committees)
   E. Information Technology

F. Risk Management/Medical-Legal Issues
G. Facilities Management Data Management Productivity

III. Personnel Management (26%)
A. Motivation
B. Staffing/Scheduling
C. Performance Standards/Evaluations
D. Counseling/Disciplinary Action
E. Education & Training/Continuing Education
F. Job Descriptions
G. Wage & Salary Administration
H. Personnel Negotiations
I. Conflict Resolution

IV. Marketing Management (12%)
A. Product Development
B. Consumer Relations/Customer Service
C. Market Research/Planning
D. Managed Care

All Board of Registry examinations use conventional units for results and reference ranges. You will need to bring a non-programmable calculator to the examination.

END OF CONTENT GUIDELINE Diplomate in Laboratory Management

Management Examination for Clinical Laboratory Directors and Supervisors

National Credentialing Agency for Laboratory Personnel
PO Box 15945-289
Lenexa, KS 66285
(913) 895-4613
nca-info@goamp.com
Contact information: http://www.nca-info.org/study/materials.asp
[connect July 30, 2007]

CONTENT OUTLINE

http://www.nca-info.org/pdfs/Management%20outline%20with%20ref.pdf
[connect July 30, 2007]
[reprinted with permission]

I. PERSONNEL PRACTICES

A. Manage Human Resources

1. Allocate and / or utilize resources and expertise

2. Monitor and / or evaluate productivity and efficiency
3. Provide for or perform employee supervision
4. Develop and / or utilize position (task) analysis within the following parameters:
   a. regulatory requirements
   b. knowledge / education requirement
   c. responsibility and accountability
   d. judgement(sic) levels and decision making
   e. standards of performance
   f. technical abilities

B. Determine Employee Selection

1. Develop recruitment criteria
2. Perform employee selection including the following:
   a. legal and regulatory requirements (e.g., EEOC, ADA)
   b. screening protocol
   c. interview protocol
   d. reference / qualification standards
   e. hiring decision

C. Develop and / or Utilize an Orientation Program, Including

1. Organizational policies including problem solving (grievance) mechanisms
2. Position description and organizational chart
3. Fire, safety, and disaster plans
4. Laboratory policies and procedure manuals
5. Rotation schedule through the laboratory
6. Employee checklist to ensure topic coverage
7. Process for competency documentation

D. Implement Disciplinary Procedures

1. Utilize appropriate documentation
2. Provide and / or perform disciplinary counseling

E. Perform and Implement Performance Appraisals

1. Develop a performance appraisal system to include the following
   a. performance standards
   b. performance rating
   c. scaled-rating
   d. competency assessment
2. Implement performance appraisal including
   a. appraiser selection
   b. evaluation interview
   c. documentation
   d. provision for employee comments
   e. deficiency correction plan
   f. future goal planning

F. Develop and / or Implement Staffing Systems

1. Determine scheduling of personnel
2. Determine job organization and delegation
3. Enforce disciplinary policies

4. Adhere to labor relations requirements
5. Monitor compliance with labor laws and regulations

G. Develop and / or Implement Staff Development and Education Program

1. Assess training needs
2. Develop training / continuing education program
3. Implement self-improvement and professional development programs
4. Monitor compliance to regulatory requirements for education and competency
5. Provide clinical instruction to staff, students, and others
6. Design / select instructional goals, objectives, learning activities, and evaluation tools used in clinical teaching

II. MANAGING THE BUSINESS

A. Management Philosophies and Practices

1. Delegate responsibilities and duties
2. Demonstrate leadership qualities
3. Practice accountability activities

B. Business Practices and Marketing

1. Strengthen laboratory public relations
2. Develop customer relation skills

C. Planning and Forecasting

1. Implement objectives from long-range or short-range plans
2. Evaluate policy development within the institution and the laboratory
3. Implement systems designed for the movement of specimens, employees, patients / clients, and results
4. Evaluate the physical limitations of the facility
5. Participate in organizational planning (e.g., committees, teams)

D. Financial Management

1. Prepare and / or utilize the following budgets
   a. monitor and evaluate capital acquisition expenses
   b. monitor and evaluate operating expenses
2. Adhere to payroll systems and deduction practices
3. Implement a materials management / inventory systems
   a. develop and / or utilize supply ordering process
   b. evaluate efficacy of standing orders, casual orders, and volume purchases
   c. evaluate inventory systems, establishing order levels
4. Negotiate and select supply order contracts
5. Evaluate and select equipment
6. Authorize purchases
7. Comply with institution or practice purchase contracts

E. Information Management

1. Record and retrieve information and data as required by accreditation and regulatory requirements
2. Develop and monitor reporting guidelines
3. Evaluate methods of storage and retrieval

4. Select laboratory information systems
5. Implement laboratory information systems
6. Evaluate laboratory information systems

III. QUALITY ASSESSMENT

A. Quality Improvement

1. Detect, monitor, correct, and prevent problems in risk management in the provision of laboratory services
2. Develop and monitor competency assessment of employees
3. Ensure that testing systems provide quality at the pre-analytic, analytic, and post-analytic phases
4. Participate in Total Quality Management or other improvement activities
5. Develop and maintain procedure manuals according to NCCLS guidelines

B. Performing Quality Control

1. Perform and evaluate correlation and validation studies on new methods
2. Select, evaluate, and monitor methods including accuracy, linearity and precision
3. Calculate and evaluate QC statistics
4. Determine reference ranges for laboratory procedures
5. Devise corrective action for procedure or equipment problems
6. Detect sources of laboratory errors
7. Perform and evaluate turnaround time studies
8. Coordinate proficiency testing (e.g., evaluate data, respond to supplier concerning deficiency, implement corrective action for deficiency)

IV. REGULATORY COMPLIANCE

A. Safety Management

1. Write / establish guidelines for safety
    a. biologics, blood borne pathogens, and infection control
    b. chemicals, OSHA, and "right to know"
    c. fire, fire-fighting equipment, and evacuation plans
    d. sharps, needles, and glassware
2. Conform and monitor compliance to guidelines for safety
    a. biologics, blood borne pathogens, and infection control
    b. chemicals, OSHA, and "right to know"
    c. fire, fire-fighting equipment, and evacuation plans
    d. sharps, needles, and glassware
    e. compressed gases

B. Institutional, Regulatory, and Accrediting Agency Compliance

1. Interpret, implement, and monitor compliance to federal, state, and local requirements (e.g., Medicare, ADA, CLIA, FDA, NLRB)
2. Interpret, implement, and monitor compliance to voluntary accreditation guidelines (e.g., AABB, CAP, JCAHO)
3. Comply and implement institution / facility requirements (e.g., personnel, safety, equipment, employee)

V. GENERAL LABORATORY SKILLS

A. Specimen Collection and Handling 5 4 0 9

1. Develop and implement specimen collection guidelines to include venous, arterial, capillary, throat cultures, urine, feces, seminal fluid, and other body fluids or specimens
2. Instruct patients / healthcare providers in the proper procedures for the collection of blood samples (venous, arterial, capillary), throat cultures, seminal fluid, urine, feces, and other body fluids or specimens
3. Develop and implement criteria for specimen acceptability to include labeling, patient preparation, specimen preservation, quantity, and appropriate transport and storage requirements
4. Evaluate acceptability of specimens based on adherence to labeling, patient preparation, specimen preservation, quantity, and appropriate transport and storage requirements

B. Instrument Operation, Maintenance, and Calibration

1. Develop and implement instrument operation, maintenance, and calibration procedures as required by practice standards and guidelines
2. Establish record storage and retrieval guidelines for maintenance and calibration records per practice and regulatory standards

C. Reagent Preparation, Storage and Handling

1. Develop and implement reagent preparation, labeling, and storage guidelines
2. Monitor reagent preparation, labeling, and storage guidelines

END OF CONTENT GUIDELINE NCA Management Examination for Clinical Laboratory Directors and Supervisors

---

Index

(*for this edition* — see ***Contents*** [*pp. xii — xxviii*] at the beginning of the book for an outline of each chapter's content with coordinated pagination).

ASCP Board of Certification

1-800-267-2727 opt 2.1